D0898048

SPEECH AND REASON

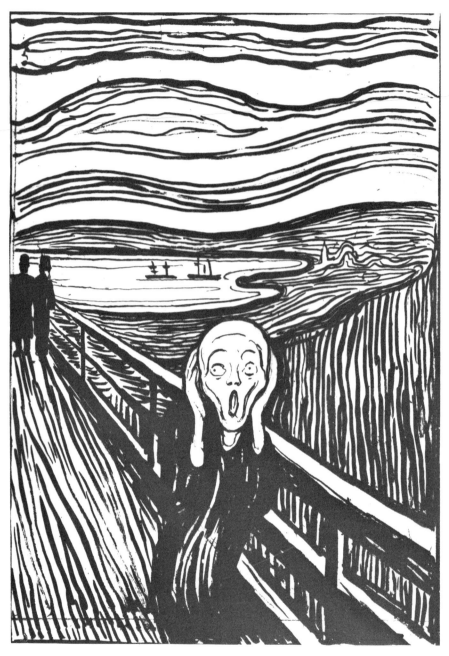

MUNCH, Edvard. *The Shriek*. 1896. Lithograph, printed in black, 13 15/16 x 10 inches. Collection, The Museum of Modern Art, New York. Matthew T. Mellon Fund.

SPEECH AND REASON

Language Disorder in Mental Disease

D. WILFRED ABSE, M.D.
University of Virginia

a Translation of

The Life of Speech

PHILIPP WEGENER

THE UNIVERSITY PRESS OF VIRGINIA

Charlottesville

THE UNIVERSITY PRESS OF VIRGINIA
Copyright © 1971 by the Rector and Visitors
of the University of Virginia

First published 1971

ISBN: 0–8139–0344–0
Library of Congress Catalog Card Number: 72–163981
Printed in the United States of America

To Elizabeth

Acknowledgments

I WISH to acknowledge the help I have had from numerous sources in producing this volume. First I want to thank Mr. David C. Hackett for the hard-core work of initial translation from the German while he was a postgraduate student in the Department of Germanic and Slavic Languages at the University of Virginia. For a short while Miss Elizabeth Hölscher (now Mrs. Douglas Day) assisted in this work. Professor William L. Little and Mr. John F. Reynolds of the Department of Germanic and Slavic Languages, University of Virginia, helped in important ways. Mr. Reynolds was powerfully effective in the arduous work of translating adequately many of the most difficult passages in Wegener's lectures. Mrs. Marianne P. Bonz assisted me in some stages of the work. Professor Norbert Fuerst of the Department of German, Indiana University, directed my attention to reviews of Wegener's work by his contemporaries, and has been generally a source of help and encouragement. Professor F. Kudlien of the Institut für Geschichte der Medizin und Pharmazie der Christian-Albrechts-Universität, Kiel, was able to obtain for me some details of Wegener's work and career.

I am indebted to my secretary, Mrs. Barbara Ann Carney, and to Miss Nancy Dunham, both of whom assisted in the preparation of the manuscript. In completing the book, a task demanding much problem-solving and some winnowing of chaff, I owe a great deal to Mrs. Virginia Kennan of the Department of Psychiatry for her excellent editorial work.

It was Professor Ian Stevenson of the Department of Psychiatry, University of Virginia, who first helped to get the translation under way; and later Dr. David R. Hawkins, the chairman of the Department of Psychiatry, University of Virginia, afforded further help. To both these colleagues, whose professional activity demonstrates their insistence on the supreme importance of meaning in language, I extend my thanks.

Finally, I wish to thank the National Translation Center of the Ford Foundation, and its Director, Mr. Fred Wieck, for a grant-in-aid which enabled the completion of this volume.

Charlottesville, Virginia　　　　　　　　D. WILFRED ABSE, M.D.
September 1970

Contents

Introduction

COMMUNICATION technology now permits people to speak directly to us from around the world and even, on occasion, from the moon. No spot is so remote that it is inaccessible to human speech. The prime minister seeking word about world events joins the illiterate laborer who simply likes the company of the electronic voices; both listen to the stranger exhort, cajole, inform, modify. At the same time, "communication" seems to many deeply troubled men to offer the only hope of reconciliation with others—often of the same culture or of the same household—who threaten and oppose them.

Beyond a doubt, we are flooded by words. It is time to question the leaching away of the power of words to evoke images, emotion, or concepts that are predictably related to reality and the common experience. Language used in the repetitions of special pleading begins to fall on deaf ears. Words coined in special deviant cultures depart weirdly from an understood frame of reference and remain as ambiguous as they are familiar. Some writers hold that the usefulness of verbal exchange will disappear before long in favor of a more immediate onslaught upon our sensors. In the performing arts those who seem to "speak" most loudly to the young maintain that words obscure everything that matters; these artists offer their followers a vocabulary of monoremes expressive of force, despair, lust, and tenderness. Young intellectuals, entirely familiar with the finely proliferated possibilities of speech, are inept in its use. Pressed to define and to defend, they helplessly repeat "Y'know!" Searching passionately—so they say—for "communication," they are themselves mute, except in echoes of tribal idiom without individuation or evidence of assimilation.

Language, seen as symbolic verbal behavior, has always been an important aspect of human psychology, although its present possibilities of misuse, and even extinction, seem unique. Yet Wilhelm Wundt's psychological approach to the scientific exploration of language at the turn of the century met with more or less intense opposition from most philologists. This early rift separating linguistics from psychology, a rift which generally widened during this century, was bridged until quite recently by only a few anthropologists. It now seems remarkable that as early as 1885 Philipp Wegener, a scholar well-versed in the comparative philology of the Indo-European languages, attempted a profoundly psychological approach to the study of language published as *Untersuchungen ueber die Grundfragen des Sprachlebens* (*The Life of Speech*).

Wegener, unlike Wundt, observes language as an experiment of nature without the encumbrance of artificial conditions in the laboratory. He understands that word language is the eventual instrument of needs and wishes and that its early development is pragmatic and functional. This understanding is deepened by his observations of the basic communication developed by the dependent child with his parents, and later with teachers and others. Moreover, Wegener's understanding of the importance of "prime movers"—the drives and associated affects—amplified by his developmental approach, is deepened by the concept that the psychic life moves along a continuum of interacting conscious and unconscious processes. Here Wegener anticipates the depth psychology of Freud and, in regard specifically to human speech, supplements and augments his findings. Lest this statement be misunderstood, it should be added that it is especially in Wegener's view of the development of the logical and structural aspects of language that one is forcibly reminded of Freud's account of the increasing structural differentiation of the ego from the id, of the characteristics of the preconscious, and of secondary process.

The scientific value of Wegener's approach to language study has already been recognized; decades ago Susanne K. Langer, the outstanding American linguistic philosopher, referred extensively to his work in her major contribution to modern thought, *Philosophy in a New Key*. Yet in spite of this recognition, the version of Wegener's lectures which I present here is the first English translation to be made of any of his writings.

As a psychiatrist and psychoanalyst, I have found Wegener's views helpful in understanding the disorders of communication associated with neurosis and psychosis. In my commentary, "Language Disorder in Mental Disease," I try to illustrate the usefulness of a clinical application of Wegener's ideas. It is my hope that my colleagues will share this interest. The extraordinarily entangled obfuscations of the language studies of modern existentialists and the difficulties of their dense and allusive style, will not, I hope, be allowed to prejudice the case presented here for a clinically well-grounded study of language in conjunction with a reconsideration of Wegener's work. The fact that many of these modern authors avowedly address themselves to some kind of concept of the unconscious in their theories of language must not become a source of confusion and deterrence. It is also my hope that outside the medical domain there will be interest in those aspects of linguistics which seem useful to a psychiatrist beset daily by the practical problem of understanding his patient. Such a focus may be of salutary value in a field which now seems to be the scene of fierce intellectual argumentation.

LANGUAGE DISORDER IN MENTAL DISEASE
D. Wilfred Abse, M.D.

Who could hope to disentangle the fabric of our inner life with its thousandfold complexities, if we were willing to pursue its threads only so far as they traverse consciousness?—Ewald Hering ("On Memory as a Universal Function of Organised Matter," Lecture to the Imperial Academy of Sciences, Vienna, 1870)

1 Freud and Wegener

THE twentieth century has seen several new approaches to the study of language. Not least are those represented by structural linguistics and by behavioral psychology. Indeed these two approaches comprise to a very large extent what is now termed *psycholinguistics*. After all, the study of language, as of history or politics, is necessarily grounded to a large extent in social psychology, and it really always has been. We hardly need such barbarisms as *psycholinguistics* or *psychohistory*, except perhaps as a clumsy reminder to apply the knowledge and methods afforded by modern scientific endeavor in psychology to the renewed study of language or history.

Work in psycholinguistics has, of course, considerable interest for the clinician and the educator. Some tests designed as instruments for the assessment of language development in children are of particular clinical importance. For example, the Illinois Test of Psycholinguistic Abilities (McCarthy and Kirk 1963), based on a pattern analysis and designed to meet a pressing need for a comprehensive instrument to estimate linguistic development in children, particularly those of preschool age, now supplements older tests of the picture identification type and normative surveys of language development. Then there are the few valuable studies on kinesics and paralinguistics, including those of Birdwhistell (1952), Trager (1964), Weston LaBarre (1964), Ruesch and Kees (1956), and Critchley (1939). Philipp Wegener was already aware in 1885 that communication is much more than the words of speech. Besides conventional forms of movement, he was concerned with all those which convey individual strivings and feelings. Moreover, long before the present development of techniques of phonemic analysis of living speech, his theory comprised and demanded a closer study of accentual phenomena—stress, pitch, loudness, and other aspects of tone of voice. Indeed, Wegener, in showing how language is rooted in the traffic of men with one another, concerns himself with the coordinating value and mutual influence of the entire extralinguistic series of behaviors with the words of speech.

Other than studies of patterns of speech development (kinesics and paralinguistics for the most part), the yield of recent psycholinguistic studies does not seem so far to have included very much that is central to the speaker's psychological situation or to the hearer's response; that is to say, very much that is of interest to a psychiatrist. On the other hand, Freud's contributions to language theory include much that illuminates our living experience. And so it is too with Wegener's scholarly *Untersuchungen ueber die Grundfragen des Sprachlebens*, published in 1885, which, until this time, has not been available in English. It is remarkable that Freud, the clinician, and Wegener, the schoolteacher, share so many ideas. Of course Freud may actually have read Wegener's book.

However, it is of more than historical importance that Freud's formidable work, throughout which his contributions to language theory are scattered, should be supplemented by Wegener's small book. Whether or not this book directly stimulated some of Freud's ideas, it remains a source of stimulation from which further psychoanalytic work can benefit. I hope to illustrate here its value in the elucidation of problems of hysteria, the sphere in which Freud emerged as a pioneer of mental science, as well as to pursue further considerations relating to thought and language, imagery, dreaming, and schizophrenia.

Freud (1923) stated that the criterion of being mentally conscious or mentally unconscious "is in the last resort our one beacon-light in the darkness of depth psychology." By means of this key concept of unconscious mental processes Freud was progressively enabled to find psychical continuities between observed phenomena, including the mental experiences reported by his patients. Yet his key concept developed side by side with attempts to understand and explain, or even to describe adequately, disorders of human behavior *without* invoking the unconscious. In 1895, ten years after the first publication of Wegener's studies concerning the basic questions of the life of speech, Freud was engaged in an attempt to construct a psychology composed of concepts entirely borrowed from neurology, an attempt which issued in the unfinished and abandoned torso we now know as the *Project for a Scientific Psychology*. As James Strachey (editor's note 1957, in Freud 1915) writes:

This astonishing production purports to describe and explain the whole range of human behavior, normal and pathological, by means of a complicated manipulation of two material entities—the neurone and "quantity in a condition of flow," an unspecified physical or chemical energy. The need for postulating any unconscious mental processes was in this way entirely avoided: the chain of physical events was unbroken and complete.

Rather, we prefer to say, *would* have been so avoided, had the explanatory power proved sufficient for the clinical task.

In *The Interpretation of Dreams* (1900), especially in the seventh chapter, Freud integrated those concepts borrowed from his studies in neurology with psychodynamic aspects including the key concept of the unconscious. In this way, he achieved a theory anchored in clinical experience and more useful as a guide in practice.

In his early days, Freud was exposed to the teachings of J. F. Herbart. According to Ernest Jones (1953), a textbook embodying the Herbartian principles was in use at Freud's secondary school. Moreover, his teachers in medical school, insofar as they were at all interested in psychology, were influenced by Herbart's writings, which notably included a recognition of the existence of unconscious mental processes. In his *Lehrbuch zur Psychologie* (1816) and his *Psychologie als Wissenschaft* (1825), Herbart endeavored to bring pedagogical practice into harmony with his own system of psychological principles. Wegener also is dependent upon Herbart for some of his basic assumptions, such as that "ideas" (both percepts and thought-formations) are dynamic entities, struggling with one another for a place in consciousness and interacting according to definite quantitative principles.

J. C. Flugel (1933) writes of Herbart:

It is obvious that, since consciousness was describable in terms of ideas not themselves present in consciousness, or at any rate not wholly so, Herbart's psychology extended beyond the realm of the conscious to that of the unconscious. In this, as in many other respects, Herbart has much in common with Leibnitz, whose *petites perceptions* constituted the first clear statement of anything approaching the modern doctrines of the unconscious. In fact, Herbart distinguished three degrees of consciousness: the focal ideas which are apperceived or clearly apprehended. . .the marginal ideas, which are dimly and unclearly present; and in the third place those ideas which are forced out of consciousness altogether. For an idea that has suffered inhibition (or repression, *Druck*) does not thereby cease to exist. It merely joins the vast company of ideas that have gone from consciousness, but may return—either through a weakening of opposite ideas or by cooperation with an ally, the combined forces being able to overcome resistances that were formerly too strong.

Flugel goes on to note the obvious resemblances to Freud's later and more developed concepts but points out differences too, namely the a priori stamp of Herbart's theories and his more intellectual bias. More particularly, this concerns

the reason for opposition between ideas. With Herbart the opposition seems on the whole to be an intellectual one; with Freud it depends upon an opposition in the sphere of desire; certain desires are incompatible with other dominant tendencies of the personality, and for this reason are banished to the unconscious.

Wegener's whole conception of a child's speech development conforms remarkably to Freud's emphasis on cognitive elements being largely in the service of striving, conation, and accompanying affects. Speech in the child, Wegener saw clearly, develops first of all from the need to influence the will of the one spoken to in a manner which appears valuable to the child—in commands, questions, hints, and challenges. The imperative admonition early expresses the will; velleity pervades developed speech.

One of Wegener's major findings is that the logical predicate (that segment of the sentence which carries more emotional tone, the accentuated part, often but not necessarily coinciding with the grammatical predicate) is the key element of the sentence. All that remains is exposition, a concession to the listener to secure his understanding. It seems that in the oldest diction the predicate stood foremost. This, Wegener informs us, remains evident in the older Indo-Germanic languages' manner of structure, verb and nominal inflection, compounds, attributive connections, appositives, and subordinate clauses. In all these instances the auxiliary word elements that follow the novel predication are subsequent revisions or expositions originating in attempts to secure correction of observedly deficient presentation. In modern language formation this is no longer so; for the most part the exposition now stands foremost. Thus we find, by contrast with the old language formations, both logical and ethical advancement. Wegener shows how the expectation of a new message remains an important element enabling the listener to join together words to understand their purpose. He tries to trace some forms of revision which finally became firm language forms, whose origins the "language-consciousness" now has long forgotten.

II Hysteria and Metaphor

Historical considerations

THE word *hysteria* is derived from the Greek *hystera* meaning "womb." This simple etymological fact reflects a reiterated view in ancient Egyptian and later Graeco-Roman medical thought, namely that disorder of the female generative system resulted in emotional instability and physical disease. The name "hysteria" was given to disease phenomena characterized by mobility and fugacity, especially when in conjunction with emotional storms. The theory asserted that wandering of the womb produced disturbances of mental and physical health (Abse 1966).

In the second century A.D., Soranus of Ephesus in Asia Minor refused to accept the idea that the womb was capable of wandering about like an animal within the abdomen. He insisted that hysteria was a disease of stricture, emanating from the uterus but affecting the whole body. As Ilza Veith (1965) records, Soranus, because of his dissenting view, criticized all previously recommended therapeutic procedures, scornfully explaining that

. . . the majority of the ancients and almost all followers of the other sects have made use of ill-smelling odors (such as burnt hair, extinguished lamp wicks, charred deer's horn, burnt wool, burnt flock, skins and rags, castoreum with which they anoint the nose and ears, pitch, cedar resin, bitumen, squashed bed bugs, and all substances which are supposed to have an oppressive smell) in the opinion that the uterus flees from evil smells. Wherefore they have also fumigated with fragrant substances from below, and have approved of suppositories of spikenard [and] storax, so that the uterus fleeing the first-mentioned odors, but pursuing the last mentioned, might move [back] from the upper to the lower parts.

Galen of Pergamon later in the second century also denied that the womb wandered about, agreeing in this respect with Soranus, but he developed his own etiological theory. He believed that a secretion similar to the semen of the male could be produced and retained in the uterus, and that retention of this substance, just as retained menses, could corrupt the blood and eventually irritate the nerves. Veith (1965) puts it this way:

In pursuing this theory, Galen offered the following further hypothesis: if repressed semen, i.e., abstinence or lack of sexual relations, gave rise to trouble in women, it was logical that a similar cause would lead to analogous disorders in men. Thus ran his explanation of the existence of male hysteria. His recognition of a syndrome resembling hysteria in males was a most significant contribution. He noted that such states also followed sexual abstinence, and he therefore assumed that they were caused by retention of sperm. From this he derived his frequently reiterated conviction that failure of spermatic emission was more deleterious even than failure of the menstrual flow.

Galen eloquently wrote (1541), "hysterical passion is just one name; varied and innumerable, however, are the forms which it encompasses." Within the quaint anatomical and physiological idiom in which the ancient theories are couched,* and more explicitly sometimes in the circumfluent language, is an emerging understanding of the basic psychological difficulties of the victims of these protean disturbances. Freud's cathartic experiments eventually yielded his theory that hysteria was derived from a disturbance of sexuality, yet, as he later wrote in *An Autobiographical Study* (1925b), at the time of formation of this theory he was unaware that in deriving hysteria from sexuality he was going back to the very beginnings of medicine. We can readily discern that the ancient physicians were concerned with the frustrated libidinous urges and with the enhanced tension, anxiety, rage, or depression which the frustration engendered, that is, with the concealed disorder of the sexual life. Study of these theories convinces us that the more perspicacious of the physicians of times long past partly understood the symptoms of their hysterical patients as defensively concealed information that their patients were unwilling or unable to impart verbally. Since Freud's work, we are familiar with the fact that these patients themselves *unconsciously* resist the expression and communication of their frustrated wishes because of inner conflict. Even in the simplest cases discussed by Galen, he was required first to evaluate non-verbal behavior as manifested in symptoms of physical distress by collating this with verbal productions, then to penetrate the palimpsest of the words. In his own idiom, he accomplishes this penetration to some extent.

It is therefore of considerable interest that, as briefly detailed elsewhere (Abse 1966), resulting from the development of the sciences of anatomy, physiology, and organic pathology, those views that were flavored with psychological concepts had become largely discounted in the nineteenth

* It is noteworthy that this idiom adheres closely to that of hysterical body-language, *but in a basic word-language.*

century before Pierre Janet and Freud. All mental as well as physical phenomena of this disease were interpreted by most nineteenth-century physicians exclusively in terms of a diseased brain basis. In order to begin to understand this partial retrogression in the understanding of hysteria—one which obstinately persists among some twentieth-century physicians—we have to consider the fact that the investigative focus of nervous disease shifted in the eighteenth and nineteenth centuries. Already in the seventeenth century, Thomas Willis had carefully studied the brain and described the arterial circle at its base. He had seen that the nerves were made up of fibres by which some influence passed from the brain to the rest of the body, but he disputed the notion propounded by Descartes that they were tubes through which "animal spirits" flowed. Luigi Galvani in the eighteenth century showed that muscle contraction was associated with electrical discharge. Later both Sir Charles Bell and François Magendie showed the distinction between predominantly motor and sensory nerves, and Bell even added a sixth sense (kinaesthetic sensation) to those described by Aristotle. Later still in the nineteenth century, the localization of central nervous system functions began to be clarified by Pierre Flourens's experimental work with pigeons, after the provocative oversimplifications and confusions of the phrenologists. Soon Paul Broca (1861) contended that one lesion among others he found post-mortem, in the inferior frontal convolution of the left cerebral hemisphere, was responsible for the speech disability of a man who had in life had this impairment for many years. Such discoveries and interpretations were the result of work founded upon the gathering momentum of the scientific outlook in medicine, an upshot itself of the success of scientific method in the investigation of the inanimate physical world. The impetus of this kind of scientific approach was also spurred by a reaction against superstitious and magical thinking which had previously suffused the practice of medicine, based otherwise on a poorly organized empiricism.

It was in this context of burgeoning scientific knowledge and related technological advances, the pace of which has accelerated enormously in our own time, that physicians acquired new thinking and language patterns which enabled them to map more adequately territories of experience with many human diseases. They struggled to divest themselves of former modes of thought and language which they came to consider as totally futile, even as beneath their dignity, and as not at all respectable. Wrapped in the "grammar" of science, their professional thinking was exclusively focused on physical evidence. It was this focus, together with regarding as unsound other modes of thinking about human beings in distress, that set limits to their attempts to unravel the problems presented by hysterical disorders.

As the language of everyday life is adapted to the focus of an area of scientific investigation, not only are new words coined to refer to previously unperceived facets of reality, but other words shift in terms of their reference, both denotative and connotative, so that their informative value in the context of a particular study is changed; moreover, some words are even more sharply nomadic under such conditions. It is also important to realize that a particular approach tends to confine itself to a special scale of observation. It is a matter of different levels of abstraction, as students of general semantics use the word. Rather one should say of *selection*, for the exhibited levels of concreteness and abstraction may range widely within a particular focus. More important, from a psychoanalytic viewpoint, are the multiple determinants which operate to motivate this focus and to resist shifts in focus sometimes necessary for problem-solving to become more effective. More generally, the limiting aspects of a special language have been emphasized by Benjamin L. Whorf (1956), who shows that a particular linguistic order may not encompass adequately all symbolic processes, all processes of reference and logic:

Actually, thinking is most mysterious, and by far the greatest light upon it that we have is thrown by the study of language. This study shows that the forms of a person's thoughts are controlled by inexorable laws of pattern of which he is unconscious. These patterns are the unperceived systematizations of his own language—shown readily enough by a candid comparison and contrast with other languages, especially those of a different linguistic family. His thinking itself is in a language—in English, in Sanskrit, in Chinese. And every language is a vast pattern system, different from others, in which are culturally ordained the focus and categories by which the personality not only communicates, but also analyzes nature, notices or neglects types of relationship and phenomena, channels his reasoning, and builds the house of his consciousness.

We find ourselves in very complex pathways if we ask how Freud was able to break through the prevalent medical semantic environment of the nineteenth century, the stereotypes of medical language and thought in which he had his own growth as a medical investigator, to approach more adequately the problems presented by the numerous patients he encountered who suffered from hysteria and hysteriform disease. As already stated, he himself later recognized that his approach took him back to considerations similar in some respects to those which permeated the thought of physicians of the ancient world. Now John Dalton's resurrection of the ideas of Democritus, who originally gave the name "atoms" to particles of matter, was founded on his own, and Robert Boyle's and others', experiments concerning especially the behavior of gases. Indeed Dalton of England in 1803 recognized the priority of Democritus of Abdera, who had first contributed this important concept (later to be modified since the indivisible particle that "atom" denotes became divisible) by using the word *atoms* in his theory. Dalton's theory was, of course, more detailed, based on careful observations, and led to further revolutionary advances in chemistry and physics, both techniques and conceptual schemata. Just as Dalton's views in chemistry harked back to the disputations of the ancient Greeks, so Freud's theory of the emotional disturbances in hysteria harked back to the physicians of the ancient world. Similarly, Freud's theory was based on more accurate observations—his own, Josef Breuer's, and others'. It was stated in more precise language than anything by his ancient predecessors and it actually became enormously more productive. In order for this advance to a psychoanalytic approach to occur, first there had to take place a partial reversion from the prevalent language of scientific medicine of the nineteenth century, a reversion to the thinking and language of everyday experience. Then ensued a specialization of this language in a direction of its own, especially in important particulars. *In this process what had to be paid attention to was the language of the patients themselves.*

Metaphor in the language of the patients

An important part of the story of this process begins in 1880 when a young woman was tirelessly nursing her dying father. One night while she was under this emotional stress there appeared to her, emerging from the wall, a large black snake which proceeded to move slowly toward her father. In her horror at that apparition her right arm suddenly became completely paralyzed, and the prayer which came to her lips could not be uttered in her terror. By the time her physician, Breuer, again came to see his patient (since renowned as Anna O.), she was temporarily mute, with paralyzed limbs twisted by contractures. The case history of Fraulein Anna O. is reported by Breuer in the book *Studies on Hysteria* which he wrote jointly with Freud (1895). This work is replete with many very interesting observations and seminal principles from which, for our purposes here, we will select a few. Breuer writes:

This regular order of things was: the somnolent state in the afternoon, followed after sunset by the deep hypnosis for which she invented the technical name of "clouds" [this word in English in the original], . . . I used to visit her in the evening, when I knew I should find her in her hypnosis, and I then relieved her of the whole stock of imaginative products which she had accumulated since my last visit. It was essential that this should be effected completely if good results were to follow.

Here Breuer was referring to the observations that her symptoms were remarkably alleviated if she were given the opportunity to discuss her thoughts and feelings, including her phantasies, and he inferred many sorts of connections between particular events, "imaginative products," and particular symptoms. He writes further: "She aptly described this procedure, speaking seriously, as a 'talking cure,' while she referred to it jokingly as 'chimney sweeping.'"

The patient's metaphors in describing her experiences, for example, "clouds" as a word to describe her periodic unclear state of consciousness, and "chimney-sweeping" as a means of describing her experience of relief in the treatment process, gave rise to the concepts named "hypnoid states" and "abreaction" in the evolving theory of the two physicians. In brief, Breuer and Freud were paying attention to what the patient said, and the patient was cooperating as much in the evolution of theory as in the cure. The metaphoric statements of the patient were related to the conceptual thought and language of the two physicians which became incorporated in the evolving theory. These particular phrases represented concepts elaborated from her inner perception of herself, or as we would now say, by her observing ego in the therapeutic alliance.

Considering the relationship of Anna O. and Breuer from a broader viewpoint, Frederick Bram (1965) notes:

It was, therefore, a matter of letting one other person sit in the wings of her "private theatre." The drama was a view to the functioning of the mentality of human-kind perhaps never before as clearly displayed to the eyes of a man of science. It clearly disclosed that even the most seemingly meaningless symptom indeed had meaning. It portrayed beyond doubt that there are memories that influence one from beyond awareness, that there therefore must be two levels of mind-conscious and unconscious. These were the *gifts* of Anna O. along with one other, the route to which the "private theatre" might be reached, catharsis which was the primordium of psychoanalysis.

He proceeds to ponder the question of her motivation, thereby contributing to our understanding of the Anna O.–Breuer relationship.

It is noteworthy that, so far as Breuer was personally concerned, this relationship provoked intense inner conflict. In 1880, in Vienna, it was quite a novel procedure to observe closely and treat psychologically a single patient over a two-year period. Nathan Schlessinger et al. (1967) write:

The theoretical chapter in the *Studies* documents further consequences of this conflict. Strachey has noted the paradox that Breuer, who had devised a psychological treatment for hysteria, wrote a physiological treatise for the

Studies on Hysteria. His work was full of references to intracerebral excitations and analogies between the nervous system and electrical conduction phenomena.

Many of Breuer's early concepts, however, were incorporated into later psychoanalytic theory, which remains biologically based. One of the negative results of Breuer's intense inner conflict was that he was inhibited from breaking through, as adequately as Freud later did, the prevalent medical semantic environment of the nineteenth century. Freud also began by adopting the neurological method of describing psychopathological phenomena, attempting in the *Project for a Scientific Psychology* (1895) a "psychology for neurologists." But as Strachey (1957) points out, Freud the neurologist was overtaken by Freud the psychologist. It became more and more obvious that ". . . even the elaborate machinery of the neuronic systems was far too cumbersome and coarse to deal with the subtleties which were being brought to light by 'psychological analysis' and which could only be accounted for in the language of mental processes."

Early in the course of his investigations with Breuer, Freud (1895) came across a series of metaphoric phrases in the statements of Frau Cäcilie M. while she was in psychotherapy with him. These metaphoric phrases were connected with different somatic symptoms. For example, in one phase of his work with her she reached the recollection of the scene of an emotionally stirring quarrel with her husband; concomitantly, the symptom of facial neuralgia was reanimated. Freud pressed his patient to describe the conversation with her husband which had been painfully humiliating for her. As she did so, she put her hand to her cheek and in this instance used the simile: "It was like a slap in the face." At another time she was afflicted with a violent pain in her right heel, a shooting pain at every step she took, that impeded walking. Freud (1895) writes:

Analysis led us in connection with this to a time when the patient had been in a sanatorium abroad. She had spent a week in bed and was going to be taken down to the common dining room for the first time by the house physician. The pain came on at the moment when she took his arm to leave the room with him; it disappeared during the reproduction of the scene, when the patient told me she had been afraid at the time that she might not "find herself on a right footing" with these strangers.

In each instance it is obvious that the metaphoric expression has a relationship to her somatic symptom, as well as to her complex dependency-independency conflicts, associated as these are with severe separation anxiety, and anxiety about being hurt. Let us bypass at this time any further analysis. It is sufficient to note that these statements, comprising figures of speech, are concerned with strong and painful feelings; in the first instance, feelings about being insulted by her husband, in the second, feelings of anxiety about steering herself adequately in a group of strangers.

Recent case illustration

To illustrate further the importance of metaphoric statement for affective communication, here is an example from my own experience. Mrs. X., thirty-five years old, and physically very attractive, was admitted to the medical department of the University of Virginia hospital, referred by her family physician for "repeated fainting spells and severe pain in the neck." At the time this patient was interviewed she had already undergone rigorous physical investigation. She was in bed, constrained by a sort of traction apparatus which pulled on her neck muscles, despite the failure of attempts to reveal any basic organic pathology. Her neck muscles were in severe spasm; certainly there was severe functional disorder as well as pain. In the first interview, as I sat at the bedside of this intelligent and attractive woman, she told me that despite the apparatus and the various medications that had been tried she still had a severe pain in the neck. She proceeded to say that before admission to the hospital, in addition to the neck pain which had progressively worsened, she had experienced alarming "black-outs." I asked her what she meant by "black-out," and the patient proceeded to tell me that she fainted, looking at me with some surprise as if puzzled by my apparent ignorance of the vernacular. Of course, I said, I understood she meant fainting spells, but she had said "black-outs." Had she herself thought of using this expression? It seemed the patient was not at all sure who had first applied this term to her fainting attacks, her husband, herself, or one of the doctors. I then asked whether, when she was "out" in the faint, she saw black. Hesitating a moment, the patient stated thoughtfully: "No, in fact, I pass out and see red." In further conversations the patient gave a restrained account of her widowed mother-in-law who was living at her home, and whose only offspring was the patient's husband. We had a talk about the mother-in-law's attachment to her only son, and the possible difficulties to which this might have led. The conversation became increasingly animated, and at one point I told the patient that despite her conciliatory and laudably understanding attitude toward her mother-in-law, in fact this lady had begun to give her a pain in the neck, and the first occasions when she had seen the mother-in-law breakfasting alone with her husband had made her see red.

As the emergency psychotherapy progressed in later interviews with this patient, more adequate affective expression of her rage against and jealousy of her mother-in-law was attained, as well as expression of guilt feelings. These strong feelings were the affect indicators of strong conflictual trends, which had roots, it was later revealed, in her early family drama with a tyrannical mother who very much excluded her even from expectable communication with her father as she was growing up.

Certainly metaphors are not merely ornaments of speech. They may mediate the direct unreflective expression of strong feelings on the one hand, and on the other, as indicated in the case of Anna O., they form an essential part of the development of discursive exposition. As pointed out by Charles Sherrington (1941) in his Gifford lectures, where knowledge falters the mind has recourse to metaphor. Analogical thinking conveyed through metaphor is a basic requisite in the acquisition and imparting of knowledge. Again and again where knowledge is inadequate metaphor is enlisted. To object to arguments because they are based on "metaphorical thinking" is quite unjust. As Wegener's lectures make clear, we have certainly at the least to use *faded* metaphor to keep our thinking afloat at all in discursive language. The legitimate question is whether the metaphors employed represent useful similarities with consequent adequate reference to things, processes, and relationships. As for the sort of metaphoric language which functions largely to convey feelings, its adequacy depends in a similar way upon how well it performs this function. Often in the preliminary retranslation of hysterical somatic symptoms into metaphoric speech, the language conveys feelings only slightly less dramatically than do the symptoms themselves.

III Emendation and Metaphor

IN THE case of the married woman who suffered the severe pain in the neck and saw red in her fainting spells, we were shortly able to see that her wish for her mother-in-law to live elsewhere, if she were to live at all, came into conflict with her sense of duty. This simple inference, which expresses her psychological plight very mildly, was confirmed time and again by the patient herself in the psychotherapy. Indeed this was the first step that she took. Once there were beginnings of translation of her symptoms into affect-laden metaphoric language, she protested that she ought to be able to get along with her mother-in-law, whom she respected, though the presence of this lady disturbed her feelings of well-being. Yet she acknowledged that she herself *had* thought what a pain in the neck the good woman was, and sometimes she *had* made her see red. This translation of her symptoms into word-language was but a retranslation back to the unspoken language of her own thoughts, thoughts which had later become forbidden. The conflict was found to have many ramifications, including the fact that it was but a reedition of an older unresolved conflict with her own mother; correspondingly, much more language was involved in a fuller retranslation of her symptoms.

The point to be made here is simply this. Sometimes a preliminary retranslation of part of the meaning of somatic symptoms to metaphoric language facilitates access to the emotions of the patient, including those emotions associated with repressed drive derivatives which are defended against because they come into conflict with how the patient thinks he *ought* to be motivated, how he *ought* to feel and to behave. In the process of unconscious defense the patient loses effective communication *within the self*. Both inner self-related means of expression and communication and the other expressive and communicative efforts toward others become progressively more distorted—beneath a shell of rationalization which, together with the somatic symptoms, are eventually offered to the physician for his consideration.

Before proceeding to a more general discussion of the role of metaphor in linguistic development, a discussion which provides background for understanding further the disorder of communication which is part and parcel of hysterical disease, we must guard against some immediate possible misunderstandings. Not all conversion symptoms are translatable into such readily recognizable metaphors of speech as "seeing red" or "a pain in the neck." Consider the following case.

A middle-aged Negro woman whose life had become one of increasing hardship, economically, socially, and sexually, developed a confused mental state associated with peculiar movements of the arms and fingers. She was referred to University Hospital for a thorough neurological investigation including air-encephalography, to test for a brain tumor or a presenile organic dementia. Here I will not go into any great detail about this woman's life or the clinical investigations which, before psychiatric examination, yielded no positive findings. By the time I saw this woman at the request of a resident in psychiatry she had already been interviewed while in amytal narcosis. At that time she had, among other matters and in a vague and disconnected way, discussed her father's encouragement of her education and her once-upon-a-time interest in the piano. At first sight of this woman, I said to the resident who had, while walking to the ward, reported the amytal interview, "But she is now playing the piano." (Of course, no piano was in the room.) In the short interview I had with her, the patient, with some initial direction, went into considerable and vivid detail about her father. Frequently he would look at her admiringly as she practiced her piano-playing. How proud he was of her at this time during her school years! I will not elaborate beyond stating that in response to adverse life circumstances this patient had retreated to a time of maximal happiness in her life, a time effectively symbolized by her piano-playing with an encouraging, admiring, and affectionate father at her side. Clinically, this case was a hysteriform borderline state, the most conspicuous features being a hysterical pseudodementia and apparently weird movements of the arms and fingers. These movements were in fact pantomimic in their essential nature.

In discussing hysterical symptomatic attacks, Freud (1909) wrote, "When one psychoanalyzes a patient subject to hysterical attacks, one soon gains the conviction that these attacks are nothing but phantasies projected and translated into motor activity and represented in pantomime." It sometimes also happens that there is a revival in memory of actual events, rich in associated phantasy and feeling, a revival which in a truncated way is pantomimically expressed in body movements, as in the piano-playing of the patient in the severe dissociative reaction briefly described above.

In order to gain some perspective about the role of affect-laden metaphor as it emerges in the retranslation of hysterical somatic symptoms

The "word-sentence,"* being insufficient, is thus supplemented by more and more words. Appositives, then relative clauses, and so on, are added as corrections of deficient presentations. Grammatical structure evolves by *emendation* of an ambiguous expression. All these auxiliary utterances Wegener sees as the exposition of the one-word sentence, providing in part or wholly a verbal context to supplement or substitute for the implicit context which is deficient as far as the hearer is concerned. In this way full-fledged speech begins to emerge.

All discourse, according to Wegener, involves the verbal or practical context and the "novelty" presented by the speaker. In connection with this novelty we encounter the second principle of language, namely, *metaphor*. When a precise word is so far lacking to designate the novelty, another word is used. This word usually already denotes something else. A word symbol, already a symbol for a thing, a process, or a relation, is used for this new purpose, on the basis of some suggested analogy. The context makes it clear that the word is not referring to the first thing, process, or relation, that this is not literally denoted; hence the word must mean something else. For example, one might say of a fire: "It flares up." One might say too: "His anger flared up." In the second use of the word *flare* we know that this does not refer to the physical flame but connotes the idea of "flaring up" as a symbol for what his anger is doing. As Langer (1942) writes of such an instance: "The expression 'to flare up' has acquired a wider meaning than its original use, to describe the behavior of a flame; it can be used metaphorically to describe whatever its meaning can symbolize. Whether it is to be taken in a literal or metaphorical sense has to be determined by the context."

Wegener shows that if a metaphor is used often, it fades to a literal significance. We take the word *literal* to mean that which all its applications have in common. Constant figurative use generalizes its sense. It comes to have again a literal significance, but a different one from its original specific meaning. He shows that all general words are probably derived from specific appellations by metaphorical use, so that our literal language is a repository of faded metaphors.

So far I have tried briefly to follow Wegener in order to suggest that the structure of language grows from the one-word sentence by gradual emendation and to point out that another essential element of discursive language, generality, is achieved through the fading of metaphor. Before language acquired faded metaphors to buttress logical thought, it could hardly do more than represent needs and feelings by a demonstrative indication of them in immediate experience. The process of

---

* An earlier vocal unit as described by Antoine Grégoire is the "monoreme," close to the interjection, but a one-unit referential pattern which precedes an actual word. See Werner and Kaplan (1963).

fading of metaphors is a bridge on the way from the early empractic phase of language toward the developed phase of discursive exposition.

Lest the discernment of metaphor embedded one way or another in a statement may yet seem elusive, let me illustrate further. Take this statement from Arthur M. Schlesinger's *A Thousand Days*: "But with all the problems and frustrations, Kennedy had gone far toward infusing a new energy into American diplomacy and a new spirit into the conduct of foreign affairs." It is at once apparent that the phrase beginning "infusing a new energy" is a metaphor taken from its literal reference, namely, the perceptual experience of fluids being poured from one container into another, or from one channel into another, a reference which adheres to the Latin *infundere*—"to pour in" from which the word *infuse* is derived. More familiar may be its other literal reference which appeared perhaps a little later in the history of the English word—that of steeping a soluble substance in a liquid. These are indeed two distinct processes, but the word came to mean either according to the direction given by a particular context. Both these literal references are absorbed in the metaphor concerning Kennedy's behavior vis-à-vis diplomacy. Now let us take one word, *spirit*, in the same statement as another example. This word is etymologically an adaptation of the Latin word *spiritus* which denotes breathing—an experience we all continue to have. Of course, it is apparent that the clause beginning "Kennedy had gone far . . ." sets forth a spatial metaphor.

Metaphors are derived, as reflection reveals, from the sensory-motor foundations of immediate experience. Experience is based on energy changes inside the body, changes which may be initiated inside or outside the body. The ego is equipped *eventually* to discriminate the source of stimuli as preponderantly external or internal, and also to distinguish between stimuli emanating directly from the body and those from its own psychic organization. Thus arise, as Wernicke (1906) expounded, concepts of the outside world, of the personality, and of the body—"allopsychic," "autopsychic," and "somatopsychic" concepts. This progressive differentiation is selectively disrupted in hysteria. In the ravages of communication wrought by a hysterical flight into illness there is, in selected instances of crucial emotional importance to the patient, a regression of metaphoric speech to its sensory-motor foundations. Then it is found that these metaphors are rooted in the exteroceptive, interoceptive, and proprioceptive patterns of perception which in childhood succeed the partially fused sensations of infancy (see Figure 1).

It is remarkable how perspicuously Wegener deals with the semantic movement and the development of general meaning through metaphor. He emphasizes the initial embedment of metaphor in the context of a situation which must be understood in order to grasp the meaning of the spoken word. He accomplished this intellectual feat independently of Michel Bréal (1897), whose "Essai de Sémantique, Science des Significations" became so well-known and enhanced so considerably the serious study of meaning.

Later we will discuss the special psychiatric importance of the disruption of metaphoric symbolism in schizophrenic language disorder. In connection with language disorder in the psychoses, Wegener's studies comprise an awareness of the depth-psychological involvement in language of the ethical and aesthetic impulses. These find expression, he shows, in the development of speech, and we find their recession in the dissolution of spoken language in psychosis.

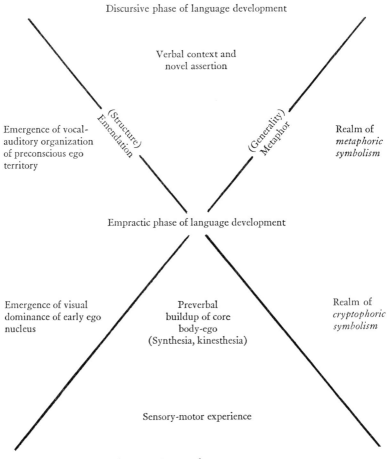

Discursive phase of language development

Verbal context and
novel assertion

(Structure)
Emendation

(Generality)
Metaphor

Emergence of vocal-
auditory organization
of preconscious ego
territory

Realm of
*metaphoric
symbolism*

Empractic phase of language development

Emergence of visual
dominance of early ego
nucleus

Preverbal
buildup of core
body-ego
(Synthesia, kinesthesia)

Realm of
*cryptophoric
symbolism*

Sensory-motor experience

Fig. 1. Development of semantic speech

IV Metaphor, Thought, and Language

IN THE *Poetics*, Aristotle (translation 1952) defines metaphor as "the application of an alien name by transference either from genus to species, or from species to genus, or from species to species, or by analogy, that is, proportion." Thus Aristotle recognizes the concept which is the reference of the word *metaphor*—first, that the word signifies "to carry change" (*Meta* = change and *phora*, from the root "to carry") and, secondly, that this change of meaning of a word or phrase functions by means of replacement of a part for a whole or a whole for a part; usually it is a shared part or common attribute that is involved in the transfer of the name to another object, process, or relation. As Wegener indicates, discursive language in its development tends to move away from the image of what can actually be perceived toward more problematical references.

The examples offered by Aristotle may be used to demonstrate Wegener's deeper insight. In illustrating "transference from genus to species," Aristotle offers: "There lies my ship." For, states Aristotle, "lying at anchor is a species of lying." Obviously here the word "lying" had first already acquired generality before transfer. We would suppose that this more general quality had arisen from numerous repeated specific uses in phrases such as "lying in bed." From the name for the experience of reclining the body, a more general transference had first occurred before the same word could be applied to the relatively motionless ship at anchor. We would, of course, agree with those who maintain that a particular naming is already a step on the road to generality, and we see no need to enter into obsolete arguments as to the priority of particulars or universals. These arguments seem to be resolved by the notion of circular dynamic effects (feedback and feed-forward mechanisms, in the language of cybernetics) which build up a quality of heightened generality. Wegener postulates an especial increment of "generality" as a metaphor fades to a literal significance. Constant figurative use in various applications, he shows, precedes the heightened generality of sense by the grasp of a common denominator, a shared part, in all the figurative uses. First then must be "the transference from species to species" in a figurative way, time and again, before the fade to a literality and a distinctive increment of general significance. As Wegener more clearly points out, this quality of generality must be engendered before a word can become adequately understood for use in the verbal context (logical subject). Since the context of an assertion tells us whether we should interpret the metaphor (of the logical predicate) literally or figuratively, it follows that the context itself must (in speech) be literal, for it has not in turn a context to give direction to its sense, to resolve ambiguity.

We have chosen above an example of metaphor offered by Aristotle which suggests, as we would have it, the semantic movement from the experience of the body itself to that of outer objects and events, a movement illuminated by observation of the distortion of word language in mental disease (cf. Schilder 1950). Here we may draw attention to another important element of the characteristic difficulty intrinsic in severe schizophrenic thought and language disorder (see below, Section VIII). In schizophrenic communication there is a gross impairment of the capacity to resolve ambiguity. The dynamic interaction between context and novel assertion becomes chaotic both because figurative meanings are not always suitably subdued to literal generalities and because literal specificities often suddenly blossom into figurative meanings. Harold F. Searles (1965) has especially clearly discussed the schizophrenic difficulty of stabilizing a differentiation between metaphorical and literal meanings, and the confusion to which this gives rise.

In his example of "transference from species to genus," Aristotle more closely approaches Wegener's principle of generalization of sense through the vicissitudes of metaphor. Thus Aristotle quotes: "Verily ten thousand noble deeds hath Odysseus wrought,'" and he comments, "For ten thousand is a species of large number, and is here used for a large number generally." It has to be borne in mind that in his treatment of metaphor Aristotle is concerned with the varieties of poetry and not directly, as was Wegener, with the genesis of discursive language. In poetry, the semantic movement is often reversed, that is from the abstract, or at any rate from the more general, toward or actually to the specific sensuous concrete image. However, the image all the more forcibly now alludes, in our formed organization of word and thought, to the more general, even the universal.

Sometimes in poetry, as in some aspects of the evolution of discursive language, there is not a movement in the concrete-abstract axis at all; it is simply that a more familiar image is replaced by an unexpected one, thus giving additional impact to the message. In discussing this phenomenon, Aristotle again approaches one of Wegener's views, this time Wegener's major contention, namely, that when there is no word, or when a precise one is lacking to designate a novel thought, metaphor is enlisted. In connection with the phenomenon of unexpected imagery, Aristotle writes:

For some of the terms of the proportion there is at times no word in existence; still the metaphor may be used. For instance to scatter seed is called sowing; but the action of the sun in scattering his rays is nameless. Still this process bears to the sun the same relation as sowing to the seed. Hence the expression of the poet "sowing the god-created light."

When we approach the function of live metaphor, as opposed to faded metaphor, in its use of, or evocation of, sensuous concrete imagery, we are confronted with the accompanying surge of emotion. Emotions signify to us primarily not the nature of things but rather our subjective reactions to things (See Abse 1966). In the terminology of general semantics, they are of more *intensional* than *extensional* value. Where affective communication is sought, as especially in poetry and drama, vivid sensuous concrete imagery is necessarily utilized. If we are to be constrained by the rhetorical categories, it will be evident immediately that not only metaphor and simile in the strict sense but allusion in general are often associated affective devices. If I refer to New York as a modern Babylon, the reference to a luxurious city steeped in sinfulness and doomed to destruction helps to convey some of my feelings about that city. Much of irony, pathos, and humor depend upon the enlistment of metaphor, simile, and allusion to arouse conflictual feelings. Poetic language, as opposed especially to scientific language, condenses multiple references which diffuse again in the minds of the audience. Philip Wheelright (1962) puts the matter thus:

Poetic language generally, by reason of its openness, tends towards semantic plentitude rather than toward a cautious semantic economy. The power of speaking by indirection and by evoking larger, more universal meanings than utterance taken in its literal sense would warrant, is one species of semantic plentitude. But it may also be that the tenor of an image or of a surface statement is not single; the semantic arrow may point in more than one direction. When two such diversely intended meanings are sharply opposed, the result is paradox. But even when the doubleness of meaning is not pushed to the point of contrariety, it may often be the case that more than one meaning is suggested simultaneously by a certain word or phrase or image. Or, more characteristically, there may be a group of verbal symbols put together in a certain syntax and suggesting certain images, some more overtly than others with the result that the interplay of meanings and half-meanings is far more copious than any literal paraphrase could ever formulate. The greater instances of such plurisignation do not lend themselves to brief exposition, for they usually require patient analysis of an entire poem.

In the symptoms of hysteria, semantic plenitude, paradox, and plurisignation generally are pushed to extremes on account of the extraordinary dominance of primary process. In the "retranslation" of these symptoms to words as part of the process of psychotherapy, we encounter the imagery, metaphor, and affects of poetic language, though, of course, these are recaptured in comparatively unorganized form. Retranslation in psychoanalytic treatment is accomplished through dissolution of resistance or, to simplify further to the essential point relevant here, through derepression. The constantly repeated clinical experience of transformation of symptom symbols into word symbols which approach poetic language suggests further extrapolation. The assumption is that in the evolution of discursive language the fading of metaphor, essential to enable progress in generality and thus an adequate basis for abstract thinking, involves a further complex contrary process of repression. There is a partial repression of the original mnemic image of the percept, of closely related conceptual elaborations, of directly connected (aroused) instinctual derivatives and emotional reactions, and to a lesser extent, of the figurative reference which had continued to carry elements of the former. The double repression is partial, for some elements are retained and resynthesized for higher order word-symbolism.

Higher order word-symbolism finally secures secondary process thinking of which it is itself an initial reflection. It fosters the more definitive thought differentiation of similarity and contrast, a differentiation which, when adequate, facilitates both the recognition or patterning of common attributes (generality) and the separation of categories on the basis of varying criteria. There seems to be a continuing "dialectical" relationship between thought and language, which periodically approaches unity in the more firmly established "secondary process" of abstract thinking which human beings, alone of all living creatures, achieve. This achievement is critically based upon the metaphoric symbolism of speech.

It is not denied that abstract thinking can take place independently of verbal connections; it can even be shown that abstract thinking (at a lower level) takes place in animals. Although the efficiency of abstract thinking is enormously enhanced through word-symbolism, there is the testimony of eminent thinkers (e.g., Galton and Einstein) that they do not think in words. It is evident that other symbolic modes, that is, modes of thought without words or with only minimal support of words, can be extraordinarily effective, as symbolic logic and other mathematical modes attest. In such instances, some thought formations may be achieved which are apparently not translatable either into our more usual word-symbolism or into visual or other imagery.

Experience in psychoanalytic therapy suggests that live metaphor arises via a flexible and regulated derepression and regression ("in the service of the ego" [Kris 1952]) to sensorial imagery with subsequent establishment of word connections. The liberated word symbols or spoken metaphors afford a discharge vehicle for drive derivatives and related feelings of the speaker and effect vivid communication with the auditor. On the other hand, in the course of the development of speech and the closely related vocal-auditory preconscious organization of the ego, via a regulated repression, original metaphors fade and provide a basis for abstract thought and language. At this level thought and language become inseparable; live metaphor, comprising the change from literal to figurative word symbolism, has itself become subdued, and faded metaphor, the resultant, has become the bridge to logical abstract thinking.

Further understanding of metaphoric symbolism can only be reached through a study of its foundations in imagery and unconscious symbolism, a study which necessarily must exceed the limits of Wegener's thought and incorporate that of Freud.

V Imagery

FREUD (1920) proposed that the perceptual apparatus of the mind could be usefully conceived of as consisting of two layers, behind which was a third and complex layer comprising the memory system. The first of the two layers consists of an external protective shield against stimuli, which diminishes the strength of incoming excitations. The surface behind this shield, the second layer, receives the stimuli and is designated Pcpt.-Cs. The system Pcpt.-Cs. forms no permanent traces so that it remains free to react to every new perception. Permanent traces of the excitations aroused in this system are preserved in the mnemic system lying behind it. Earlier, Freud (1900) had discussed some of the complexities of mnemic subsystems which comprise the memory bank in the seventh chapter of *The Interpretation of Dreams.* Some of the ideas therein, and ones developed later, had their origin in his work with Breuer. For example, Breuer had stated in the "theoretical" chapter of *Studies on Hysteria* (1895) that the basic essential of the perceptual apparatus is that its *status quo ante* should be capable of being rapidly restored; otherwise further perception would be impaired. On the other hand, Breuer pointed out that the essential of memory is that permanent changes are wrought. He suggested that these two contradictory conditions could not be met by a single apparatus.

Freud (1925a) compared a small toy writing tablet called the "Mystic Writing Pad" with the hypothetical structure of the shielded perceptual system superimposed on mnemic systems. This layered writing tablet provides both a shielded and ever-ready receptive surface and a layer for permanent traces of notes made upon it; the later engraphic effect is upon this deeper layer which is visible through both the celluloid shield and the delicate receptive surface. Freud (1925a) wrote:

We need not be disturbed that in the Mystic Pad no use is made of the permanent traces of the notes that have been received; it is enough that they are present. There must come a point at which the analogy between an auxiliary apparatus of this kind and the organ which is its prototype will cease to apply. It is true too that once the writing has been erased, the Mystic Pad cannot "reproduce" it from within; it would be a mystic pad indeed, if, like our memory, it could accomplish that.

Through the portals afforded by vision, hearing, touch, kinaesthetic sensations, smell, and taste, under certain conditions of attention there is a rapid exteroperception which leaves memory traces. When these traces are revived later in consciousness, the corresponding previously perceived objects are reexperienced, in a modified form, as images.* Under usual adult waking conditions, this new experience carries with it the qualification that the objects are not felt as immediately present to the senses. Indeed a testing with regard to "immediacy" is inextricably involved in the testing of outwardly produced perceptions.

In the differentiated psyche of the adult, side-by-side with the perception of the external world, interacting with it in varying degrees of forcefulness, there remains a self-involvement which includes a body-core, instinctual drive derivatives, and affects. The complete act of perception of the outer world by an adult remains influenced, although generally less so than in earlier phases of the life-cycle, by the drive-affect state operative at the time of perception. Under calm conditions primitive introjective-identifications and projective-identifications are purposefully controlled, and affects are either reduced to signals or modulated for useful cognitive steer. The prevailing orectic state may be reinforced, modified, or even completely changed, as in surprise, in the beginnings of the act through the influence of the drive-organized memory system. Later, the images "reexperienced" are remodeled on the basis of another orectic state of the individual in a different situational context. Thus the "reexperience" can never be quite congruent with the earlier perceptual experience, though it might approach it closely. An example of especially close approach, even as to small details, occurs during hypnotic rapport and trance when the operator insists on review. Generally, however, the "reexperience" has similarity rather than identity.

Besides the lack of complete congruence, there is the other qualification mentioned above—a part of the gap between "experience" and "reexperience" is the negative sense that the recollection does not convey the feelings of objects "out there" and happenings in outer reality. There is also the positive sense of "inner" location, perhaps partly cued

* It is advisable to distinguish the supposed "reexperiences" of infants from those of children and adults, and perhaps to designate the former simply as "representations" of their perceptual impressions rather than as images. In the undifferentiated psyche of the infant, it seems that perception is synaesthetic and that inner and outer worlds are merged to begin with. As this only slowly changes, representations in early infancy must be vastly different from those, such as images, which occur at a later period of development. It must be mentioned too that even the word "representation" would be avoided in this connection by some psychologists who reserve this word for representations more like their own and denied perhaps by others who would place representation even of a primitive kind as later than early infancy.

by the negative, that makes this an entirely inward experience. In health, memory images, however vivid, are not usually confused with an outwardly produced perception. The function of reality-testing has developed to avoid such confusion, which would, of course, be maladaptive (militating against survival). Reality-testing relies essentially upon motor action which affords the criterion of elimination of an ego-experience. Freud (1917) states: "A perception which is made to disappear by an action is recognized as external, as reality; where such an action makes no difference, the perception originates within the subject's own body—it is not real."*

The condensed account given above of the nature of revived experience is supported by a series of ingenious experiments which also led F. C. Bartlett (1932) to the view that remembering is an imaginative reconstruction of past experience rather than a mere replica of it. Indeed in the process of imagining, as compared with simpler imaging, there is an increased distancing from actual perceptual experience. Revived representations of images are, to a varying extent, condensed or disjointed and displaced, creating new combinations. The mnemic residues of recent perceptual experience are often combined with older memory images in this process. If, as briefly noted, imagery is partly ordered under the influence of drive and affect organization, in the realm of imagination this influence is vastly enhanced. Imagination entails the release of an increased interaction between recent memory ordered by present motivation and feelings and drive-organized memory traces of the more remote past. This increased interaction contributes imaginative products, some of which achieve conscious presentation.

Imagining is indeed characterized by a shift in the balance of secondary and primary process in favor of the latter, as is hinted above (cf. Varendonck 1921, and Rapaport's comments in Rapaport 1951). The dominance of primary process becomes especially emphatic in dreaming consciousness; recent and childhood sensory experience is often condensed in the manifest content, which takes the form generally of visual hallucinosis. Under the conditions of dreaming, the negative qualification mentioned above in regard to memory images—that the objects are not felt to be immediately present to the senses—does not usually obtain. Only occasionally in our dreams do we rally to assure ourselves that these are only dream images (Freud 1900). Then again, in many pathological mental states (with the breakdown of reality-testing), vivid imagery with full sensual force results in hallucinations. Some psychologists (Jaensch 1930) have distinguished eidetic images

---

* The meaning is clear, though the language quoted may arouse some objections. "Real," for example, in this case refers to external reality; of course there is the psychic reality of inner events such as imagination produces as well as external stimuli.

from the usual memory images. These images are especially vivid, like those in dreams and in pathological hallucinosis, but have a more direct and less distorted connection with perception, in this respect like the more usual memory images. Eidetic imagery is mainly confined to young children. E. R. Jaensch (1951), the originator of the term, states:

Optical perceptual (or eidetic) images are phenomena that take up an intermediate position between sensations and images. Like ordinary physiological after-images, they are always seen in the literal sense. They have this property of necessity under all conditions, and share it with sensations. In other respects they can also exhibit the properties of images. In those cases in which the imagination has little influence, they are merely modified after-images, deviating from the norm in a definite way, and when that influence is nearly, or completely zero, we can look upon them as slightly intensified after-images.

In *Education Through Art* (1943) Herbert Read writes:

Such people [adults who claim eidetic imagery] are generally artists—visual artists like painters, but sometimes also poets and musicians. It may be that such eidetic individuals are more self-analytical than an eidetic individual without creative gifts would be, but the theory has been put forward by Jaensch and others that such persons are creative artists *because they are eidetic.* . . . A certain amount of evidence has been collected by Dr. Rosamond Harding. She quotes statements by the painters William Blake and W. Northcote, writers such as Charlotte Brontë, Charles Dickens, Thackeray, Alphonse Daudet, Shelley, Coleridge, and one musician, Elgar. All these statements point to the presence and use of eidetic imagery, and are sometimes very specific. For example, Medwin, in his *Life of Percy Bysshe Shelley*, relates that the poet could throw a veil over his eyes and find himself in a *camera obscura*, where all the features of a scene were reproduced in a form more pure and perfect than they had been originally presented to his external senses. It should be recalled that Shelley suffered from hallucinations, which sometimes had a disastrous effect on his life. From a less romantic source, evidence may be quoted which shows the high value which the artist places upon such images when he commands them.

Read then quotes from *An Anecdote of William Hogarth,* wherein the artist relates how he became dissatisfied with copying, and instead fixed forms and characters in his mind to revive them at the time of applying himself to his canvas.

According to Gordon W. Allport (1924) the genetic function of eidetic imagery is performed in the earlier years of mental development when, by preserving and elaborating sensory data, it enhances the meaning of the stimulus situation for the child and enables him to perfect his adaptive responses. This kind of consideration buttresses the argument of Read, who puts forward far-reaching claims for the place of art in the educational system and contends that a too-exclusively logical ideal has been imposed on early education. However, Allport's notion does not include any chronological precision; and anyway it does not justify such extensive claims as Read makes.

Indeed, Read (1943) takes an extreme view of the relevance of cultivating imagery, especially visual imagery, to adequate human development. An aphorism of Bernard Shaw adorns the title page of his book and briefly summarizes his own message: "I am simply calling attention to the fact that fine art is the only teacher except torture." This extreme view is challenged by the work of Jerome S. Bruner, et al. (1966) at the Center for Cognitive Studies. Bruner insists, taking an opposite position, that it is highly important to help the child to achieve freedom from an early preoccupation with the vivid, and more superficial, attributes of things. We are here, it would seem, dealing with questions of optimal timing in education. Presumably the interventions that Bruner might encourage could take place too early for a particular child, whereas the methods which Read strongly advocates might hinder another from developing his full capacity for abstract thinking. These considerations touch especially upon the supremely important role of language in cognitive growth. Language is the principal means of achieving and expressing conceptual thought, as Wegener's investigations of the life of speech emphasize.

Francis Galton (1907) reported in 1883 that he had found a wide variation in the power of visual imagery among a hundred men (of whom nineteen were Fellows of the Royal Society) and that the scientists clustered for the most part at the lower end of the scale. He found, too, that the power of visual imagery was generally higher in women and in schoolboys than in men. He considered that where advancing years were accompanied by a growing habit of "hard abstract thinking" that the faculty of visual imagery was further impaired. Clementina Kuhlman (1960), as reported extensively by Bruner et al. (1966), found that children with high imagery were better than those with low imagery at tasks concerned with the association of arbitrary verbal labels and pictures. On the other hand, the child with low imagery excelled when challenged to form a concept by recognizing the shared attribute of a set of pictures. She remarks, "A functional attribute or a complexly patterned perceptual attribute is frequently criterial for the meaning-categories [concepts], and hence for the correct use of language." In conceptualizing, choosing the correct shared attributes and generalizing therefrom are sequential mental operations. The inferior conceptual performance of children with imagery preference was found to be the result of their use of surface features in grouping and not a failure to generalize labels—a failure, in other words, in their awareness of the bases upon which generalizations are usefully made.

The findings afford some experimental support for William James's (1890) view of two stages in the development of reasoning; in the first stage similarity merely operates to call up cognate thought; in the second the bond of identity between the cognate thoughts is noticed. Abstract reasoners, men of science and philosophers, are those who notice the bond, whereas, according to James, men of intuition, even those of genius, do not. James (1890) writes:

At first sight it might seem that the analytic mind represented simply a higher intellectual stage, and that the intuitive mind represented an arrested stage of intellectual development; but the difference is not so simple as this. Professor Bain has said that a man's advance to the scientific stage (the stage of noticing and abstracting the bond of similarity) may often be due to an *absence* of certain emotional sensibilities. The sense of color, he says, may no less determine a mind away from science than it determines it toward paintings. There must be a penury in one's interest in the details of particular forms in order to permit the forces of the intellect to be concentrated on what is common to many forms. In other words, supposing a mind fertile in the suggestions of analogies, but, at the same time, keenly interested in the particulars of each suggested image, that mind would be far less apt to single out the particular character which called up the analogy than one whose interests were less generally lively. A certain richness of the aesthetic nature may, therefore, keep one in the intuitive stage. All the poets are examples of this.

Later James adds a comment which perhaps could temper the enthusiasm of those who too one-sidedly advocate the training of children in conformity with ideals of logical language:

A man in whom all the accidents of an analogy rise up as vividly as this, may be excused for not attending to the ground of an analogy. But he need not on that account be deemed intellectually the inferior of a man of drier mind, in whom the ground is not as liable to be eclipsed by the general splendor. Rarely are both sorts of intellect, the splendid and analytic, found in conjunction.

Indeed, as Galton (1907) already indicated in 1885, it would seem that the best method of developing and utilizing imagery, without prejudice to the practice of abstract thought in word symbols (which develops from it), is a considerable educational problem.*

* William James's (1890) discussion of two stages (or types) of reasoning is preceded by consideration of man's superior association by *similarity*, as compared with animals in whose mode of association *contiguity* dominates. He makes it clear that the capacity to attend to abstract characters depends on this basic superiority. As originally stated by Aristotle, the laws of association of ideas are that of similarity (or contrast) and that of contiguity (in space or time). Roman Jakobson (1946) points out that two fundamental verbal operations are word selection and word combination, the former based on similarity and the latter on contiguity; adequate verbal communication requires both, though more of one than of the other for different purposes.

It is now necessary to turn our attention from imagery of the outer world to the imagery of the body itself in which symbolism, as we will later expound, has its other root. Freud (1923) maintained that the infant ego becomes differentiated from the id not only by the direct influence of the external world acting through the infantile perceptual apparatus, but also through the impingement on that apparatus of excitations and discharges emanating from the infant's own body. He writes:

Another factor, besides the influence of the system Pcpt, seems to have played a part in bringing about the formation of the ego and its differentiation from the id. A person's own body, and above all its surface, is a place from which both external and internal perceptions may spring. It is *seen* like any other object, but to the *touch* it yields two kinds of sensations, one of which may be equivalent to an internal perception. . . . Pain, too, seems to play a part in the process, and the way in which we gain new knowledge of our organs during painful illnesses is perhaps a model of the way by which in general we arrive at the idea of our body.

The direct observations of an infant by T. W. Preyer (1882) are relevant. He observed that the infant was intensely preoccupied with his body during the first year of life, and this diminished in the second year. As soon as he could see well enough, the infant watched his arms and legs in motion, much as he would a strange moving object. He looked at his own grasping hands as attentively as at another person's moving fingers. Later he would observe himself and touch himself in his bath, especially the feet; he would press his hand on the table like a toy. Gradually the infant became able to distinguish his own body from other objects. In this development, Preyer emphasized the importance of pain experience.*
    Willi Hoffer (1950) writes;

We feel on firm ground, however, as soon as we think of mental processes which characterize the spread of the feeling of the self over the infant's body, in which the self is housed. When the body is seen—after sight has been sufficiently developed—it is perceived like any other object reaching the infant's mind, by the organ of vision. Quite different is the perceptual effect when the infant touches his body. Here two sensations simultaneously yield an experience, and this may arise very early in life, perhaps even in the intrauterine state. Our own experience when touching the body makes us think of one part of our body, the hand, for instance, actively approaching another part which passively experiences being touched. There seems no simple justification for assuming that the same happens in early infancy. Coming in touch with its own body elicits two sensations of the same quality

---

* He also discussed, as did S. Bernfeld (1925), the importance of the obedience of the organ to motor striving as a further basis of ego differentiation.

and these lead to the distinction between the self and the not-self, between body and what subsequently becomes environment. In consequence this factor contributes to the processes of structural differentiation. Delimitation between the self-body and the outer world, the world where the objects are found, is thus initiated.

K. W. Dix (1923) emphasizes the importance of pain experience in the delimitation of the infant body from the outer world. It is notable that a ten-month-old child may injure his head with little pain reaction, and a bleeding skin wound may provoke little crying. At this age, however, pain reactions to disturbances in the internal organs, for example, to colic, are much stronger. It seems likely that the weaker reactions to injury of the outer part of the body are nonetheless important in reinforcing the gradual formation of the ego boundaries.

Hartmann and Schilder (1927) point out that, as far as direct adult experience goes, we know nothing of the organs inside our bodies; all that we are actually aware of is a heavy mass. However, experience of psychophysiologic disorder, as adumbrated elsewhere (Abse 1966), leads to the hypothesis of an early infantile mouth-breast-visceral ego, a forerunner of the mouth-ego which later develops into a fuller body-ego. It is certainly true, as Schilder (1964) states, that the sensations which become part of our subjective experience as adults relate predominantly to the surface of the body or to the immediate subsurface, including the body openings which are experienced only a small way under the surface. In children and adults, as distinct from infants, bodily sensations, except that of weight, are concentrated on the surface. Thus what we know of our organs is largely acquired intellectual knowledge. Certainly, normally, our sensations would not disclose to us at all clearly the existence of heart, lungs, and intestines. One's direct experiences of his own body are generally based on visual and tactile impressions, on perceptions of the weight of the body and its various parts, and on the happenings on the sensitive surface, as Schilder maintains; whereas under regressive conditions, as even normally in dreams, the insides of the body may more easily influence imagery. Moreover, it is quite clear that the development of the outer body schema progresses *pari passu* with sensorimotor development. Thus in young children's drawings there is a lack of synthetic relations, parts of the body are simply juxtaposed as an eye next to the head, or some parts are omitted, and so on. Of this, Schilder (1964) writes:

Of course, drawing is a rather complicated psychic activity and it may be difficult to determine whether this synthetic deficiency is at all based on sensory difficulties or whether it is due to motor incapacities. But the child is completely satisfied with his drawings, and therefore I believe that the way in which children draw human figures really does reflect their knowledge and sensory experience of the body image. They express at least the mental picture they have of the human body, and the body image is a mental picture as well as perception.

Mention of the fact that in dreams, as in earlier life, the insides of the body may more easily and directly influence imagery brings us to a consideration of K. A. Scherner's view that the material with which the dream-imagination accomplishes its "artistic" work is provided by organic somatic stimuli, including the "moi-splanchnique," usually so obscure to adults in the daytime. According to Scherner (1861), the preferred way of the dream to represent the organism as a whole is a house. On the other hand, a row of houses may indicate a single organ; for example, a long street of houses may indirectly represent stimuli from the intestinal tract. Yet again, separate portions of a house may stand for distinct parts of the body; thus in a dream accompaniment of the sleeper's headache, imagery included the ceiling of a room covered with disgusting spiders. Freud (1900) commented that the preoccupation of the imagination with the subject's own body is not peculiar to dreams and added:

It is true that I know patients who have retained an architectural symbolism for the body and genitals. . . . For these patients pillars and columns represent the legs (as they do in the *Song of Solomon*), every gateway stands for one of the bodily orifices (a "hole"), every water-pipe is a reminder of the urinary apparatus, and so on. But the circle of ideas centering around plant life or the kitchen may just as readily be chosen to conceal sexual images.

It is, indeed, evident that images which pass into all the major categories, mineral, vegetable, and animal, may be used in dreams to replace other images.

VI Symbolism

THE means of representation in dreams are principally visual images and not words. For this reason, Freud (1913b) compared the interpretation of dreams to the decipherment of an ancient picto-graphic script such as Egyptian hieroglyphs. Some of the pictographic elements of dreams are distinguished from others as the bearers of an *unconscious* order of symbolism. This order of symbolism is not con-fined to dreams and, in accordance with Flugel's suggestion (recounted by Jones 1916), may be designated as cryptophoric.

A small boy five years and three months old, while dressing one morning with his mother's assistance, reported that he had had a frightening dream. He had dreamt that he was swimming, that he and others had to go through a circle in the water into a cave, and that he did not want to go because he might be drowned. Taken at face value, the word-symbols of this report simply communicated recall of dream experience; for both dreamer and auditor the words referred only to the imagery, feelings, and thoughts of the manifest dream. As Freud (1900),* Wilhelm Stekel (1911), and others have repeatedly shown, such verbally reported imagery may also be taken as a series of symbolic references of quite another order. In this example of a boy's dream, the swimming would thus refer to sexual movements of the body, the circle to the female genital, the cave to the womb, and then, of course, the anxious feelings and thoughts immediately have another dimension of significance. Indeed, in this case, the symbolism con-densed the boy's sexual wishes and those of returning to the womb in the context of the sway of an intense Oedipus complex, and the dream also comprised the attendant castration anxiety, and anxiety of being overwhelmed. The five-year-old boy in his dream used a primitive mode of expression although he, like an auditor who took it at face value, did not know the undercurrent of meaning just adumbrated. This other order of symbolism is cryptophoric, concealing unconscious contents, inasmuch as by its translation we are helped toward an understanding of ideas repressed from both the boy's waking and his dreaming con-

---

* In fact, the material on dream symbolism was only added in the 1909, 1911, and 1914 editions of *The Interpretation of Dreams*. Now it is all found in Chapter VI, E.

sciousness but expressed in the latter through this cryptophoric kind of symbolism.

Reflection concerning these two orders of symbolism, "preconscious" and "unconscious," that is the verbal report of the dream which refers to conscious ego-experience and the dream imagery itself which additionally refers to unconscious strivings, makes it evident that we confront a complex epistemological problem. As Freud (1916) writes:

In the first place we are faced by the fact that the dreamer has a symbolic mode of expression at his disposal which he does not know in waking life and does not recognize. This is as extraordinary as if you were to discover that your housemaid understood Sanskrit, though you know that she was born in a Bohemian village and never learned it. . . . Hitherto it has only been necessary for us to assume the existence of unconscious endeavors— endeavors, that is, of which temporarily or permanently, we know nothing. Now, however, it is a question of more than this, of unconscious pieces of knowledge, of connections of thought, of comparisons between different objects which result in its being possible for one of them to be regularly put in place of the other. These comparisons are not freshly made on each occasion; they lie ready to hand and are complete, once and for all. This is implied by the fact of their agreeing in the case of different individuals— possibly, indeed, agreeing in spite of differences of language.

In the next chapter, I shall describe how these peculiar comparisons are utilized by the essential dream-work with the later emergence in dreaming consciousness of one of the terms as an image; such connections of thought are a constituent also of mythopoeic ego activity.

The visual cryptophoric symbolism of dreams pertains, to a very large extent, to the expression of sexual strivings, the symbols substituting for sexual objects and relations. The philologist Hans Sperber (1912) put forward the view that sexual designations have played a large part in the origin and development of speech. The evolved word-symbols, however, for the most part have denotative and connotative values removed from sexual significance; the denotative semantic arrow and many connotative arrows point away from sexuality. The cryptophoric symbolism of dreams, on the other hand, only assumes adequate meaning when translated back into its sexual reference. Sperber conjectured, on the basis of finding so many linguistic roots which had sexual significance, that originally these sexual root words were expressed during the course of cooperative activity by primitive men. He suggested that rhythmically repeated utterances probably accompanied joint work so that sexual interest could be effectively attached to work. Man made work more acceptable, the more he could emphasize its joyous similarity to sexual activity. The words enunciated to fulfill this function during work in common came in this way to have two

references: they denoted sexual acts as well as associated working activity. In the course of time, the words became fixed to the work and
detached from the sexual meanings in waking consciousness. As in
later generations new sexual words were applied to other types of work,
an additional number of verbal roots formed. These subsequently also
lost (to consciousness) their sexual meanings, despite their sexual origin. We here come across the notion of *symbolic transformation*, which
inspired Langer (1941)* to establish a "new key in philosophy." There
is a very considerable gap between the cryptophoric symbols comprised
of visual imagery which form part of the text of the manifest dream and
the phonetic symbols which are the words we use in daily communication. On the one hand, the dream work is concerned with disguised
expression, and it would be an artifact to assume a higher level of awareness and communication inwardly and interpersonally. The Talmudic
precept that a forgotten dream resembles an unopened letter is already
on a high level of sophistication but ignores the natural function of the
dream. On the other hand, discursive word language is a function of
more highly organized ego activity and is concerned largely with *communication*. Sperber's ideas enable us to understand that dreams preserve in visual imagery the basic "thing-similarity" upon which the
ancient verbal (phonetic) identity was erected. Later the word meanings became polarized. To give an example: According to R. Kleinpaul
(1893), the word for *plough* in Latin, Greek, and Oriental language
was customarily used to denote the sexual act as well as the agricultural
one. Indeed, the Greek word for *field* also denoted the female genital.
Sometimes, a reversion to archaic bipolar reference induces an increment of emotional intensity and dramatic effect. Thus in Shakespeare's
Pericles, Boult, about to deflorate the recalcitrant Marina, declaims:
"An if she were a thornier piece of ground than she is, she shall be
ploughed." To use an example already offered to illustrate a more
complicated evolution and the undoing of the polarization usually
maintained in discursive language: an image of a cave in the manifest
dream is a cryptophoric symbol for a womb in the unconscious; both
have the common quality of being *hollow*—whence indeed etymologically the English word *cave* derives its meaning.†
   It is not only in relation to more narrowly conceived sexual body

* Whereas the emphasis in Langer's work is on the transformation of the raw data of
experience into a symbolic mode, here we are discussing as well the way in which the
symbol changes its meaning.
   † At the end of the 1887 edition of his *Etymological Dictionary*, W. W. Skeat gives a
list of Indo-European roots. Root 74 in this list signifies both to swell out and to take in;
also to be strong and to be hollow, to contain. It is present in *cave, ceiling celestial,* and
church. This seems also an example of K. Abel's thesis (1884) of the antithetical meanings
of primal words.

parts, processes, and relations, so extensive in dreaming, but in relation to body parts, processes, and relations *generally* that symbolism actually takes root. The primary importance of the arduous construction of the body image in the very first year of life as a prelude to, and accompaniment of, the infant's orientation to the outer world is now well established. Lying behind exteroperception there is a continuous, even circadian, lifelong process of construction, destruction, alteration, and reconstruction of the body image, a process sometimes dependent upon actual physical growth and alteration as well as upon other, especially emotional, vicissitudes of the personality. Lawrence S. Kubie (1953) writes:

. . . early in its formative process every concept and its symbolic representatives develop two points of reference, one internal with respect to the boundaries of the body, and one external. This dual anchorage of every symbol in the constellation "I" and the constellation "Non-I" is inherent in the process by which we acquire knowledge and by which we orient ourselves both to ourselves and to the outer world.

In the case of our example here of the visual image of the cave as a symbol of the womb, one (the "inner") of its two poles of reference had become inaccessible to consciousness in the ordinary course of individual developmental events, or else phylogenetically, or at least with a phylogenetic reinforcement.

It is to be noted that we are discussing something actually prior to what has been wittily described as "The Original Word Game." The original word game for each individual is played out as an encounter with a group psychological product—a particular language with its ready-made words and with implicit rules for their usage. As a group-historical process these words were created as symbols for things, processes, and relations by individuals in interaction in groups. For the most part, the individual finds the creative task already accomplished; he has to learn to converse in the language of those around him. "The Original Word Game," Roger Brown (1958) writes,

. . . is the operation of linguistic reference in first language learning. At least two people are required: one who knows the language (the tutor) and one who is learning (the player). In outline form the movements of the game are very simple. The tutor names things in accordance with the semantic custom of his community. The player forms hypotheses by trying to name new things correctly. The tutor compares the player's utterances with his own anticipations of such utterances and, in this way, checks the accuracy of fit between his own categories and those of the player. He improves the fit by correction. In concrete terms the tutor says "dog" whenever a dog appears. The player notes the phonemic equivalences of these utterances, forms a

hypothesis about the non-linguistic category that elicits this kind of utterance and then tries naming a few dogs himself.*

This conscious learning and, extending through adult life, preconscious learning of words as symbols for things, processes, and relations,
of course presuppose capacities already matured and acquired. Brown
says that the concepts of space, time, causality, and the enduring object
are formed, with little assistance from language, as basic referent categories during the first two years of life. This kind of orientation of the
self in the world depends heavily, as previously noted, upon the building
up of the body image, which is associated closely with events of libidinal development. The later acquisition of language continues to be
heavily influenced by the libidinal structure of the postural model; every
disturbance in the emotional life will react on the body image, and
libidinal disturbances which provoke changes in the image of the body
markedly influence speech development and the acquisition and use
of language.

For example, in one case of severely stunted physical stature associated with chronic anxiety, the patient's adaptive and defensive formations included working as a fireman and impressing his reference group
by his large vocabulary. It was also notable that his choice of words was
studiously polysyllabic; even when quite short words were entirely
adequate this patient worked hard at replacing them with larger ones.

Just as the (visual) symbolic elements of dreams lost from consciousness one pole of reference, so did, in Sperber's conjecture, the (phonetic)
word-symbols for sexual concepts, which thus came to have a unipolar
nonsexual alloplastic reference in most contexts in the communal language. Vital nonsexual parts of the body, as noted, also influence considerably the growth of language; the words to which they give rise
may secondarily acquire a genital sexual significance in some contexts,
though for the most part without polysemy.

Many years ago, an Indian soldier was hypnotized. He had been
suffering severely following traumatic experiences in battle. In the
hypnotic trance he said, "Sir, I entered battle with a large heart." Later
he went on, "after each battle my heart grew smaller and smaller, smaller and smaller." With this metaphor, the man ruefully acknowledged
his progressive loss of courage. The word *courage* (the Latin *cor* =
heart) is itself a faded metaphor. The abstract quality of character
(courage) is denoted by a word which has come to have its concrete,
bodily reference subdued; the Indian soldier merely reverted to its

* It should be mentioned that it is only very exceptionally that a high level of fluency
can be achieved in any language other than the mother tongue, and even moderate fluency
can only be achieved in a strange tongue with long, hard work.

foundation in live metaphor. In the English word *courage* the reference is shifted so far that the word symbol further loosens its pole of reference in the body image. More than this, there is *no* other *concrete* pole of reference, as we have previously noted that there is with cryptophoric symbolism. The cryptophoric symbolism of dreams often replaces a part or function of the body by the visual image of an external object. Thus, the male organ may be replaced by a snake or airplane, the female breasts by peaches, the female genitals by a jewel case, and so forth. There is an even more primitive type of cryptophoric symbolism (Ferenczi 1913), of which tooth and eye symbolism are notable examples, in which a part of the body may be replaced by another part of the body in a dream or a neurotic symptom. In losing concrete points of reference faded metaphor departs the farthest from cryptophoric symbolism. Thus metaphor is enlisted to engender both generalization and abstraction (see Cassirer 1944, Chapter 8). Of course the process may undergo special and complicated reversals. For example, the word *courage* may be sometimes used as an indicator of sexual potency, as when a man solemnly informs his psychiatrist that in recent months he has lost his courage.*

Sandor Ferenczi (1913) discussed those symbols that apparently have a logically inexplicable and ungrounded affect, an affective overemphasis due to repressed unconscious identification with something else to which the surplus of affect really belongs. He thought that in this way the upper half of the body, "as the more harmless," attains its sexual symbolic significance bringing about displacement from below upwards, a phenomenon often observed in hysterical disability (see Abse 1966). Kubie (1934) observed a bodily dramatization of castration-anxiety in a different direction. He writes:

It was necessary to perform a lumbar puncture on a young man of twenty-six. Some years earlier this young man had been subjected to the same procedure, and at the time had suffered intense pain. As a result, he was excessively apprehensive, and consented to the lumbar puncture only on condition that it be performed under a general anaesthetic. He was admitted to the Neurological Institute and the lumbar puncture was made under nitrous oxide-oxygen anaesthesia. As the equipment was wheeled into his room his terror mounted visibly, and he began to do a rather peculiar thing: although

---

* Regarding moral character, it is remarkable that in all languages there are a large number of *physiognomical* terms to be found; that is, emotional expression, as it is revealed facially with the play of expression, comes to have a powerful determining force in the choice of words and phrases defining character. There is always a tendency to confuse internal character with that external form evident in the countenance. Physiognomic judgments, so important in later life, are grounded in the importance of the mother's face and facial expressions for the infant in the preverbal period of life. For an interesting eighteenth-century account, see G. C. Lavater (1783).

normally modest, despite the presence of the nurses, he made quick impulsive gestures which would repeatedly expose his genitals. Then, to our amazement, as he began to be affected by the anaesthetic, but before he was completely relaxed, he did exactly the reverse: that is, he reached out for all the bedclothes that he could grasp, for his bathrobe, for a pillow, for anything which his groping hands chanced to touch, and piled a protecting mountain of clothes and bedding over his genitals.

Kubie raises the question why an "attack" on one part of the body (in this case the backbone) is reflected in the patient's mind in such a way that it apparently represents to him an attack upon his genitals. Later he writes: "The phenomenon of 'displacement upward from below' is only a special instance of this phenomenon; and it might be better to speak of centrifugal and centripetal displacements, that is, of displacements away from or towards the instinctive zones."

Metaphor is preeminently concerned in the semantic movement from a sensuous concrete image to a more problematic referent. In this complicated process the imagery of the body plays a weighty role beside that of exteroperception. Quoting again the example offered by Aristotle (on Poetics),* "There *lies* my ship," we can agree with the ancient philosopher that "lying at anchor is a species of lying" but would suggest that the analogy he discusses makes its impact on the basis of ego-experience in the recumbent position of the postural model of the self and then of others. It would seem that the displacement originally occurs from the body image to images of others, including animistic projection to inanimate external objects. These kinds of unconscious displacements which underlie metaphor are also an essential part of cryptophoric symbolism. Symbolism in general also depends on condensation: images of things are first brought together in a "thing-identity." Later, one thing (usually bodily) is repressively detached from another, which then achieves heightened conscious representation through the capture of some of the original interest in the former. In some instances, as in the abstract concept of courage, it is the emotional (basically visceral) experience, with its foundation in cardiac sensations when fear and anger are both aroused and controlled, which shapes the semantic arrow so that a particular word becomes the verbal symbol of communication. In other instances, such as Homer's "sowing of the god-created light," the concept has been obviously shaped in exteroperceptive experience— by the observation of scattering seeds in the earth—but we cannot here ignore its resonance with sexual body imagery and phantasy, which remains unconsciously active and which was important in the pre-stages of language.

It is necessary to understand that usually when a "thing-identity" or

* Quoted previously in Section IV.

a "sensation-identity" occurs in a phase of condensation, then a "verbal-identity" follows (sometimes, however, a reverse sequence accounts for etymological difficulties and complications.)* It is after this doubling of identity that the repressive process enables a polarization of metaphoric symbolism, thus repeating a process which occurred at an earlier and more primitive level with cryptophoric symbolism. Metaphor, however, comes to supersede the sphere of cryptophoric symbolism which is entirely restricted to the replacement of one "concrete" image by another. Metaphor emerges as an instrument of thought which enables imageless abstractions. We have to agree with the Fowlers (1931) that "Strictly speaking, metaphor occurs as often as we take a word out of its original sphere and apply it to new circumstances. In this sense almost all words can be shown to be metaphorical when they do not bear a physical meaning; for the original meaning of almost all words can be traced back to something physical."

* The verbal identity which culminates in so-called traitor words or *faux amis*, that is, words identical or appearing the same in *two or more* languages with totally different meanings, is one of the curses of tongues. For example, when you are embarrassed about something in Spain, do not use the word *embarazado*—it means "pregnant." *Desconcertado* is the appropriate word to use (see *The Curse of Tongues*, Douglas Busk, Pall Mall Press, London, 1965). This particular example itself merits psychoanalytic scrutiny. Perhaps it is sufficient to indicate that the end results of the organized sounds we know as words are subject to a variety of shifts, both phonetic and semantic. For another example, the reader is referred to Wegener p. 124 below.

VII Dreams and Speech

The "dream-work"

FREUD (1900) described many processes which comprise the
dream-work, that is, the transformation of the unconscious *latent*
dream thoughts into the text of the dream, the *manifest* dream. Mobili-
zation of memories, condensation, displacement, pictorial representation, and symbolization all occur from the time that the repudiated
wish, the "child of the night," is transferred to the day's residues, to the
time that the dream is perceived. Secondary revision may then reorder
this perception. Freud (1933) writes:

Let us go back once more to the latent dream thoughts. Their most powerful
element is the repressed instinctual impulse which has created in them an
expression for itself on the basis of chance stimuli and by transference on to
the day's residues—through an expression that is toned down and disguised.
Like every instinctual impulse, it too presses for satisfaction by action; but its
path to motility is blocked by the physiological regulations implied in the
state of sleep; it is compelled to take the backwards course in the direction of
perception and to be content with a hallucinated satisfaction. The latent
dream thoughts are thus transformed into a collection of sensory images and
visual scenes. It is as they travel on this course that what seems to us so novel
and so strange occurs to them. All the linguistic instruments by which we
express the subtler relations of thought—the conjunctions and prepositions,
the changes in declension and conjugation—are dropped, because there are no
means of representing them; just as in a primitive language without any
grammar, only the raw material of thought is expressed and abstract terms
are taken back to the concrete ones that are at their basis. What is left over
after this may well appear disconnected. The copious employment of symbols, which have become alien to conscious thinking, for representing certain
objects and processes is in harmony alike with the archaic regression in the
mental apparatus and with the demands of the censorship.

The dissociated dream ego nucleus and the nocturnal ego

As expounded by Freud (1900, Chapter VII), the dream-work consists
topographically of a general progressive-regressive ("zig-zag") rhyth-

mic series of cathectic events within the component parts (psi-systems) of the mental apparatus during sleep, events which culminate in the hallucinatory experience which may later, in the waking state, be verbally reported upon, that is, the manifest dream. The culmination of the dreaming experience is itself a partial awakening of the pre-conscious and conscious systems, in order that the state of sleep may *for the most part* continue in all systems. This usual consequence of the dream-work may be an expression of its major purpose: to preserve sleep. The dream-work issues in the discharge, for the time being, of unconscious excitations in harmless hallucinosis, which excitations would otherwise press forward for fuller arousal of the (conscious and preconscious) perceptual and motor systems. The wish to sleep, deriva-tive of somatic need, is thus served by the dream-work, just as it also serves to gratify other and unconscious derivatives in the disguised ex-pression they achieve, despite censorship, in the overdetermined oneiric experience. For this intermediate purpose of compromise (essentially between (1) the wish to sleep, (2) forceful unconscious wishes, (3) the continuing, though lessened, unconscious repressions, and also (4) un-discharged preconscious tensions) the dream-work relies upon the man-agement of primary process, that is to say, unconscious processes of condensation and displacement, upon dramatization in visual terms, and upon a cryptophoric symbolism. It is not altogether clear in Freud's accounts whether the purpose of ensuring sleep is superordinate, or whether the partial discharge and binding of some unconscious excita-tions otherwise blocked from expression in waking life is of equal importance. Recent experimental work concerned with both sleep and dreaming seems to favor the latter hypothesis.

This brief consideration brings into sharp relief important features which seem clearly to lead to a *structural view* of the dream-work as an ego-activity, a piece of organization effected by an unconscious ego apparatus. The question arises as to whether this special collocation of ego functions—the dream-work—proceeds only during sleep when there are special cathectic conditions within the sphere of the ego (rela-tive derepression, heightened narcissism, regression from phonetic sym-bolism to visual imagery and cryptophoric symbolism) or whether it *also* proceeds in the waking state. From Freud's accounts of the "trans-fer" of the unconscious wish to the day residues, it seems that the dream-work is partially accomplished during the preceding day, and even sometimes during longer preceding intervals (Freud 1900). It can be hypothesized that there is a dissociated ego-nucleus which prepares the ground for the time when general regressive alterations in the ego (in sleep) facilitate further dream-work. At this time, that is during the night, the regression toward more primary process (condensation and displacement) is purposefully utilized by the dreaming ego as a means of evasion of remaining censorship, the trail of the superego-ego organization of the day.

Recent experimental work on sleep and dreaming suggests strongly that dreaming occurs throughout the mammalian kingdom; it is not confined to man or even primates (Hawkins 1966). Thus it is possible that the unconscious ego apparatus which continuously performs the dream-work is the phylogenetic representative in man of a mammalian "dream-organizer." For adaptive purposes in mammals lower than man in the evolutionary scale, focus on data-processing for survival during wakeful activity may have been more efficiently rendered when shelving of immediately irrelevant internal stimuli became possible—to be dealt with, at least partially, later through dreaming when in repose. This may have been a prelude to man's heightened consciousness,* superior preconscious (and language) system, and repressive capacity. Yet this earlier method retains its utility for man too; perhaps he is even dependent upon it to a much higher degree than other mammals.

In any event, the dissociated ego-nucleus of the day would seem to "know" of its preparatory task for the nocturnal ego, much as occasionally one of the dissociated partial personalities in multiple personality may know of the dominating personality's needs, though the latter may know nothing at all about its auxiliary.

This view of an ego-nucleus preparing latent dream thoughts to have ready-to-hand for the altered nocturnal dreaming ego happens also to fit very well with Freud's later expulsion of "secondary revision" from the core dream-work; obviously secondary revision is accomplished by the waking and the awake ego as an extension of the dream-work. This may be partly already occurring during the latter part of the actual oneiric experience and partly later during recollection and reporting.

The latent dream thoughts of most importance for the dream-work are those which require dream distortion—the proscribed dream thoughts. The essential dream-work uses and distorts them especially because they already represent the psychic material which carries the essential dream-constructor: the repressed infantile wish. "It is this unconscious wish that gives the dream-work its peculiar character as an unconscious revision of preconscious material" (Freud 1900). If this (primary) revision is largely accomplished by day, the task at night is mainly to achieve access to consciousness under the altered conditions of the state of sleep. Essentially, the additional task of the nocturnal ego,

---

* It is to be borne in mind that, according to Freud, man's consciousness may be described as a sense organ with two sensory surfaces: one directed toward perception and the other toward the preconscious thought-processes (the pcs having developed the mnemic system of indications of speech).

which now incorporates the formerly dissociated ego-nucleus, is this achievement of perceptual consciousness while the evasion of censorship is sustained. Of course, the task is facilitated when (1) outside stimulation of perceptual consciousness is absent or minimal and (2) the other surface of consciousness, that toward the preconscious thought processes, is especially depleted of stimulation by the decathexis of those mnemic subsystems which afford phonetic symbolic foundations for thinking.

That part of the dream-work which consists of regression from phonetic symbolism to visual imagery and cryptophoric symbolism has some interesting results. It follows, as Freud insists (1900), that the dream-work cannot actually *create* speeches. "However much speeches and conversations, whether reasonable or unreasonable in themselves, may figure in dreams, analysis invariably proves that all that the dream has done is to extract from the dream-thoughts fragments of speeches which have really been made or heard." While Freud makes some modification of this statement, he insists that whatever stands out markedly as speech, with acoustic and motor accompaniments in the dream, can be traced back to real speeches. But Freud goes further in another place (1901) and does not allow that the dream-work is creative at all:

If we keep to the definition of "dream-work" as the process of transforming the dream-thoughts into the dream content, it follows that the dream-work is not creative, that it develops no phantasies of its own, that it makes no judgments and draws no conclusions; it has no functions whatever other than condensation and displacement of the material and its modification into pictorial form, to which must be added as a variable factor the final bit of interpretive revision. It is true that we find various things in the dream-content which we would be inclined to regard as a product of some other and higher intellectual functions; but in every case analysis shows convincingly that *these intellectual operations have already been performed in the dream-thoughts and have only been taken over by the dream-content.* A conclusion drawn in a dream is nothing other than the repetition of a conclusion in the dream-thoughts; if the conclusion is taken over into the dream unmodified, it will appear impeccable; if the dream-work has displaced it onto some other material, it will appear nonsensical. A calculation in the dream-content signifies nothing more than that there is a calculation in the dream-thoughts; but while the latter is always rational, a dream-calculation may produce the wildest results if its factors are condensed or if its mathematical operations are displaced onto other material. Not even speeches that occur in the dream-content are original compositions; they turn out to be a hotchpotch of speeches made, heard or read, which have been revived in the dream thoughts and whose wording is exactly reproduced, while their origin is entirely disregarded and their meaning is violently changed.

The question remains, however, whether or not under other less usual and routine conditions the dream has any part in creativity. If we postulate the daytime preparatory unconscious ego apparatus which performs the dream-work, incorporated later into the dreaming ego, and usually dissociated from the waking ego with its vast preconscious system (a large part of which territory is composed of mnemic systems subserving word connections), then we can postulate unusual conditions when this dissociation no longer fully obtains or even is to a considerable extent superseded. Under these unusual conditions, in a hypnoid state, there would ensue an unusually free interplay between verbal (phonetic) symbols and acoustic and visual imagery. Out of the resulting ideational ambiguity and plasticity, quite novel predications could arise. Further consideration of creativity would, of course, take us far afield.* Yet it does seem that Freud's basic argument is well justified usually both phenomenologically and theoretically. For as we take a stricter definition of the *essential* dream-work, with possibly its own special brain-basis, it would follow that it operates upon auditory residues as it does upon other perceived and stored "psychic material," that is, entirely in the service of guarding sleep and affording discharge of some unconscious excitations.

We have already noted that during sleep (1) outside stimulation of perceptual consciousness is absent or minimal and (2) the other surface of consciousness, that toward the preconscious thought processes, is especially depleted of stimulation by the decathexis of those mnemic subsystems which afford phonetic symbolic foundations for thinking. We must now add, as was originally discussed by Wegener, that the foundations which enable discursive language include a repository of faded metaphors. Upon this racial repository, learned and somehow incorporated in the child's later mnemic subsystems, generality and adequate understanding of the novelty of statement depend. The collocation of ego functions which performs the essential dream work is *of itself* and *by itself* inadequate for creative adaptation since it is without adequate metaphoric symbolism. In brief, before language had faded metaphors to buttress logical thought it could not render a situation by any other means than a demonstrative indication of it in present experience. Essentially the dream-work utilizes this device through regression to visual imagery and, to boot, employs a primitive cryptophoric symbolism alien to our usual more fully awake mode of thought. However, it would seem possible that the dreaming ego has its own kind of

---

* Some considerations relating to aesthetic appreciation, creativity states, and fascination and trance are discussed in Chapter VII of *Hysteria and Related Mental Disorders* (Abse 1966).

awareness (including that of this cryptophoric symbolism) which can escape the censorship of the more fully integrated psyche to a very considerable extent. The remarkable preponderance of genital symbols exhibited in dreams can only be accounted for by the nuclear position of the Oedipus complex in man's psychosexual development and indeed in the development of the kinds of civilization within which he is bound to seek his daily satisfactions.

The superego and the dreaming consciousness

Phonetic symbolism is built upon the body-ego, not only crucially developing the organization of the ego and heightening its capacity for consciousness but enhancing the differentiation of conscience. "Then the Lord spoke to you out of the midst of the fire; you heard the sound of words, but saw no form; there was only a voice." Thus spoke Moses to all Israel, according to the Fifth Book. Later it is recorded therein that he said, "Take heed to yourselves, lest you forget the covenant of the Lord your God, which he made with you, and make a graven image in the form of anything which the Lord your God has forbidden you." It seems that the auditory basis of the superego is both dramatized and emphasized in this way in the Old Testament. There are times in dreams when the superego makes a considerable contribution to direct speech; often these are occasions when the dream imagery is additionally censored for its forbidden character. This oneiric situation is explained by Robert Fliess (1953) who sums up: "It is the ego that fantasies under the impulsion of the return of the repressed from a time when there had not yet been a superego; it is the superego that enters the fantasy in a speech expressing rejection."

The Market Dream of Freud's young woman patient illustrates the considerable contribution which the superego makes to direct speech in the manifest imagery. Freud (1901) relates the dream as follows:

She dreamt she was going to the market with her cook, who was carrying the basket. After she had asked for something, the butcher had said to her: "That's not obtainable any longer," and offered her something else, adding: "This is good, too." She rejected it and went on to the woman who sells vegetables, who tried to get her to buy a peculiar vegetable that was tied up in bundles but was of black color. She said: "I don't recognize that; I won't take it."

The remark "That's not obtainable any longer" was closely related to Freud's explanation to the patient a few days earlier than the earliest memories of childhood were "not obtainable any longer as such." Her own speech in the dream occurred in an entirely different connection. On the previous day she had reproved her cook, who incidentally also appeared in the dream, with the words: "Behave yourself properly! I don't recognize that!" meaning that she did not understand and would not put up with her defiant behavior. Only the latter exclamation had entered the manifest dream as acoustic imagery.

Freud writes that while the more innocent part of her speech entered the dream content, in the dream thoughts the other part played an obvious role. "For the dream-work," he notes (1901), "had reduced to complete unintelligibility and extreme innocence an imaginary situation in which *I* was *behaving improperly* to the lady in a particular way. But this situation which the patient was expecting in her imagination was itself only a new edition of something she had once actually experienced." Fliess (1953) amplifies the idea that the suppressed phrase, the imperative admonition, is an utterance easily traceable to the superego. However, this phrase, "Behave yourself properly!" which would obviously have applied if someone had ventured to make improper suggestions and had forgotten "to close his meat shop," might have too easily betrayed the forbidden sexual meaning of the dream. Even so, the dream utterance, "I don't recognize that; I won't take it!" is a defensive objection instigating repression at the behest of the superego. These considerations indicate the complexity of the dream-work which strives to guard sleep; in pursuit of this aim, it must avoid a development of the censor into more of a superego than would be compatible with the state of sleep.

Actually, of course, there is another option besides total *arousal* by the reestablished superego in the dream, namely masochistic compliance to the superego in a manifest punishment sequence which permits sleep to continue, usually provided the punishment is not too severe. Mostly in these instances no direct speech enters into the dream. The partial insertion of the superego through direct speech is sometimes negotiated by the nocturnal ego in order to avoid either arousal or definitively punitive imagery.

A middle-aged divorced woman dreamed that she entered a building and heard solemnly intoned the words: "The end of truth is the singing animal." In association, she quoted: "The Bird of Time has but a little way to flutter—and the Bird is on the Wing." These words from Edward Fitzgerald's *Rubaiyat of Omar Khayyam* somehow had to do with the strange assemblage of words she had heard in the dream. She then recalled that in the dream she had revisited her lover. She proceeded to discuss conventional doubts about having sexual intercourse before remarriage, and her mother's cautionary admonitions. It soon became apparent that she was nonetheless about to accept fully the invitation to visit the distant city from which she had received a telephone call the day before.

The location in the dream was felt as benevolent, indulging, exonerating, and the diction as ex cathedra. It is thus also evident that the superego may sometimes be invoked for support of wish fulfillment and that this may be rendered in direct speech during dreaming.

VIII Language and Schizophrenia

IN THE *Project for a Scientific Psychology* Freud (1895) suggested that the social function of speech is a secondary acquisition. The innervations of speech are at first a discharge mechanism for the stored excitations in the "retentive neurones"; this path of discharge then secondarily acquired the highly important function of establishing human contact. The infant screams and thus attracts attention to his distress; then, afterwards, the cries serve to bring understanding with other people and are gradually absorbed into speech associations.

It is likely that this notion of the passage from a physiological to a psychological level of organization and interpersonal interaction, while reflecting an important element of truth in the chronology of both ontogenetic and phylogenetic development, is a simplification. The development, which builds upon a biological and maturational foundation, is actually much more complex and includes feedback and feed forward systems in interaction. From the psychological standpoint it is evident that the expressive and communicative aspects of vocal events in infancy are, for the most part, already inextricably intertwined before the appearance of any distinctive word which symbolizes both a thought formation and a referent. Wegener's studies show that, in speech, communication proper develops out of the need to influence the behavior, and therefore the mind, of another person. This development occurs along lines which radiate from the stark imperative "one-word sentence" but which, whatever else may be implicit or explicit, retain implicitly the naive demand that another person experience congruent elements of consciousness. Wegener states that the listener comprehends by means of conclusions drawn from the situation, from the speaker's linguistic indications, and from the various expressions of the speaker's emotion. In a basic (originally maternal) form of communication the listener infers the speaker's state of suffering (or discomfort) and feels motivated by the ethical force of sympathetic feelings to help the suffering one in the inferred manner. "Thus," writes Wegener (p. 270 below)

he obeys the deduced commands, thus he answers the posed question, thus he looks at the perceptive picture indicated, thus at the picture of consciousness, a pattern; and according to the extent that the speaker knows how to arouse the sympathetic feelings of a listener, to this extent is cultivated his interest and the clarity and vividness of the images summoned to consciousness.

We have previously considered how in hysterical disorder, primarily as a result of mental conflict, the speaker is himself unable to accept and thus to clarify consciously his own more important forbidden wishes. Consequently, without a listener specially engaged in the task of decipherment, as in the process of psychoanalysis or analytic psychotherapy, communication is bound to remain affectively inadequate and to miscarry in some important ways. In the various forms and phases of schizophrenic disorder the derangement of communication is more extreme. Verbal communication may break down altogether; the patient may be withdrawn and mute, or suffer disfigurements of speech among accessory symptoms. Even when these symptoms are minimal or absent, it frequently happens in schizophrenia that the patient's "verbal exposition" is entirely inadequate. It is as if the speaker assumes that the listener should understand from a word or two even when the physical and social context offers no clues; thus there ensues a gross miscarriage of "empractic" speech. Then again, the listener's usual experience of purpose in his own speech and actions, and of sympathetically understanding the purpose in those of others to whom he is accustomed, does not often provide him with criteria for expecting the predications emerging in the schizophrenic's utterances; he therefore finds it difficult to sustain his attention. Such expectations as he tentatively generates successively become disappointed; patience falters and anger gathers. We shall see that there are other gross deficiencies in the supports to purposeful dialogue which Wegener described.

Agrammatism: thought and language in disarray

In describing a case of schizophrenia of hebephrenic type in the sixth edition of their textbook, Henderson and Gillespie (1944) quote the remarks of a young woman, twenty years of age, who had been employed as a nurse before admission to the mental hospital. At the time of these remarks her condition had become gradually worse. She wandered about restlessly and, when the physician visited the ward, would clutch him by the arm, only eventually being detached with difficulty. Her thought processes were blocked and her speech incoherent, "her sentences being composed of detached words and phrases which have no relationship to each other, except for an occasional superficial association," according to the authors of the textbook. They offer this example:

Losh, I don't know what it is. You see—she says—I don't know, I'm sure. There's Cinderella. There is a much better play than that. "I don't know," I said. He is an awful idiot. Oh dear God, I'm so stupid. That's putting two and two together—saying I really don't know—saying Cathie, and so I observe and—flowers. An orange and shoe laces. The gaberdine skirt. Pettigrews and the jazz-band with cream cakes. She says no. They like my hair bobbed, but I'm so stupid. Contrary Mary. Statues at Copland and Lyes. "Oh," I said, "Yes, yes, yes." I'd go off to sleep immediately afterwards. I said, "I know quite well." I said, "Nothing." I forget all that I saw next. The next thing was—eh? The poor man's mad. They'll be chopping off our heads next and—calendars tied with blue ribbons. Oh dear God. Contrary Mary again. What period—that's right. I don't like acting the goat at all. A cream-sponge sandwich. My memory is so slow, that all I'm sure. It was caramels then and fruit cakes. "Well, well," I said, "I can't help it"—I don't want to help it, and well, I don't care. Contrary Mary again, and says— Nurse Grant—dogs barking. What's the matter with me anyway? I'm so terribly stupid. I'm fed up with this place—that's all. Sago pudding. She looks pale and tired often, but not—I know that. [Sings] "Take me over there, drop me anywhere, Manchester, Birmingham, Leeds, well I don't care!" I should like to see my best girl—Mrs. Patrick, she says—"Though it's time for parting, that's it, Jean, and my tears are starting!" I've got the Kruschen feeling—blue belts and medals—three eggs for tea. No, that won't do. Oh, dear God, I'm so stupid. I won't see my way—white rabbits. "Back home in Tennessee." That's the way it's spelt. Oh, I don't know what I'm going to do now. It's all wrong. Dear God, I'm so silly. It's killing, isn't it? Cream cakes, French cakes and méringues. Flies, fleas, butterflies.

The sample shows clearly what Emil Kraepelin (1905) designated as agrammatic disturbance. Confusion is caused, as far as the listener is concerned, by the fact that ideas indicated by correctly chosen words are distorted by the structure of a sentence and by the juxtaposition of sentences which do not logically belong together. Moreover, topics are introduced without adequate exposition (verbal context). Again and again, expected predications do not arrive; they are omitted sometimes in elision and sometimes because of sudden thought-deprivation in a withdrawal of attention and redirection to another logical subject. That aspect of the distortion designated agrammatism by Kraepelin (1905) represents the abrogation of Wegener's first principle of support to full-fledged speech: the grammatical structure has not evolved sufficiently by *emendation* of an ambiguous expression to support purposeful dialogue. All those auxiliary utterances, evolved in the process of exposition of the early one-word sentence, which provide a verbal context to substitute for the deficient implicit context, are conspicuously absent in much of this sample. In that respect it is as if the patient had reverted to the notion that few speech indications *must* be sufficient as far as the hearer is concerned. The impression created in the auditor in such instances is that excessive brevity is the soul of witlessness.

If we look carefully at the sample provided by Henderson and Gillespie (1944) and are prepared to utilize our experience and professional knowledge, including closer study of similar hebephrenic Ophelias, we notice features which group themselves in our minds, though disjunctively presented. There are fifteen or sixteen interspersed assertions revealing that there is a great deal of self-observation relating to her awareness of disturbed thought and conduct—I'm so stupid, silly, don't like acting the goat, idiot, and so on. Then there are half-a-dozen or so further self-observational assertions, also interspersed but connected with the above category, concerning her negativism—Contrary Mary, I don't want to help it, and so forth. Another category features erotic and ambitious phantasy (Cinderella) and persecutory anxious phantasies (madman, chopping off heads, dogs barking). Then there are many interspersed references to bonnes bouches, such as caramels, fruitcakes, and meringues, which represent a regression away from the conflicted and problematic wishes hinted at in the preceding category.

Finally, also in a regressive direction, there are several whimsical statements, some included as songs and others only partially realized: pettigrews and the jazz-band, blue belts and medals, white rabbits. These may be hilarious in emotional tone, and perhaps condense pleasurable sounds and sights in childhood and adolescent shopping and dancing experiences—they may, too, symbolically refer to lost "innocent" pleasures that she is trying to recapture. In any case it is evident that, despite the agrammatism, tentative expectations about what she is (deficiently) saying are readily aroused in experienced psychiatrists. However, there is here no immediate relevance in pursuing further the meaning of her disorganized speech.

Acataphasia and disturbance of metaphor

As a second example of speech disturbance in schizophrenia, we will consider the case of paranoid schizophrenia reported by Carl G. Jung (1906) in *The Psychology of Dementia Praecox*. In this case we will also encounter severe disturbances relating to Wegener's second principle of language, that regarding metaphor (see Fig. 1, p. 22). Jung's patient was investigated partly by using the word-association tests which Jung had then recently invented. A middle-aged seamstress, she spontaneously verbalized fleeting delusions of grandeur and of persecution, claiming to be a millionairess and complaining that in the night her bed was filled with needles. In 1888, a year after she was admitted to the Burgholzli Hospital, Jung (1906) described her speech as becoming "more and more disconnected and her delusions less understood." Nevertheless, he understood that she felt that she had a mysterious "monopoly," and by the aid of her peculiar gestures eked out by a few words he gleaned that a certain Rubinstein from St. Petersburg sent her money by the wagonload. He commenced simple word association tests to the first item of which, the stimulus word "pupil," the patient responded with "Now you may write: 'Socrates.'" Jung (1906) thought that this was "a quite striking reaction for a seamstress," that it looked very affected, and pointed to a complex of emotionally accentuated ideas. In regard to this response, as well as to others, including neologisms such as "groundpostament" (given as the 67th stimulus item on later occasion), Jung attempted to learn what the patient had meant. This attempt was a failure, for in response to requests for explanation the patient produced a series of fresh neologisms comprising a word-salad, though she "spoke in a self-confident tone, as if she were perfectly clear about the meaning of her words, and seemed to think what she said was an explanation" (1906). Thereafter, Jung moved to the method of continuous associations in order to try to elucidate the meaning of her strange responses. He asked the patient to say all that came to her mind when he presented her successively with her own responses as fresh stimuli. Presented with "Socrates," she responded as shown below. Jung (1905) states that, "As the patient spoke very slowly in reference to her delusions and was constantly disturbed by 'thought-deprivations,' her production could readily and literally be transcribed." He therefore reproduced the tests verbatim, omitting, however, the repetitions:

Socrates—scholar—books—wisdom—modesty—no words in order to express this wisdom—it is the highest groundpostament—his teachings—had to die on account of bad people—falsely accused—sublimest sublimity—self-satisfied —that is all Socrates—the fine learned world. [long pause] No thread cut—I was the best tailoress, never had a piece of cloth on the floor—fine artist world —fine professorship—is doubloon—twenty-five francs—that is the highest— prison—slandered by bad people—unreason—cruelty—excess—rudeness.

Jung (1906) further writes:

The thoughts did not follow smoothly, but were constantly inhibited by "thought-deprivation" which the patient designated as an invisible force which always takes away just what she wishes to say. Thought-deprivation appeared especially whenever she wished to explain something conclusively. The conclusive thing was the complex. Thus we see from the above analysis that the essential element appears only after having been preceded by a number of obscure analogies. The object of the test was, as the patient knew, to explain the neologisms. If it took her so long to reproduce the important phrase ("no thread cut"), her imaginative faculty must have suffered from a peculiar disturbance which can be best designated as a *deficiency in the faculty of discrimination between important and unimportant material.* The explanation of her stereotype, "I am Socrates" or I am Socratic," lies in the fact that she was the "best seamstress" "who never cut a thread" and "never had a piece of cloth on the floor." She is an "artist," a "professor," in her line. She is tortured, she is not recognized as a world proprietress, etc. She is considered sick, which is a slander. She is "wise" and "modest." She has performed the "highest." All these analogies to the life and end of Socrates; she therefore wishes to say, "I am and suffer like Socrates." With a certain poetic license, characteristic in a moment of strong affect, she says directly, "I am Socrates."* The pathological part of this lies in the fact that her identification with Socrates is such that she cannot free herself from it. She takes her identification somehow as self-evident, and she assumes so much reality for the metonymy that she expects everybody else to understand it. Here we distinctly see a deficient capacity to discriminate between two ideas. Every normal person can still differentiate between an assumed role or a metaphoric designation and his real personality, even if a vivid phantasy, with an intense feeling-tone will for a time firmly adhere to such a dream or wish-formation. The connection does finally come with a diminution of feeling and a readaptation to reality.

From Jung's account, it would seem that the patient became involved, at any rate fleetingly, in the false belief, the delusion, that she actually was Socrates. From her standpoint (as long as we assume what seems evident from Jung's report, that she had read about the historical, or the Platonic Socrates' persecution and death) Socrates, like herself, was a perfectionist; he too (but metaphorically) did not cut the thread, for he adhered to his commitment to pursue the truth by his dialectic method however much threatened. His exalted status as a philosopher likewise is analogous, from her standpoint, to her exalted position as "World Proprietess," as having performed "the highest." She and he are alike in being in captivity and slandered, as she sees it. Her imaginative faculty is disturbed in a way which can be specified more narrowly than in Jung's assertion that the deficiency is "in the faculty of discriminating between important and unimportant material." Certainly, it is important that Socrates was a man and that he died in the year 399 B.C.; these two conditions are different from her own. In her mind, they are overridden by the important respects in which she feels she resembles

---

*Motives for using metaphor are: poverty of language, emphasis, and circumlocution. Emphasis sums up poetic use; circumlocution sums up defensive use; and poverty of language describes the word need which results in the creative expansion of discursive language.

him. It is, of course, in the *completeness* of the identification that her imaginative faculty is disturbed. The trial identifications, part of the experiments of thought, which are controlled and integrated in the total process of reality-testing, often become quite uncontrolled in schizophrenia under the influence of strong emotion. In particular, as Freeman, Cameron, and McGhie (1958), following Paul Federn (1952), have elaborated, there is a basic weakness of ego boundaries so that ego-feeling may become invested heavily in one of these identifications. A regression to primary identification, to that sort of identification which preceded the formation of ego boundaries, then readily occurs under conditions of arousal of strong emotion.

Harold F. Searles (1965) in discussing the increasingly stable thought differentiation in two treated and recovered schizophrenic patients states:

Thus, although it is correct to say that without the establishment of firm ego boundaries, a differentiation between metaphorical and literal meanings cannot take place, it would seem equally correct to say that metaphor, at least, could never develop if there had not once been a *lack* of such ego boundaries—if there had never been, as we believe there always has been, in infancy, a relatively unimpeded flow between the areas of experience which come, later, to be felt as inner world and outer world.

The two examples of speech disturbance in schizophrenia so far discussed were chosen to illustrate two fundamental aspects of this disorder. In regard to the disorder of metaphoric symbolism, which a consideration of the "Socrates" response of Jung's patient elucidated, it is to be noted also that we were led directly to the most radical aspect of this disorder of word symbolism. This radical aspect concerns disrupted ego functioning, including thought and language, which at the level of metaphoric symbolism are inextricable. Similarly, in the example of Gillespie's patient, we were confronted with that havoc which reversion to an empractic form of speech, when employed inappropriately, can create in the process of emendation described by Wegener. The patient's speech specimen obviously shows an "intra-psychic ataxia" (Stransky 1929), consisting of the expressing of poorly repressed and regressive forbidden wish-fantasies, meeting with sudden interruptions—thought-blocking—and then sudden tangential shifts in the total process of defense. This adds, of course, to the telegrammatic impression and to the confusion which one-word sentences or longer phrases with inappropriately exiguous exposition themselves create. It is obvious, however, that underdeveloped exposition makes its contribution to the agrammatism that Kraepelin (1905) separated from acataphasic disturbance, that part of the disorder in which the patient does not speak a particular language according to the usual meanings of its words and phrases in his community. Besides the disturbance in metaphoric symbolism there are other contributions to acataphasia, though these are not so pervasive. One of these contributions consists in those neologisms constructed by schizophrenic patients to reflect and designate concepts for which our usual language is not well suited. Eugen Bleuler (1919) writes in this regard, "Particularly the hallucinations, the persecutions and everything connected with them must be characterized by *one* word by the constantly preoccupied patients. Thus to 'snortie' means to talk through the walls." The changed experience of the patient demands words which designate *his* experience, not those provided by the vernacular. In Bleuler's example above the patient would not be satisfied with "auditory hallucinosis" for the very reason that he does not regard himself as hallucinated in our sense.

In some chronic forms of schizophrenia, and sometimes in a relatively quiescent phase of schizophrenia of recent onset, there is an inability to discuss topics of a personal nature. Any approach to these topics is met by an anxious effort to change the subject and to withdraw into silence, if not actually to depart suddenly. This symptom, commonly encountered, is known as "dys-symbole," following the work of J. Skottowe (1939) and S. J. Thomas (1940). As long as the patient discusses topics remote from his personal life and usually also thus fairly remote from any stimuli which evoke "complexes" in Jung's original sense, his speech may remain quite well organized, with no faulty emendation or disorder of metaphoric symbolism. If the conversation is drawn into the arena of more personal discussion despite the mounting anxiety of the patient, speech itself may be greatly disordered. The topic to be discussed may, say, be one concerning the patient's loss of a friend or relative; despite the anxiety evoked, and the patient's efforts to withdraw from or to change the subject, the effort to help him to ventilate his feelings may be persisted in. As sadness and a whole gamut of other feelings emerge, the patient's speech begins to show severe disorganization. Emotional flooding is obviously, in these patients, the precursor to severely regressive ego functioning in the area of thought and language. These seems to have been a basic fault in the taming of affects, and the patients themselves try to avoid, or are signaled inwardly by gathering anxiety to avoid, the emergence of a storm of emotions. The avoidance of close personal relationships which arouse strong feelings is but another facet of the same basic and complicated problem.*

* A syndrome allied psychodynamically to "dys-symbole" but none the less distinct from it, especially phenomenologically, is that which Kraepelin termed *schizophasia*: in this condition, speech disturbance is prominent and takes the form of overwhelming compulsive talking, sometimes disjointedly and with interspersed composite words and

We earlier noted that symbolism is based on the primary processes of condensation and displacement. When the ratio of primary to secondary process is high, symbolism takes the form we have designated as crypto-phoric, based on its usual exhibition in dreaming consciousness and the need, from the viewpoint of ordinary waking consciousness, for its decipherment. We noted too that this primitive symbolism was an-chored in the image of the body, of parts of the body, and of functions of the body; things outside the body are perceived first in terms of the body and bodily effects. Cryptophoric symbolism depends on "thing-identity," with later one thing being repressively detached from the other and achieving conscious representation only through the recapture of some of the original interest in what is repressed. So the visual symbolic elements of dreams (e.g. snake, jewels, cave) have lost one pole of reference in waking consciousness but retain considerable affective im-portance. When the ratio of secondary process ordering to primary process is high, as is usual in waking life, reversing the direction of the ratio in dreams, phonetic (word) symbols (which originated also in a bodily context) may lose their pole of reference in actual bodily ex-perience. At this point of semantic movement we encounter metaphoric symbolism, a symbolism which from its source in affect-saturated sen-sual experience eventually reaches imageless abstractions. Though we cannot yet trace accurately all the details of this process of sublimation (which entails numerous symbolic transformations effected at enor-mous speed preconsciously), the derangements of thought and language in schizophrenia offer many clues. We will follow up a miscellany of them here. All are indicative of a more or less sustained and severe im-pairment of symbolizing capacity. Sometimes the underlying nature of the impairment is only revealed by its recurrent manifestation under conditions of emotional arousal. We are thus left with the impression that two interrelated aspects of the basic impairment are (1) wavering ego boundaries and (2) failure to respond to emotions as signals or as affective symbols tamed in a secondary process; except for anxiety which is comparatively often under some degree of control, though often only by resort to very massive and regressive defenses. We have already noted the contributions of Freeman et al. (1958) and Federn (1952) to the understanding of a basic impairment of ego structure in schizo-

clang associations, the content often being largely a running commentary on persons and objects in the currently surrounding environment. The excited schizophrenic patients who manifest this syndrome are attempting this way restitutionally to cling to the object-world, and at the same time to crowd out their own problems, conflicts, and feelings more concerned with people and things important to them—thus the syndrome also bears a resemblance to manic excitement, and may now be considered a schizo-affective disorder. A recent account of schizophasia is by J. H. Van Epen of the Netherlands in *Nederl t. psychiat.*, 11 Oct., 1969.

phrenia, one which develops before the emergence of speech (though later in various ways is partially compensated for before the outbreak of psychosis).* This impairment remains basically extralinguistic. Speech is, however, secondarily much affected; Jung (1906) originally noted its derangement when affect was released through the stimulation of "complexes." Kurt Eissler (1954 and 1953), in an intensive study of one of his patients in analysis, elucidated certain of the basic difficulties encountered by the schizoid person. This woman's emotions were "never reduced to signals"; once activated, emotion was apt to develop maximally—liking grew into passionate love, disliking into hate, anxiety sometimes into terror. Defense against these excessively intense emotions took the form of a feeling of deadness, a total damping of affect; pretended emotions would then be purveyed by the patient. It seemed there was an insufficient barrier to internal or external stimuli in the first place and a failure to differentiate adequately external perceptual stimuli from those emanating from within.

Acataphasic miscellany

1. Primary process: condensation and displacement

In the beginnings of dialogue a vocal indication in a shared physical context may be sufficient to elicit an adequate, gratifying response. Later, as Wegener points out, a word or two may be similarly sufficient. Still later, however, in changing contexts of greater complexity, with increasing range and variability of differentiated intentions and wishes, the mere one- or two-word sentence often remains far too ambiguous, even nebulous in meaning. More words are added in order to effect an adequate verbal context, one which will give direction to the expectations of the listener. With this more copious means of exposition, the more complex novel predications which emerge are comprehensible. In this general way sentences are made up by the individual from words. But, as Wegener also points out, there is a reverse process of shortening sentences to words. This, of course, reaches an extreme expression in technical terminology. Thus, in contradistinction to the expansion of empractic language, this new word-formation is reached by reducing a précis into a word. (Words with prefixes and suffixes are early examples of the process of condensation of several words into one.) The method of abbreviation, of *pars pro toto*, quite essential in symbol development,

---

* Sometimes by an especial fluency of speech, among other ways.

accompanies condensation or is part of it. Elision of all that becomes by repetition or custom unnecessarily explicit in verbal group interaction certainly makes things much harder for an intruder or newcomer in the group. However, the method achieves considerable economy in the verbal indications required of speakers who share in this word game. These speakers, of course, are bound by a mutuality of interest in particular areas of problem-solving, and it is the shared experience and interest which provide the context in which such abbreviations, elisions, and code words are most effective. In such instances of new word formations, some of which become established in a language community, it is noteworthy that the process of condensation is under the control of a regard for the listener's understanding—especially the pace of it.

When condensation is effected unilaterally, even though still under some preconscious control, communication readily founders. To give an example, a schizophrenic patient kept repeating a word which was carefully transcribed as: "ordamaysonfor." Puzzling about the meaning of these sounds resulted in tentative decipherment as *hors d'ame et sans fort,* an archaic French for "without spirit and strength." Discussion with the patient on this basis, using the words and their English equivalents, led to the revelation that he believed he was a wounded and captured knight living during the time of the Crusades. This heroic theme, it turned out, was a remodeling into glamorous terms of actual adverse experiences in life. We were able to approach these experiences, including the accompanying intense feelings, via the patient's delusions. Parenthetically, we may add here that these delusions could usefully be looked upon by the psychiatrist as a species of sustained and elaborated metaphor, though for a long time the patient remained locked in the literal meanings, unaware of allusions to and correspondences with actual biographical data.

Often primary process, that is, condensation and displacement, invades speech in schizophrenia so totally that secondary process ordering completely fails. In the instance offered above, however, though the ratio of primary to secondary process is vastly increased, there still remains a residue of ordered presentation. In the case of the paranoid patient that Jung (1906) discussed as a paradigm, we have already noted the neologism "groundpostament." This was found to refer to the attitude of kneeling down on the ground in prayerful reverence, that is to say, of posture on the ground. In this instance, displacement as well as condensation is quite evident. Here again it is to be noted that new words may be normally formed on such a basis, through a controlled employment of condensation and displacement. And such words, just as "groundpostament" in this schizophrenic patient, may move away from their immediate perceptual basis to acquire a larger semantic plenitude. In this patient, however, the process proceeds in accordance with her own complexes without adequate regard for the listener or the communal language, that is, on a heavily narcissistic basis.

2. Hypochondriacal or organ-speech

In *Bridge of San Luis Rey,* Thornton Wilder describes the twins Esteban and Manuel who are foundlings brought up in a convent under the aegis of the Abbess. In this remarkable work of fiction, Wilder writes:

From the years when they first learned to speak they invented a secret language for themselves, one that was scarcely dependent on the Spanish for its vocabulary, or even for its syntax. They resorted to it only when they were alone, or at great intervals in moments of stress whispered it in the presence of others. The Archbishop of Lima was something of a philologist; he dabbled in dialects; he had even evolved quite a brilliant table for the vowel and consonant changes from Latin into Spanish and from Spanish into Indian-Spanish. . . . So when he heard one day about the secret language of the twin brothers, he trimmed some quills and sent for them. The boys stood humiliated upon the rich carpets of his study while he tried to extract from them their *bread* and *tree* and their *I see* and *I saw.* . . . . Long shocked silences followed each of the archbishop's questions. . . . The priest thought for a while that they were merely in awe before his rank and before the luxury of his apartment, but at last, much perplexed, he divined the presence of some deeper reluctance and sadly let them go.

Wilder tells how secret language was the symbol of their profound identity with one another and their way of showing their separateness from a hostile world—the usual communal speech around them was for them "a debased form of silence." It is not infrequently the case in fact in an identical twinship that a secret separate language is elaborated, though perhaps seldom as independent of the mother tongue as in this fictive instance in *The Bridge of San Luis Rey.* Such a twinship often epitomizes the phenomena pertaining to narcissistic object-choice. Wilder's twins also demonstrate their aversion for and rebellion against the *mother* tongue. The neologisms discussed previously are the cryptic results of the pronouncedly narcissistic position of the libido in phases of schizophrenia before complete disorganization sets in or while it is indefinitely suspended by restitutional events. Another phenomenon associated with the characteristically pathological narcissism in schizophrenic disorder is hypochondriacal or organ-speech. Schizophrenia is often ushered in with symptoms of hypochondriasis and exaltation, both phenomena associated with deepening narcissistic withdrawal; that is, the libido withdrawn from the environment is reinvested in the self. Sometimes, as Freud (1915) illustrated in a case of incipient schizophrenia, "organ-speech" is evident. A young woman in mental distress after a quarrel with her lover was brought to the clinic of Dr. Victor Tausk, Freud's pupil. She complained that "her eyes were not right, they were twisted." Later, she amplified this strange remark in more coherent language, saying "she could not understand her lover at all, he looked different every time; he was a hypocrite, an eye-twister, he had twisted her eyes; now she had twisted eyes; they were not her eyes any more; now she saw the world with different eyes."

It is to be noted that in German *Augenverdreher* (literally, "eye-twister") has the figurative meaning of "deceiver," a point which Freud does not emphasize. It would seem in this instance to be of great importance, for here, once again, not only is there the literal bodily reference but also the disturbance with metaphoric symbolism—a literal significance is *felt* and onesidedly elaborated. This elaboration is associated with the hypercathexis of parts of her own body brought about by the heightened narcissism.

Freud (1915) also reports another communication of the same patient: "She was standing in a church. Suddenly she felt a jerk; she had to change her position, as though somebody was putting her into a position, as though she was being put in a certain position." There followed a fresh series of reproaches against her lover.

He was common, he had made her common, too, though she was naturally refined. He had made her like himself by making her think that he was superior to her; now she had become like him, because she thought she would be better if she were like him. He had given a false impression of his position; now she was just like him [by identification], he had put her in a false position.

Freud continues:

The physical movement of "changing her position," Tausk remarks, depicted the words "putting her in a false position" and her identification with her lover. I would call attention once more to the fact that the whole train of thought is dominated by the element which has for its content a bodily innervation (or, rather, the sensation of it). Furthermore, a hysterical woman would, in the first example, have *in fact* convulsively twisted her eyes, and, in the second, have given actual jerks instead of having the *impulse* to do so or the *sensation* of doing so; and in neither example would she have any accompanying conscious thoughts, nor would she have been able to express any such thoughts afterwards.

Thus in contradistinction to conversion phenomena, though these also sometimes appear in schizophrenia (see Noble 1951), the disturbance in metaphoric symbolism remains in this patient within the psychic sphere, as is more usual in schizophrenia. Indeed the regression in conversion hysteria to the inaudible somatic foundations of speech, to body language, is focused within a narrow range and is a defense which prevents more diffuse disorder of metaphoric symbolism. In borderline cases, the conversion defense is an important means whereby ego functions in general are safeguarded—it is a sacrifice of a part of the whole, so that the remainder may continue to furnish a useful basis for coping functions. The regression in the ego, though deep, is restricted in hysteria as compared with schizophrenia. In this restricted regression the conversion phenomena, as we have noted, betray sexual symbolic references, a cryptophoric symbolism of the same order as that of the dreaming ego.

A conversion defense may at times be attempted in schizophrenia. Repression, however, fails more completely in schizophrenia than in hysteria and a restricted *regression* in conversion in an effort to counteract the failure in repression rarely puts on more than a temporary patch. In another phase of schizophrenia, the failure in repression and the regression in the psychic part of the total mental ego* results not only in a general disturbance in metaphoric symbolism but an infiltration of cryptophoric symbolism into conscious thinking. The patient whom Freud (1915) next discusses in *Das Unbewusste* is an excellent example:

A patient whom I have at present under observation has allowed himself to be withdrawn from all the interests of life on account of a bad condition of the skin of his face. He declares that he has blackheads and deep holes on his face which everyone notices. Analysis shows that he is playing out his castration complex upon his skin. At first he worked at these blackheads remorselessly; and it gave him great satisfaction to squeeze them out, because, as he said, something spurted out when he did so. Then he began to think that a deep cavity appeared whenever he had got rid of a blackhead, and he reproached himself most vehemently with having ruined his skin forever by "constantly fiddling about with his hand." Pressing out the content of the blackheads is clearly to him a substitute for masturbation. The cavity which then appears owing to his fault is the female genital.

It is certainly true that in schizophrenia words are sometimes subjected to the same primary process as that which makes the dream images out of latent dream thoughts. It is also true that the cathexis of word-presentations of objects may be retained, or even hypercathected, in a restitutional effort, when object-cathexes are diminishing. These two propositions of Freud remain unaffected by the fact that in his discussion of examples he has overlooked the important part played by a

* The ego, of course, is entirely mental, consisting of the core mental representation of the body and the psychic superstructure.

regression in the symbolic process itself. This regression may result in both a display of disturbance of metaphoric symbolism and an infiltration into waking consciousness of cryptophoric symbolism, normally relegated to dreaming consciousness. Wegener concerned himself with the evolution of metaphor and its contribution to discursive language, that is, with the preconscious evolution of word language; he failed to discern the roots of metaphor in more primitive unconscious body symbolism, though he reiterates that language is rooted in the depths of the unconscious.

In rare cases, words are so highly cathected and the psychic experience of the patient so remote from that of his entourage, that he actually attempts the feat of inventing a new language. Like Rudolf Carnap's (1937), his "ideal language" has its "logical syntax," though this, as in ordinary language, cannot be formalized in mathematical symbolism. Like Wittgenstein (1953), the patient tries to discover the *Verbindung* between language and reality—as he experiences reality. The efforts with words, especially abstract words, sometimes reach extraordinary proportions, while the basis for a sound abstract attitude (Goldstein 1934) is being steadily eroded.

Often such restitutional efforts gradually become impaled upon mere "verbalization." These efforts run counter to the general direction of regression of the libido. The regression in the ego which usually follows in the wake of the narcissistic withdrawal often results finally in much attention being focused on assonance, alliteration, rhythmic repetition, and rhyming. Silvano Arieti (1959) discusses the regressive events directly related to language as follows:

Although the healthy person in a wakened state is concerned with connotation and denotation of a symbol, he can shift his attention from one to another of its three aspects (connotation, denotation, verbalization); the regressing schizophrenic, however, is concerned more and more with denotation and verbalization, and experiences a partial or total impairment in his ability to connote. This is what I have called *reduction of the connotation power*. For example, when regressed schizophrenics are asked to interpret the proverbs, they do so literally. (A patient asked to explain the proverb, "When the cat's away, the mice will play," replied that the mice felt free to play when the cat was away. He could not give the word "cat" the special connotation, "a cruel person in authority.")

Kurt Goldstein (1934) had earlier termed this kind of restriction of the meaning of words to specific instances as a reduction to the "concrete attitude." On the other hand, in schizophrenia, it is also the case that the metaphorical is heavily utilized without awareness of its being metaphorical. This is especially evident in relation to affect-laden wishful phantasies when the literal truth may be quite excluded. Here is another justification, and an important one, of Bleuler's name for the disease which consists in a complex disorder of symbolism, including that of metaphor.

Kubie (1953) insists that there is always a preexisting neurosis out of which major aspects of a psychosis may evolve. Every psychogenic psychopathological process results in symptoms or symptomatic behavior which constitute an unconscious symbolic language for the expression of repressed intrapsychic conflicts. Illness begins "as the conflict engenders a repressive-dissociative process which obscures the links between symbolic constructs and the percepts and conceptualizations which represent the body and its needs and conflicts; i.e., the 'I' pole of reference." Alone this produces the neurosis. "In the psychotic process," writes Kubie (1953), "there is an additional specific distortion in the relationship between the symbol and its pole of reference to the outer world: i.e. to the 'non-I.'" The distortions of the symbolic process to which Kubie draws attention are evident in the localized embodied metaphors of conversion hysteria, and in the tendency in schizophrenia either to become lost in the metaphor entirely or to avoid any involvement in it at all; also in the localized sexual symbolic references of the bodily symptoms in hysteria, and in the more diffuse sexual symbolism evident in schizophrenic mental disorder.

3. The invention of a new language

Words may be very highly cathected by schizophrenic patients in their efforts at restitution of reality-relatedness. Jung's patient, discussed above, called some of the words that she herself coined "power-words." She said of herself: "I am double polytechnic irretrievable." It eventually became evident that for her "polytechnic" meant the highest skills which she possessed and the commensurate rewards which were her due. Thus in this word she distilled the essence of many ideas about herself. The sentence now becomes comprehensible, though her use in it of other words as qualifiers is unusual: she means, of course, to emphasize her perfection with "double," to put the matter mildly, and by "irretrievable" that no one else can possibly reach out so far as to acquire such perfection. Moreover, the concern with the words as such, the "verbalization" aspect, their assonance and rhythm, seems as important as the message. The mood of mystery which she invokes is no less evident. Anyway, the word "polytechnic" has as its reference a diffuse concept; and it has its physiognomic aspect too, that is to say, its acoustic qualities seem merged with the meaning.

Heinz Werner (1948) points out that in advanced forms of mental activity thought processes may be quite detached from the concrete sensorimotor perceptual and affective sphere. In more primitive thinking, thought processes are more or less fused with functions of a sensorimotor and affective type. "It is this absence of a strict separation of thought proper from perception, emotion and motor action which determines the significance of so-called concrete and affective thinking" (Werner 1948). Thus, according to Werner's criteria, we would have to regard the diffuse concept achieved in the word "polytechnic" by this patient as a primitive type of abstraction, a type which certainly retains considerable vitality and which indeed plays a large part in the speech of older children. When schizophrenics attempt to reach higher levels of abstraction as they often do in extraordinarily intense restitutional efforts, they then become even more confused and confusing. Of course, when we think in abstractions there is a danger that we too may, in Freud's words, "neglect the relations of words to unconscious thing-presentations," and our philosophizing may then begin "to acquire an unwelcome resemblance to the mode of operation of schizophrenics" (Freud 1915).

The interspersion of quantities of "power-words" and other neologisms is common in schizophrenia but the actual construction of an entirely new language is rare. Karl Tuczek (1921), Bleuler (1918), and Lucie Jessner (1931) have each described a case of an extensive attempt at new language formation.

Many of the new words formed by the woman suffering from catatonic schizophrenia described by Tuczek (1921) were arrived at by naming objects for a constituent feature of the total situation in which the object so named participated. Thus she designated the object *bird* by the word "song." The word "cellar" was changed to "spider" and then to "tearable." This sequence may be understood from the fact that spiderwebs are often found in cellars and that the patient had experienced them there. She subtracted "web" and gave "spider" at first and then, since webs are palpably tearable, used "tearable" instead to denote the cellar. The doctors she called "the dance" because during their visits "they were dancing around the professor." It is notable that she named according to what impressed her vividly, sensually—she selected as a name a part of the situation in which the object was actually involved in her own experience and that part which she found most affect-arousing and sensually impressive. This reflects the narcissistic stance. The word arrived at is holophrastic, that is, it is a word-sentence concerning the object. The object is treated as the logical subject of a logical predicate, and it is this predicate that is partially indicated in the selected word.

This patient's way of thinking may be further elucidated by some of her other verbal responses. For the word "zero" she substituted "name early le le." When asked about this, she responded, "In the morning a mother must ask her boy whether he has been to the bathroom. Zero is a testicle which looks like a zero." It seems that early in the morning she had been wont to ask her boy whether he had urinated ("le le"). "Zero" is understood in this instance by her as a whole sentence: "Early in the morning I ask my boy whether he has urinated." It captures the action of a reminiscence suffused by an interrogative address to her son and by the image (remembered or imagined) of his genitals; maybe too zero = o, which is a pictograph for the bladder. It would also seem that onomatopoeia plays a part in her expression for micturition. Of more importance is the overt evidence of an uncontrolled infiltration of consciousness by cryptophoric sexual symbolism.

Wegener's views of the life of speech are amply illuminated by Werner and Kaplan (1963) in their book on *Symbol Formation*. They write that the spheres of connotation of the linguistic vehicles which schizophrenics often employ in naming, as in the above instance, are

(a) . . . suffused with highly personal themes and hence are egocentric-idiosyncratic; (b)they lack contour and hence tend to leak into other spheres and to assimilate other spheres to themselves; they thus may undergo sudden alterations, expansion, mergings, transformation, etc.; (c)they are global-holophrastic, cutting across, between and around the meanings expressible via the communal lexicon; and (d)they are affective-connative-imperative, containing the fears, wishes, commands, etc. of the speaker.

In certain phases of schizophrenia this kind of acataphasia and of agrammatism is prevented by the avoidance of all topics of a personal nature—so-called "dys-symbole" (Skottowe 1939, Thomas 1940); in other forms and phases of schizophrenia one word, even one only remotely connected with a personal theme, is enough to arouse an acataphasic response.

Werner and Kaplan (1963) introduce the term *monoreme* to designate single vocables of a referential nature, neither words nor any part of speech, which are uttered by the infant prior to any syntactic differentiation. They point out that many utterances of schizophrenics are remarkably similar, formally, to infantile monoremes. Wegener first showed how the word in early childhood communication stood for a sentence. These authors trace this phenomenon to the immediately preverbal stage of vocal utterance and then cite similar instances in schizophrenia, such as the following. One of Walter Gerson's patients (1928) would utter the monoreme "schum" (probably derived from the slang term *schumrig* = cozy). This was used to express the comprehensive wishful thought of taking her boy in her arms and embracing him, and also

of having him close to her. It does not seem to me that the formal similarity is really sufficient to justify calling this kind of schizophrenic utterance a monoreme, since it differs from the infantile monoreme; the
neologisms are constructed, however partially or tenuously, on the basis
of previously learned word symbols. However this may be, the examples
we have given of Tuczek's patient may be sufficient to awaken memories of *Through the Looking-Glass* (Carroll 1872):

"When I use a word," Humpty-Dumpty said, in rather a scornful tone,
"it means just what I choose it to mean—neither more nor less."

"The question is," said Humpty-Dumpty, "which is to be master—that's
all."

Martin Gardner (1960) has pointed out that proper names seldom
have a meaning other than the denotation of an individual object,
whereas other words have general, universal meanings. In Humpty-
Dumpty's realm the reverse is true: ordinary words mean whatever
Humpty wants them to mean, whereas proper names like "Alice" and
"Humpty-Dumpty" are supposed to have general significance. Arguing
with Alice, Humpty is negativistic and will even contradict himself in
order to contradict Alice, so that the reversal noted above is just another
"un-birthday present." At one time he insists on pointing out that words
are physiognomic ("my name means the shape I am."); at another he
indicates their arbitrariness and their polysemy and so on. These con-
trarieties are, however, correct. The author's extraordinary insight about
language is complemented by his understanding of Humpty-Dumpty's
character—his colossal pride and liability to fall to pieces.

Capricious qualities of language and of the self may be partially sur-
mounted by those schizophrenic patients who create a whole new language in their fragile and excessively proud rebellion against the communal lexicon. This effort was confined to a childlike modification of
Swiss-German by Bleuler's (1918) patient who claimed to have constructed an "artificial language" with new words for the whole language. On the other hand, Jessner's (1931) patient constructed a new
language which, according to the professor of linguistics at the University of Koenigsberg was not closely related to any other living tongue.

Bleuler (1919) in commenting generally on the phenomenon of an
"artificial language" wrote:

The neologisms may still be discernibly based on words in common usage,
or they may be entirely new creations, often obviously pretending to imitate
a specific language. In that case, the patients may themselves designate their
language as French, Chinese, etc. Sometimes, at least, it may be shown that
identical words are always used to express certain concepts. For the most
part, however, the "artificial language" seems to be a product of the moment,

and is soon replaced by another. It cannot always be determined just how seriously the patients take these "languages"; they often seem to have the meaning of a joke or mystification. However, in a few cases the patients really believe that they have expressed themselves correctly; they believe they are speaking their usual or another existing language; or they may be conscious of their new creation.

As stated, Jessner's (1931) patient constructed a new language, not closely related to any other known living tongue. It does, however, contain isolated word stems from Latin which are related in the manner of borrowed words in German. The patient herself indignantly denied that she had created the language. "It would be idiotic," she said, "to construct a language for oneself; there are enough languages already." She described her language as "that of Hippocrates, old-Roman, also related to Esperanto." Dr. Jessner (1931) comments:

This spontaneous language has a double significance for the patient. On the one hand it is a language of love—it is used for spiritual understanding with her beloved. . . . On the other hand, however, it is a scholarly language—similar to the language of the Middle Ages—in which the scientists of all countries can make themselves understood without being understood by laymen.

The vocabulary has great range, but limited content. It is drawn mainly from two areas which form the center of the patient's psychotic experience: the erotic and the scientific. Jessner (1931) states:

Thus we find on the one hand an abundance of love-words, expressions of affection, and sexual terminology, and on the other hand, medical, pharmacological, botanical and physiological designations. Words for everyday use, such as furniture, tools, food, if not related to either area, are lacking. Abstracts far outweigh the number of concrete objects.

There is a system to this language, though this is not evident immediately. The same words are not consistently used for the same meaning, but it can be shown that this phenomenon is not owing to forgetfulness or playfulness, but to the fact that each word has a different nuance or that the intended concept can be broken down into several distinct terms—placing this spontaneous language close to the languages of some primitive peoples.

An intensive infatuation, a transference introjection of one of her doctors, is evident in the two themes elaborated in the language, namely that of love and that of the medical scientific. This introjection is later distanced, dissociated, for the patient claims that in the spring of 1929 she arrived at "Hengonelosie" (foreign languageness) through becoming the medium of her lord and master—she heard his voice then, and periodically later, dictate the language for her. As the erotic motif retreated, her thinking shifted for a while from a predominantly concrete, diffuse, and erratic style to an abstract, systematizing, scientific one. The affect, Jessner states, "then became drier, cooler and fainter." The events included auditory hallucinosis during which the language was trans-mitted; then it was optically transmitted, as well as by means of "tele-graphic writing," according to the patient; and later still, elements of the language came "inspirationally," as a religious expression. In all this, it becomes evident that as the narcissistic identification with the doctor proceeds, she feels elevated from her humble station, one in which she had suffered severe disappointment and humiliation.

A year or so later, when she was first investigated by Dr. Jessner, she claimed that she no longer occupied herself with the language; how-ever, all the documentation about it including her dictionary and gram-matical rules were available for study. The patient's activity at the time was mainly concerned with drawing. She claimed she was training to become an artist. Upon request on one occasion, she took out of her dress a stack of drawings, of stylized animals in a fantastic landscape. Some of these drawings bore inscriptions in a spontaneous language akin to, but not identical with, the earlier language. The patient herself stated that this was "African" and had nothing to do with the former "Latin language.'" For the most part the patient refused translation, but she did make an exception of an inscription on one sketch which showed a unicorn shot to death. She said that the inscription meant "death" (*Tod*) and was at the same time an epigram which she was not permitted to repeat. Dr. Jessner writes:

We believe that a new language principle has appeared, since, namely, one word represents an entire sentence. We assume that we are dealing with a primitive language and that the accurate instinct of the patient designated this language as African and the earlier as Latin.

Finally, then, when investigated by Dr. Jessner, the patient was in-terested in another language, in a primitive tongue which reduced to few words her complex ideation. There was an extraordinary regres-sion to the "one-word sentence" type, from which, as Wegener taught, discursive dialogue emerges. It is noteworthy too that at this time she was more interested in the visual mode of expression and communica-tion than in the acoustic.

4. The influencing machine and speech

The "Influencing Machine" is a well-known delusion encountered in paranoid schizophrenia. In the present era of advanced technology, the apparatus may be conceived of as an electronic device rather than merely as an electrical instrument, as it was until recently; no doubt it assumed other guises in earlier days. The device or instrument is believed to deploy marvellous power, perhaps making the patient see two-dimensional pictures against his will, or producing or removing his thoughts, or stimulating motor or secretory phenomena, e.g., erections and seminal emissions. In various ways the patient feels he is being influenced by the machine and persecuted by means of it.

In 1919 Tausk listened to his patient Natalija A., a thirty-one-year-old student of philosophy, describe a variant of the influencing machine. She believed that she was under the malign influence of an electrical machine which had the form, for the most part, of her own body. According to the patient, her rejected suitor, a college professor, prompted by jealousy, utilized the apparatus to persecute her. Soon after the patient had refused his courtship, she felt he was forcing a friendship between her and his sister-in-law. Then she felt he subjected her mother, her physician, and her friends to the influence of this diabolical machine. Thus her physician submitted a mistaken diagnosis of her illness, thus she was alienated from her friends and relatives. Later she stated that Dr. Tausk too was under the influence of the machine and had thus become hostile toward her, and so on.

The "Influencing Machine" is itself a mechanical variant of the more prevalent paranoid delusion of chemical poisoning via food. For example, years ago, I encountered one paranoid schizophrenic patient, a captured Nazi high official, who held the firm conviction that not only was he being mentally influenced by means of subtle food poisons but his medical attendants, though well-intentioned, were also being poisoned, one symptom of this being their "glassy eyes" (Rees, 1947). In the case of Natalija A., Tausk (1919) saw a subvariant of the more usual kind of diabolical machine, one which he considered revealed a phase of its development in a disowning projection of body self-representations. He writes:

When the influencing machine of Miss Natalija A. first came to my attention, it was in a special stage of development; I was fortunate, moreover, in observing the machine in the process of development as concerned the limbs, and also in obtaining specific information from the patient herself regarding the genitalia. I assume that this process will end with the production of the typical influencing apparatus known to clinical observation.

Tausk's article contains many interesting suggestions concerning the complex psychogenetics and dynamics underlying the production of this psychotic delusion of being influenced by a machine.

As regards the development of the "Influencing Machine," he dis-

tinguishes three principal stages. First, he notes that the internal alteration of the body-image produced by greatly heightened narcissism often
results in hypochondria. In this connection he outlines the possibility
that deepened narcissistic withdrawal itself is a result of sexual challenges impinging upon a basically anxious and narcissistic (schizoid)
character structure. Second, following the hypochondriacal symptoms,
the patient complains of feelings of estrangement from the bodily self.
These are produced by rejection of the pathologically altered representations of various organs or of some of their functions which thus become
experienced as ego-alien. In this connection, Tausk draws attention
to aroused heterosexual and/or homoerotic drives anchored in these
organs and functions and elaborated in secondary delusions. Third,
Tausk (1919) points out:

the sense of persecution (paranoia somatica) arising from projection of the
pathological alteration on to the outside world, a)by attribution of the alteration to a foreign hostile power, b) by construction of the influencing machine as a summation of some or all of the pathologically altered organs (the
whole body) projected outward. It is to be noted that among these organs
the genitals take precedence in the projection.

The latter statement is not invariably accurate. In a case reported by
Edward Bibring (1929), the important projected body-part was the
patient's buttocks.

Tausk (1919) differentiates two types of projected objects in close
relation to the infernal machine. He notes that the hostile apparatus is
handled by persons who to an objective observer cannot but appear as
loving—e.g., suitors and physicians. These persons deal with the body
and are associated with sensuousness. They demand, or seem to demand, a transfer of libido to themselves. Indeed such a transfer is a
normal development. Tausk (1919) continues:

But the narcissistic libido whenever too strongly fixated, cannot but regard
this demand made by love objects as inimical, and looks upon the object as
an enemy. It is to be noted, however, that another group of love objects—
mother, the patient's present physician, close friends of the family—are not
counted among the patient's persecutors but among the persecuted, compelled
to share his fate in being subjected to the influencing machine.

To expand upon Tausk's view, it would seem that the patient remains
capable of libidinal ties only to the extent of identification within the
close reference group of those who care for him; all these people share
"goodness" with him, and the "bad" is split off. Following the splitting,
the bad is projected, regarded as outside, and includes the machine and
its manipulators. This redeployment and transference-projection of internal objects after splitting into "good" and "bad" is a desperate regres-

sive defense against a severe ambivalence which would make life with those who actually nurture the patient impossible for him. Without this paranoid defense a deeper regression into a self-supply system—an even more autistic libidinal position—would become necessary. Thus the paranoid defense enables maintenance of a lifeline of narcissistic identification with nurturing objects and also permits hate to be diverted from the self. The paranoid mechanism thus militates against further tendencies to disintegration and deterioration; these tendencies, of course, become prominent in those other schizophrenics who attempt the impossible task of autistic self-supply, turning away entirely from the external world to their self-created inner world. In this context, it is evident that the machine is based largely on "bad" body representations of the self, as Tausk emphasized; as we shall see, these are also merged with "bad" bodily representations of others with whom the patient had identified. The manipulators, on the other hand, are discredited with all the disowned genital incestuous, homosexual, and pregenital sadistic impulses with which, in the regressive surge, the patient is inwardly and conflictually confronted. Not only is much condensed in the machine itself, but persecutors, machine, and word-symbolic thought formations are diffusely conceived and confused. There is a thought-disorder which consists of diffuse concretistic thinking and includes a breakdown of metaphoric discrimination—"like" is treated as "the same."

A nineteen-year-old white male student was referred to Dr. Vamik Volkan at the University of Virginia because of severe disorganizing anxiety and was treated under his supervision by Dr. Tajammul Bhatti, resident in psychiatry. Here is Dr. Bhatti's initial account of the patient, amended only to avoid identification.

This is a nineteen-year-old white male student who was referred in through Student Health for "anxiety."

PRESENT ILLNESS: On September 14, 1968, the patient rode with the father from his home many miles away on his way to this University. The patient was noted to be anxious early in the afternoon. In the evening the patient was apparently upset by his father's excessive drinking and making a public scene. After watching television in the evening at a motel en route, the patient became upset when he found his father advancing toward his bed. (The patient's father says he was too tired and does not recall any incident.) The patient ran out to the car and sat inside it for some hours. He heard some gun-clicking sounds and also heard his father. He became frightened and drove away to his uncle's. The patient and his father were reunited the next day and after going through the registration proceedings, the patient started attending classes. He continued to be fairly anxious and was being seen in the Student Health Department. He recalls noticing the psychology teacher's gaze on him and he associates this with the words "introverted neurotic"

Also he felt that the security police were tailing him and that other people were looking at him. According to his family, he was apparently calming down until one day at his uncle's house he was going through the family book and saw a picture of his deceased grandfather giving a piece of cake to him when he was a child. He reportedly became much more disturbed that afternoon and had to be brought to the hospital.

SITUATIONAL ANALYSIS: The patient is the first of four siblings in the family, the youngest being three and a half years old. His conception is reported to have been planned and the parents are not aware of any difficulties in early childhood or early school years. At age 13 the patient recalls an incident in which he took his father's car and was with a boy coming from a family "on the other side of the tracks." He said they weren't doing anything but were seen by a policeman who reported it to his father. The patient states he was accused by his father of being a homosexual and thus deprived of all self-esteem and self-respect. While stating this, the patient broke down for the first time in the interview. (The parents stated that at that time most of the boys in the neighborhood were hanging around a particular drugstore where they were encouraged to abstain from school, spend money on cigarettes, and possibly also encouraged in homosexual activities. The patient's father had appeared to be convinced of the fact that his son was a homosexual. The mother, however, had debated the issue and had said that they really had no evidence to believe this.) During that year the patient's grandfather died and the patient recalls difficulties between his father and his grandmother on the distribution of the grandfather's assets. He regards his father's attitude as unfair and also recalls his being dictatorial and negligent of the other children in the family. (In February of 1968 the patient was involved in an automobile accident following a drinking binge in which he hit a parked car and was deprived of his driving privileges for a six month period. The patient did not relate this incident to the therapist. He spent the summer with his parents and was withdrawn and quiet most of the time.) The patient states that he was disturbed by the fact that at dinner times he was served before anybody else in the family. He elaborated this by saying that he feels his father neglects the other children and his reception of the special treatment makes him feel somewhat responsible for the plight of other children in the family. He had done fairly well at school and has no history of drug intake. (The patient's parents apparently have had arguments ever since they have been married and the wife thinks this may have a lot to do with the patient's troubles since "the children were always aware of their fighting." The father, who seems to have difficulty with alcoholism and hypertension, did not seem to think there was much wrong in the family.)

MEDICAL HISTORY: Aside from childhood illnesses, there have been no other sicknesses.

PSYCHIATRIC EXAMINATION: The patient was quite cooperative. He was frightened and showed a visible shaking. The patient had a tendency to stay in the same posture for quite a good length of time. He showed a nervous habit of pulling on his hair over the occiput where he had a four inch wide bald patch. His facial expression was close to one of being in terror. His voice, though mostly steady, tended to break down frequently. There was frequent blocking of speech and expression of his desire to return to the dormitories and he repeated, "I want to know really what's at the bottom of all this." His affect, though persistently of fear, would respond to some extent appropriately to recollections of more pleasant subjects in the distant past. The central content of his thoughts could be best described as "I guess I'm all right. I want to get to the bottom of all this." He frequently stated that he was being treated like a dog and was "in a trap." He had auditory hallucinations. He heard voices of police chasing his father and the father making derogatory comments about him. There was no overt evidence of magical thinking. There was some evidence of compulsive-obsessive thinking. Some depression was felt to be present. There was no evidence of any phobias. The patient was well oriented to time, place, and person and his memory for recent and old events appeared to be intact. The patient did not have any insight, was fairly suggestible, and agreed to stay on the ward, saying "okay, if you say so, I'll stay here." The patient was not felt to be suicidal.

DIAGNOSTIC EVALUATION AND FORMULATION: The clinical diagnosis at this time is consistent with paranoid schizophrenia, homosexual panic, and paranoid reaction. The patient's hallucinations center about his father's accusation that he is a homosexual. Later on they changed to accusations of murder, although he could not say whom he had murdered or who was accusing him of this crime. There is obvious malresolution of the oedipal complex and difficulties in sexual identity. There is evidence of some depression earlier in the summer and apparently the final precipitation came from his father's behavior on the night of the incident.

PROGNOSIS: Although guarded, is not so poor because of the rather acute exacerbation.

THERAPEUTIC PLAN: The patient is to be studied in field work case study with Dr. Volkan. A combination of supportive and uncovering therapy is needed to allay some of his anxiety and to be able to reach an understanding of the present dynamics. Tranquilizers may have to be used if the anxiety reaches excessive levels.

Later, in interview with Dr. Volkan the patient spoke of his concern about a machine, saying that if something was not done to turn it off, he would "go nuts." The patient kept complaining of the machine, which accused him of being a homosexual. He also maintained that he was embarrassed when girls (nurses) came to his room, since they could all hear his thoughts as "the machine vomited them back." Then again, it accused him of murder, of framing his father. Dr. Volkan guided the patient to talk of his experience with his father just prior to the onset of his severe anxiety. The patient then related how his father had behaved in an obnoxious and embarrassing way in a restaurant on the way, and how the waitress deftly handled the situation to get them out as soon as possible. The patient said his father, especially when he drinks, behaves like an infant and cannot be turned off. Dr. Volkan interpreted that in this he was like the machine, could not be controlled and threatened the patient.

In further work with this patient, it became apparent that the projection of the "bad father" overlaid the bodily self projection as the machine. The poorly established ego boundaries during his usual functioning prior to the decompensation resulted in a merger of father and son; later in the decompensation, there was projection of the bad part of self-father. Often in the experience of the patient at home, especially as a child, the father was turned on and off like a machine—he had reacted to stimuli without self-control, more particularly in frightening temper-tantrums and ill-disguised primitive homoerotic tendencies. The patient's own homoerotic and sadistic impulses and thoughts were dissociated and then projected; they too are machinelike dissociated parts of the self, which when turned on run their course until out of fuel, unless a superior authority intervenes.

The patient's attitude toward his own thoughts and impulses may be compared with that of a severely depressed obsessive patient. The patient, an elderly and religious widow, complained of recurrent blasphemous thoughts; among others, she later confessed with shame, was "Fuck you, God." She maintained these phrases arose in her mind as if they came from a recording machine. The point here is that the reprehensible and dissociated defiant thoughts were located within, though regarded as alien intruders. Just as with the student patient, however, the widow experienced for a time a denuding of affect, that is, an isolation defense, which furthered the machine analogy; that is to say, the machine image helped to keep emotional responses removed from awareness. Throughout her discussions of the blasphemous thoughts, the patient maintained metaphoric discrimination; she knew she was using an analogy to a machine in describing how the iterations ran on their own against her will. Nor did she believe that someone else was turning an influencing machine on and off, determining the messages emitted.

We have throughout emphasized that phonetic symbolism is built upon the body-ego, crucially developing the organization of the ego and heightening its capacity for conscious representation. It is, therefore, not surprising that the influencing machine, in its development beyond the point that Tausk described, as in the case of the student described above, comes to emit verbal messages as well as nonverbal effects. Some of these verbal messages are representations of disowned forbidden id-wishes; others are representations of superego reactions. Just as the superego makes a considerable contribution to direct speech in dreams, especially when the dream imagery is belatedly additionally censored for its forbidden character, so the influencing machine takes up the cudgels of the outraged conscience. Thus one patient complained of an influencing machine annoying him with the iteration "mother-fucker." The accusation was itself couched in obscenity, illustrating in the phonetic symbolism the closeness of the archaic primitive superego to id-processes.*

The schizophrenic patient whose influencing machine is partly to be understood as a verbal apparatus "vomiting back" discreditable thoughts to cause him shame or emitting false accusations similar to those once made by his father, much to his indignation, brings to mind some of the many complex ways in which language is an important regulating instrument. Through word language the group is enabled to regulate the individual much more effectively, and especially forcibly in the impressionable years of childhood and youth. Aside from the signified content, as Charlotte Balkányi (1968) has recently emphasized, there is early on an enhancement of the "sense of rules" through the gradual assimilation of language per se as a system of conventional signs conventionally related. Regarding the signified content, studies by Theodore Lidz (1960), by Bateson and Jackson (1956), and by Lyman C. Wynne (1958), show the possibility of the family's defective utilization of language as a cultural instrument. In the case of the developing individual who later succumbs to schizophrenia, the family network in which he is reared may beget an abuse of language, as seen from the usual viewpoint of the ambient social group.

Wegener's investigations of the fundamental role of metaphor in the development of discursive language suggest a qualification of these family studies (Lidz 1960, Bateson and Jackson 1956, and Wynne 1958), perhaps most easily demonstrable by consideration of an example of cultural contrast. In Wales the popular response to a request to explain the meaning of the proverb "a rolling stone gathers no moss" is to the effect that a man who roams about (the "philobat" of Balint 1959) will not accumulate wealth. In Virginia the response is more likely to be that the man who is ready to move around resists decrepitude or becoming moldy (as presumably would Balint's "ocnophiliac"). The same proverb thus conveys two different meanings in these two capitalistic ecosystems. Such divergence in meaning in two slightly different cultural contexts does not in either one indicate any fundamental disturbance of metaphoric symbolism. Similarly, at this level of figurative meaning,

* Obscene terms have an especially adherent physiognomic character. In this regard, Leo Stone (1954) has made a notable scholarly contribution.

family deviance from the surrounding social group would only indicate eccentricity. However, persistent and wide-ranging eccentric responses of a family may well be associated with one member's more fundamental disorder of metaphoric symbolism, as occurs in schizophrenic derangement of thought and language. The fundamental disorder in schizophrenia is not merely aberrant figurative meaning, but also the incapacity to differentiate literal and figurative meanings. A secondary disorder of persistent culture-deviant figurative meanings may become quite idiosyncratic. Here the symbolic distortion takes place at another, higher, level of development of language and does not reflect the same depth of regression in the language behavior as occurs in schizophrenia. Indeed, there is sometimes represented a considerable reorganization of language in a restitutional attempt to avoid chaotic disorganization of ego functions generally.

In our technological society we are becoming more and more conscious of the pervasive effects of ever-flowing propaganda. The technological society seems to need its propaganda machine to hold itself together; that is to say, it also seems to demand its "influencing machine." Jacques Ellul (1965) makes a trenchant distinction between "integration propaganda," which aims at getting citizens to adjust in allegedly desirable patterns of behavior, and "agitation propaganda," which leads men from mere resentment of current mores to actual rebellion against them. Integration propaganda is a development of the language of social cohesion which exists in and has always pervaded all conditions of society. But it seems that now the delusional influencing machine of schizophrenics has some degree of actuality and validity as part of the social process in modern society. Sometimes a modern bureaucracy may function in a paranoid way, availing itself of the same defenses against anxious phantasies of destruction with which we are familiar in the psychopathology of schizophrenia, expending itself in distortions of social reality, bringing about or provoking problems it apparently seeks to avoid. We are reminded of Wegener's work, of his insistence that language develops first of all from the need to influence the will of the one spoken to in a manner which appears valuable to the speaker, beginning with the imperative one-word sentence of the child and the imperative admonitions (often also in one or two-word sentences) of the child's mentors, originally those of his mother. These first words are there to transfer certain elements of *consciousness* from one mind to the other, and this coercive quality remains always with words; there is a natural tendency, once elements are brought to consciousness, for action to ensue. Sometimes the action is confined to minor attitudinal changes. Sometimes there is action in the outer world. Sometimes the former prepares for the latter. And sometimes this process is inhibited or qualified—the implicit coercion is thwarted. Often this latter process commences with a "no." In any event, we see that from the beginning language is, as Wegener showed, an "influencing machine," influencing thought, emotion, and striving in the auditor (though not always in the way desired by the speaker). The propaganda of modern states is obviously concerned with influencing attitudes and actions rather than stirring rational reflection, and a "no" may be required before rational reflection can take place.

Thus there is the inflexible, irrational, automatic "no" response of the schizophrenic, who sometimes manufactures a concrete machine out of what remains to us as only a useful metaphor. In so doing he indicates an underlying intensity of emotion without being completely overwhelmed by it.

IX Pre-Stages of Language

Etymology and the repressed unconscious

THE investigation of language disorders in mental disease sheds light on the "life of speech," on its development and social dynamics. In this respect, study of language disorder is an important instance of the general finding that scrutinizing disease is apt to illuminate the dynamisms responsible for establishing and maintaining health. This present foray into territory already occupied by clashing linguistic scholars has been based in the first place on observations and inferences which regressive phenomena in hysteria and hysteriform disease copiously afford. The nature of these phenomena as revealed by Breuer and Freud (1895) plunged this discussion precipitately *in medias res*. The emergence of metaphoric symbolism in speech had to be considered, as this entered the dialogue of investigative efforts to understand the symptoms. On one hand, this led to consideration of Wegener's views of the complex role of metaphor in the development of discursive language. On the other hand, psychoanalytic investigation led deeper into those aspects of the symptoms which functionally resembled the cryptophoric (generally sexual) symbols of dream imagery. It seemed likely, following Sperber (1914), that this direction paralleled a retracing of some of the steps of the development of speech in the human species: some of the speech sources which had earlier reference to sexual activities later also referred to similar nonsexual forms and actions, and then the sexual meanings were subdued or nullified. Noted above too was the fact that in schizophrenia this repression was sometimes so much undone that speech itself became infiltrated with cryptophoric symbolism. Moreover, following Paul Schilder (1935) and Kubie (1952), it was necessary to observe the exposure in mental disease of the narcissistic base in representation of the body on which primitive symbolism is constructed; this body-symbolism is often enough readily traceable in word-symbolism.

As an instructive example of this kind of retracing from the word itself, Theodore Thass-Thienemann's (1968) extended discussion of the English verb *to write* may be cited. He points out the original meaning is even transparent in closely related languages. Thus in German *reissen*, from the former *rizan*, "to cut, tear, split" and in old Saxon *writan means* "to injure, cut." Thass-Thienemann (1968) raises the question "What is the origin of this aggressive component in the notion of writing?" Writing, of course, was originally epigraphy, a carving into hard material—stone, metal, wood—thus the letters necessarily were engraved by some deployment of force. Certainly it is by their roots that you may know them; yet Thass-Thienemann is not satisfied with only this reason. He points out such further primary references as "to wound," "cut the skin," "scar" and maintains that the primary material of "writing" was the human skin. The verbal forms indicate that more violent activity than actual writing was involved in their inception. He writes (1968):

The fantasies involving "writing" come from another source. This is indicated by the symbolic equation of "writing" and "plowing." It is in accordance with verbal fantasies that the "pen-man" calls himself *Arator* in Latin, or *Plowman* in early English literature. "My pen is my plowshare," the German *Ackermann*, "plowman," said. One has no difficulty in understanding when Cicero wrote to Atticus: *Hoc litterularum exaravi*—"I plowed out this little letter." The pen "plows" the paper. In fact this is the proper idiom in Hungarian. It is in accordance with these fantasies that the written lines were called "furrows." In Latin the lines were called *versus*, in English *verse*, properly something "turned over" from the verb *verto,-ere, versum* "to turn." One can even observe that the "furrow lines" were running from the left to the right and then from the right to the left in early literacy—a strange way of writing which must have had some motivation. Its Greek denotation gives the answer: it was called *bou-strophedon*, properly "oxen-turn" equating the lines with the furrows of plowing.

Thass-Thienemann (1968) develops the theme that writing was introduced to the minds of illiterate agricultural people and that the reference to "plowing" reinjects a sadomasochistic sexual element into the notion of writing. As mentioned earlier, Kleinpaul (1893) noted that the words for *plough* in Latin, Greek, and Oriental languages were customarily used also to denote the sexual act. Similarly Shakespeare incorporated images of ploughing and deflorating in *Pericles*: "An if she were a thornier piece of ground than she is she shall be ploughed!" The physiognomic perception connects two different meanings, one referring to acting on the body itself, the other extracorporeal in its reference.

The child: born to speak in a world of speakers

Wegener made it clear that he regarded further progress in linguistic studies to be contingent upon abandonment of one-sided preoccupation with dead languages, but he was not satisfied with this. He insisted on the observation of living speech, self-observation, and the observation of those around us. Wegener was especially a pioneer in the study of the child's acquisition of language. He stresses that in learning words the child is in the grip of intense feelings of pain and pleasure. These feelings influence his selection of words to imitate his beginning conceptual world. They are immediately related to the gratification or frustration of strivings for food, drink, and comforting body contact, and they are also related to delight in possession and mastery (see especially Wegener, pp. 128–130 below). In regard to these considerations, Lili E. Peller (1964) recently wrote that the earliest words are embedded in a lot of gibberish and that, in her opinion, different parents pick out different words as their child's "earliest." That is to say, the parents are selecting out of many possible early words, their child's "first" words. As Oscar Bloch (1921), the French linguist and a leading specialist in child language, wrote:

I have only slightly observed the speech of the first year and first months of the second year, or rather I have recorded little. Not only is it difficult indeed to grasp and to record the sounds that are produced, but to interpret them also entails large demands.

It is evident that if trained linguists find the first words difficult to locate, parents may be missing some and finding some others. However, the Belgian linguist Antoine Grégoire (1933) has attempted a rigorously systematic and exact phonological transcription of the child's early utterances, and his work does show the emergence of the linguistic structure.

Peller (1964) points out that the child may say "cookie" *after* he has been given one, as one of his earliest words. Early words may in this way confirm the sense of possession and of mastery, intensify pleasure, and enable the child to begin to share emotion. Thus the child's first words are not always merely wishes and requests. The Sterns (1907) report "tic-toc" as their daughter's first word. G. Church's son said "fish" to a large Japanese paper fish hung in the nursery, signifying his joy in recognition (Church 1961). "Many children," states Peller (1964), "begin articulate speech with 'No-No' or with Mama.' " Otto Jesperson (1925) insisted that early words may express, besides wishes and requests (including countermanding), the child's "joyful interest in what he beholds." It is doubtful whether modern linguists have yet surpassed the description offered by Wegener of the complex sensations which, repeatedly associated with the phonic image *milk*, enables a transition from a perceptual to a conceptual course of mental events. But regardless of the actual word which somehow becomes recognizable by observing adults following the infant's cooing and babbling phases, the work of Grégoire (1933) initiated studies which clearly confirm the view, developed by Jakobson (1942), that there is a fixed order throughout phonological development. In this respect too, Wegener was an important forerunner of Grégoire and of Jakobson et al. He not only observed that the words which children first learn are articulated very imperfectly, but he noticed the difficulties in the imitation of particular sounds, the exchanging of certain sounds heard, the 'incorrect" fusions of different sounds, and their unravelment in the further development of the child's speech (see Wegener, pp. 124–127 below).

The numerous observations of the advent of word language at about the same age in healthy children throughout the world and, more remarkable than this, the further observations that the *relative* chronological order of phonological acquisitions is everywhere the same, so far as it has been tested, support the concept that genetically determined processes of maturation underlie the human capacity for speech and verbal understanding. Of course these biological foundations of language are in continuous interaction with a human environment from which they are only removed in abstract thought. Noam Chomsky's (1967) notion of a universal (deep) grammatical structure seems a more tenuous hypothesis, an imaginative extension perhaps of Jakobson's better-grounded concept of phonological universals, bearing as well a distinct resemblance to Jung's archetype of meaning. The exaggeration may only be that Chomsky puts overmuch burden on syntax and correspondingly neglects the inner relationships of word, thought, and meaning. There are many different, though allied, paths to the same meaning, there being so many variables, and some of these can be studied in the intrinsic qualities of individual words.

Word and thing

Ferdinand De Saussure (1916) in his *Course in General Linguistics* shows that what emerges as a sound image or a word—in his terms, a

linguistic sign—is a union of "signifier" and "signified." Yet he considers, as did Aristotle, that the linguistic sign is quite arbitrary, with
no inner relationship of sound image, thought, and signified thing. He
writes: "Because the sign is arbitrary, it follows no law other than that
of tradition." Similarly, Max Black (1968) in the *Brittanica Perspective*
entitled *The Labyrinth of Language* writes: "Everybody will freely
concede that the phonemic system of a language is conventional or arbitrary. Nothing about the human purposes served by language, or about
the objective reality to which it aspires to refer, dictates the character of
the basic stock of phonemes or the nature of the rules governing their
combination." He points out that even the so-called onomatopoetic
words, those that seem to imitate the sounds they represent, vary from
one language to another. The dog may be called *bow-wow* in the English nursery and *oua-oua* in the French. Then in adult language the
animal called a *dog* in English is elsewhere a *chien*, a *sabaka*, a *keleb*
and so forth. Black further points out that the sound of a shot is rendered as *bank* or *crack* in English and as *pum* or *paf* in Spanish. Then
he asserts that "the point, though obvious, is worth emphasizing, because there is a lingering inclination to postulate some essential connection between word and thing." Indeed Professor Black compares
this "lingering inclination" to the thinking of the proverbial old lady
who thought it so clever of astronomers to discover the names of the
stars. Taking it as settled that choice of the basic phonemic elements
associated with "thing-meant" is arbitrary, Black next discusses what
he considers to be the much less settled and less obvious answers to two
questions. Is the division of reality into things nameable in a given
language also arbitrary? Do the differences between the grammars of
various languages show that morphology and syntax are as arbitrary as
phonology?

It is necessary to consider the possibility that Black's disparaging view
of "lingering inclinations" to suspect some essential connections between word and thing is not at all justified. Even more important, these
lingering suspicions may hover around the yet mysterious core of the
problem of the evolution of language in the human race and, to a lesser
but still important extent, in the individual. The more fashionable view,
reflected by Black, which partially results from recent acquisitions in
knowledge tending to refute some of the postulates of the scholarly
predecessors of modern linguistic scientists, is nonetheless an arrogant
overreaction; it throws out the baby with the bathwater.

Black himself asserts that to attempt to discuss linguistic interaction without reference to understanding and to understood meaning
is absurd. In this respect he follows the mode of Wegener. He quite distinctly separates himself from those professional linguists who pride

themselves on being able to ignore semantic problems. Yet meaning may basically and originally be connected by certain similarities of different orders (sometimes combined variously) between word and thing, similarities which we will shortly consider here.

In 1812, Samuel Taylor Coleridge asserted: "I wish our clever young poets would remember my homely definitions of prose and poetry; that is, prose—words in their best order; poetry—the best words in their best order." It is in poetry that the "best" words, those that somehow retain essential links between word and thing, most often occur, being one of several ways, of course, whereby poetry may be differentiated from prose.

In his essay "On Obscene Words," Ferenczi (1916) makes the point that the "worst" words too have a peculiarly compelling power, vividly evoking the excremental or sadistic sexual function in substantial actuality. The impact of these words may be felt as assaultive and resisted in disgust. This special character of arousing memory traces of a primitive hallucinatory and motor quality is related to their "arrest" in the context of concrete thinking. At the same time as the psychic counterforces—disgust, shame and guilt—against sadistic infantile sexuality are being formed, the impulse develops to utter and to draw obscenities. This is during a preliminary stage in the inhibition of visual sexual curiosity and exhibitionism. Later, with the advent of the latency period of psychosexual development, there is a wave of repression against primitive sexual phantasies and activities, even as manifested in the weakened form of speech. Thus the "obscene word images" are repressed at a time in the child's life when speech is still characterized by a *vivid mimicry of imagery*. In consequence, the dissociated verbal signs remain at a primitive developmental stage, whereas the rest of the vocabulary for the most part gradually outgrows its hallucinatory and motor character and is thus made suitable for abstract thinking. It is in this light that the compulsive swearing in the syndrome of Gilles de la Tourette acquires a special significance in the periodic severely regressive ego functioning evident in this mental disease (Abse 1966). The utterance of obscene words shows in high degree what is scarcely indicated with most words, namely, their original source in pretermitted action (Stone 1954, Abse 1955).

Plato, although he pushes the idea to absurdity, suggests in the *Cratylus* that words do not arise from the arbitrary choice of the gods but have a natural origin. Plato also has Cratylus say, "Surely, Hermogenes, you do not suppose that you can learn, or I explain, any subject of importance all in a moment; or at any rate, not such a subject as language, which is perhaps the very greatest of all." Thus the buried origins of many of the "best" words are hard to unearth and lengthy to explain, especially because it is not merely a matter of simple onomatopoeia, that is of the original selection of such words in terms of modified imitation of natural sounds emanating from animate and inanimate objects around. It is also a matter of sounds which other than phonetically suggest their sense through associations grounded in the very matrix of perception, *itself genetically synaesthetic and sensorimotor* in operation. As we have previously noted, in poetry there is often a reversal of the usual preconscious semantic movement from the concrete to the more general and abstract: the specific sensuous concrete image becomes a dominant element consciously, sometimes approaching a hallucinatory and motor character.

First, as an example of imitative origin, which though it remains essentially phonetic goes far beyond simple onomatopoeia, here is the case of the Zulu word *fumfuta*, meaning "confused," described by Mac-donald Critchley (1939). *Fumfu* means "blown about like grass in a wind" whereas *fu* means "a cloud." The word is build on the sound and movements of the human mouth in blowing and puffing, imitating the wind which may bring together things which do not usually belong to-gether, or separate those that usually do. That the sound of a shot is rendered as *bang* or *crack* in English and as *pum* or *paf* in Spanish does not, despite Black's objections (1968), put the onomatopoetic ori-gin of such words out of court; on the contrary, it conveys a hint of the multiplicity of variables involved in the emergence of onomatopoetic forms. Moreover, a further complexity results from *synaesthesia*, by the fact that sensations of modalities other than audition are also often involved, as already mentioned above.

The experimental investigations of Hornbostel and Boernstein on the "unity of the senses," as reported in English by Felix Deutsch (1954), led to the notion of a common suprasensory factor known as "brightness" in opposition to "darkness." The characteristic of bright-ness is shared by high-pitched tones, loud colors, penetrating odors, and sharp-pointed tactual stimuli. In these experiments, the simultaneous stimulation of one of different sense-organs—auditory, olfactory, tactual, pain-sensitive—produced an influence on visual acuity in terms of per-ception of brightness or darkness. These and similar experimental find-ings in adult subjects are connected with the developmental views of Werner, which are based on observations of infants and children. Werner emphasizes that development involves increasing differentiation and organization. When an infant is stimulated, he responds in a gener-alized, undifferentiated way with perhaps his entire body. As maturation proceeds, there is increasing differentiation of activity and cognition. Responses become more focused, less diffuse, and less stimulus-bound. With further progression, the increasingly differentiated functions are organized into levels, the earlier being subordinated to the later. The more differentiated adult psyche manifests an integration of the several sequential stages, with the later more differentiated processes ascendant and predominating. In this development the primordial synaesthetic mode of sensation is superseded but not entirely replaced.

In any account of the ramifications of onomatopoeia, synaesthesia must be considered. As a marked example of a synaesthetic phenomenon, some adults continue to experience with every auditory sensation an accompanying visual one; there are even attempts by artists to translate music into visual effects, or vice versa. In connection with such phenomena, R. Paget (1955) finds that in English the vowel sound "ah" refers often to anything which is wide open or *flat*, and "ee" often to that which is high (for example, *steeple, peak*) or little—that which is seen from on high (for example, *teeny*). In regard to the latter paradox, the antithetical meaning of primal sounds (Freud 1910) affords the beginnings of further explanation which need not be treated here. The following passage from John Moore's book (1961) well illustrates the synaesthetic basis of choosing and rechoosing the sounds to fit the sense:

In the same way, "slimy" seems to me suggestive of viscosity, and I cannot help feeling its currency demonstrates that "natural selection" among words does result in the survival of the fittest. It's an old word in English, akin to Latin *limus*, mud, mire, and possessing a lot of slimy relations, for example Greek *leimax*, a snail, and *limne*, a marsh, Old English *lim*, glue, birdlime, Old English *sliw*, a fish, Norwegian *slo*, a blindworm (whence our slowworm) and the English words slick . . . sleek, loam (sticky earth) and linament (something smeared on). The slight revulsion which most of us experience when we encounter this word *may* be due to its associations with say, snails, or eels or slugs—of which a whole genus bears the scientific name *Limax*. It may; or is there also some viscous suggestion in the sound?—

> "The very deep did rot: O Christ!
> That even this should be!
> Yea, slimy things did crawl with legs
> Upon a slimy sea."*

Actually to appreciate more fully intrinsic relationships of sound, thought, and thing, the phonetic and synaesthetic aspects have to be considered as complemented by the *kinaesthetic*. It then becomes apparent that more words than are usually considered remain anchored intrinsically despite the effects of phonetic drift, including consonant shifts and other complex factors in the natural evolution and social dynamics of language which come to obscure the earliest origins of words. They thus may come to *seem*, as Black (1968) insists they *are*, "arbitrary" linguistic signs.

* Coleridge's *The Rime of the Ancient Mariner.*

Here then is another example of a parallel between word and "thing-meant," mainly kinaesthetic. The "oo" sound, as in *room, tube, loop,* that is to say used to denote something enclosed, tubular, or elongated, is produced by lip movements which before phonation already imitate the form of the object named.

Associated with such mechanisms of origin of word sounds is the so-called "poo-poo" theory where the hypothesis is that the dominion of speech is erected upon the downfall of interjections, a hypothesis which yet may contain a solid grain of truth. An example quoted by E. B. Tyler (1873), will suffice. The Latin word *stare,* "to stand," originates, it is claimed, in the expressive sound "st" representing an interjection suggesting sudden arrest—"stop!" In such an interjection it is apparent that the movements of the lips and tongue establish a bond of similarity between process named and their kinetic patterning.

Jakobson (1942) urges that so far as the phonemic inventory is concerned, language in the narrow sense of the word, that is, as a system of conventional ("arbitrary") signs, must not be confused with sound gestures whose phonological form is motivated; nevertheless the ramifications of the evolution of the latter into adult modern languages has yet to be surveyed adequately. It is to be remembered in this connection that the development of language, in the above narrow sense of the word, is not simply a one-way linear movement. Actually, certain styles of speech may acquire infantile characteristics, for example, so-called "sweet-talk," as an adaptation to child language. Fashion can extend the use of such features and spread them throughout the whole language. Sometimes, as Jakobson (1942) himself notes, phonological changes in language arise from children, from the nursery language, not only by the adaptation of the older generation to the child, but "by the permanent reluctance of children, i.e., the new generation, to accept a certain component of their linguistic inheritance. Such sound changes from one generation to the next have been discussed and emphasized more than once in the linguistic literature" (Jakobson 1942, Cassirer 1944).

Symbolic development, from primitive symbolism through metaphoric symbolism, as it unfolds, is associated with the enhancement of the capacity for abstract thinking and by means of innumerable faded metaphors contributes to the greater use of conventionalized forms in speech communication. However, Werner and Kaplan (1963) are correct when they state in regard to symbolism:

Applied to language, this means that there would be an ontogenetic decline in the physiognomisation of verbal forms. This process of "denaturalisation" does not imply, however, that the verbal symbols at advanced levels are entirely "objective" phenomena, divorced from the formative activity of the symboliser or the listening individual. We submit that even the most conventionalised units of speech—words and sentences—are still part and parcel of the articulatory process, bodily postural activity, which through its dynamic features, links those conventionalised units to their referents.

Libidinal and ego development

The pre-stages of language are embedded in the general development of childhood, in both libidinal and aggressive development and in the associated early building of the image of the body which becomes invested with "ego feeling," that gradually achieved personal feeling of unity and continuity, of contiguity with others, and of causality.

In 1905 Freud described the progressive shifts in body zones most responsive to and most actively interacting with the environment and outlined oral, anal, and phallic phases of development. These observations were later (1913a) incorporated in the concept of successive but overlapping *libidinal organizations* in each of which different drives dominate. As René A. Spitz (1946) has emphasized, libidinal development breaks the path for all developments, and this certainly includes that of speech. The oral-cannibalistic phase dominated by the drive to incorporate is followed by the sadistic-anal phase in which the child's strivings to master his body, and all obstacles encountered, are paramount.

Peller (1964) writes:

In the first phase mouth and skin are most highly libidinised; in the second phase skeletal muscles and the ring muscles of the body openings (mouth, anus, urethra) are the executive organs. Each phase can be characterised by the changes which occur between its start and its end. At the beginning of life, the infant cannot differentiate which sensations come to him from the outside and which from the inside of his body; he only knows his comfort and discomfort. Toward the end of the oral phase, he can remember the agent related most often to the relief of tension and to positive pleasure; he has an image of the mothering person, is attached to her and has rudiments of an image of his own self. . . . He comes to perceive whatever has the greatest impact on his search for comfort—augmenting or reducing the pleasure. Through the highly libidinised incessant and tremendously repetitive motor and sensory activities of the sadistic-anal phase, the child comes to develop further the images of his body self and of his body functions. His activity creates for him the world of *things* contained in three dimensional space, and it is during this period that he forms attachments to his family. . . . In the third organisation, the oedipal-phallic phase, the child's component drives and his cognitive achievements are focussed in such a way that he can conceive of his parents as *persons*.

Throughout these developments, as Peller (1964) points out, the infant seems to experience and exhibit differing forms of megalomania, of feelings and ideas of vast power and importance, only subsequently considerably indented by the exigencies of living with reduced maternal protection. It is necessary in this connection to grasp the profound importance of *unconscious identification* upon which *imitation* is based. All is not so simple as the phrase "an instinct of imitation" might mislead one to think; identification is achieved by the child on account of a need to survive and to master, to take into himself the powers of the protecting parents in order to combat the feelings of helplessness which gives rise to anxiety at the time that ego differentiation is taking place in the anal phase. At this time, about 18 months of age, the child learns to utter words like those uttered around him. Soon, from 24 to 30 months, there is a veritable "naming explosion," so that from a few words at about 18 months and a few more until about 2 years, he comes to acquire a vocabulary of about a thousand words and understands about twice as many uttered around him.

Peller (1964) enumerates some important developments which precede language, the intensity of which are species-specific:

1. A prolongued helplessness which fosters strong attachment to the mother.
2. The early interest in and understanding of facial expressions.
3. The intense pleasure derived from the functioning of the vocal apparatus.
4. Extensive playful activity which brings about contact and motor interaction with the human and nonhuman environment. In this connection Peller rightly emphasizes the pleasure derived from responding to *self-created stimuli*.
5. The great reliance which comes to be placed on the distance receptors of sight and hearing.
6. The readiness to become aware of similarities between himself and others which, itself gradually built-up, then prepares the ground for the ability to put the self into the place of the other, and even to see oneself from a distance.

All these widely different developmental features of the human infant precede language, and some in turn through language are themselves greatly enhanced. Throughout childhood development there is this dynamic circular process which consists of feedback and feed-forward processes in a network. Thus the vocabulary explosion noted above is the result as much of the newly arising activities of the infant as of the maturation of cerebral mechanisms. Prior to this, there is one type of play where the feedback character is obvious, namely, babbling and lalling. At about six months the vowellike cooing (which has become interspersed with occasional consonantal sounds) gives place to babbling and to lalling which more clearly resembles single syllables. The deaf child soon gives up this babbling—presumably because there is insufficient feedback, no accompanying enjoyment engendered by hearing his own voice or any other. Normally this babbling and lalling play goes on for hours of every day during many months. As the Sterns (1907) pointed out, it may continue even in the dark. Peller (1964) writes:

Indispensable as this self-stimulation is, it is not enough. The infant must listen to other humans speaking—or the formative period for speech will come and go and language will not develop. . . . Incidental observations indicate that the child listens intently to his mother's voice and that *it is this listening* which enhances his babbling.

The mother's talking and the child's listening display but one facet of their mutually nurturing bond, a bond which when impaired results in the child's failure to thrive in many aspects of growth and development. It is certainly of profound significance that we speak of our "mother tongue," the language that eventually evolves from our cries when in need and our coos when satisfied. The coos emerge later than the cries, at about the sixth to the eighth week of extrauterine life, often following the smiling response.

The babbling and lalling which occur in the second half of the first year of life are often replaced by a periodic "blathering"—the recurrent protrusion and withdrawal of the flattened relaxed tongue through the lips while phonating. Blathering is also occasionally evident in the second year of life. This oral libidinal activity provides the pleasurable foundation for free tongue and lip movement, that is to say, the self-pleasing early functioning of the tongue, including blathering, becomes a means also of imitating sounds heard and later embedded in verbal communication. The importance of the tongue in early oral libidinal development has been generally overlooked, as Augusta Bonnard (1960) explains and elaborates. W. Scott (1955) has given a brief account of a blathering episode in the setting of an early maternal transference situation engendered during the treatment of a thirty-five-year-old woman.

The tongue has been "overlooked," as Bonnard (1960) insists, in its role as a primal organizer of the self in the early oral phase of libidinal development. Early on it is a means of finding and scanning the outside, and by its movements and sensations the baby begins to discriminate between the inside and outside surfaces of the mouth. It achieves, indeed, a high degree of precision and versatility of movement ahead of any other part of the baby. Moreover, the tongue always returns to its fixed, midline base, presumably aiding early orientation. Bonnard

(1960) states: "If we watch young children attempting a troublesome balancing or integrative task, including learning to write, we can often observe the tongue protruded to serve like the offsetting combination of the rudder and the center board of the boat, i.e. as the body's centering point." Corresponding with its vast importance in the early orientation of the self in the world, the area of representation of the tongue in the human cerebral cortex is very large compared with that of other parts of the body. It is probable that the overlooking of the primal importance of the tongue in the early development of the baby is due to its later major role in speech. However, this overshadowing function, this harnessing to the requirements of speech, is prepared for in its earlier orientating functions; phylogenetically this speech function follows the adoption of the erect posture.

Early on the tongue is an important sensory bridge from inside the self to the outside and to the beginning experience of external objects. Similarly the movement from self-pleasuring autoerotism to knowing and loving other people and the world we all inhabit together is promoted by the acquisition of the mother tongue. From his cries meant to restore pleasure and remove pain, from his enjoyment of babbling and lalling, to his monoreme, his one-word sentence, the infant makes a momentous transition: he recognizes the need, for his own purposes, to speak the language of those around him. In the word explosion which soon follows, he is like Adam, whom God allowed to share in the creation by naming each living creature. If at first in his magical thinking he glories in the borrowed omnipotence, yet this uniquely human capacity to conceptualize objects and to fix the concepts with names is a really potent instrument for constructing the world and finding himself and his place in it.

There are certain dissociative reactions in which the lalling which occurred in the transition from infancy (Latin *in* = not + *fari* = to speak) to childhood is regressively revived. Such *glossolalia* also often occurs in the setting of religious excitement in groups and currently is of special interest (Abse 1966) in connection with ingestion of hallucinogenic mushrooms or of d-lysergic acid diethylamide.

Ecstatic utterances are described as occurring in the religious ceremonies of the ancient Egyptians, and lalling, it would seem, formed part of the manifestations of ecstasy generated in the rites of the mystery religions of ancient Greece. The Pentecostal experience recorded in the Acts of the Apostles includes a description of the disciples "filled with the Holy Ghost" and speaking "with other tongues." Paul praised this lalling as a way to edify the spirit of the speaker in private prayer, but he worried about its abuse.

From contact perception to reliance on distance perception: ontogenetic and phylogenetic aspects.

Spitz (1955, 1965) has advanced and maintained the proposition that perception has its beginnings in the oral cavity and that this cavity serves as a bridge from inner to external perception soon after birth. Even in the foetus (Hooker 1952) and clearly in the neonate a response to stimulation in and around the mouth can be readily demonstrated, namely rotation of the head toward the stimulus, followed by a snapping of the jaws. In the nursing situation this infantile response includes ingestion of the nipple and is known as the rooting reflex; by means of a combination with the sucking reflex the infant quickly achieves *directed* behavior obviously of primary survival value. We have above, in conformity with Bonnard (1960), emphasized the role of the tongue in these early beginnings of perception and orientation for survival. The tongue, cheeks, and nasopharynx, in which are later differentiated the sense modalities of touch, state, smell, temperature, pain, and even of deep sensation, as this is involved in the act of swallowing, furnish the surfaces for early stimulation. These beginnings of perception and orientation are early on supported and amplified by the activities of the hands and labyrinths, that is, by developing prehension based on the grasp reflex and conditioned responses based on vestibular reflexes. Thus in connection with the latter, by the eighth day of life a suitable change of positioning of the baby will elicit rooting and sucking responses (Spitz 1965). These precursors of perception, brought into operation through the instrumentality of the oral cavity and of the ancillary organs (hands, labyrinths, and skin), constitute the origins of *contact perception.* This is soon to be vastly augmented by stimulation through the portals of the eyes and ears, the beginnings of *distance perception.*

An epigenetic view, that is one which takes as its perspective the life cycle, induces the conception of an endogenously unfolding program of maturation inexorably followed at its own pace, released and modified by developmental factors of an interactional order. An important part of the individual geno-genic program has its base in the history of the species, as E. Haeckel (1879) originally contended; and there is the necessary corollary that ontogeny helps to determine phylogeny. Today recapitulation and partial simulation of Lamarckian evolution by genetic assimilation and by other evolutionary feedback mechanisms remain lively issues in theories of evolution (Sol Tax 1960). It is relevant here to bring an evolutionary viewpoint, albeit briefly, on the move-ment from reliance on touch and olfaction to the predominance of vision and hearing in the history of Homo sapiens.

It is clearly by progressive increase in size and complexity of the brain that the primates emerged from among the mammalia and that man in turn transcended other primates. The complex functional change is in the nature of an increase in the powers of vision and of hearing, of rapid association of these with touch and with one another, and with muscular movements or other active responses. The increase in range, rapidity, and complexity of association and response is remarkable. Even more remarkable is the associated immense increment in the power of memory, an increment which also enables a range of higher mental activities, including reflection based on conscious recall. In man, above all other primates, memory-protection supplants excessively repeated experimentation, a state of affairs which unhappily is often offset by the destructive forces of the human psyche. In summary, we may cite the following observations. The brain of a manlike ape (gorilla, chim-panzee, orangutan) closely resembles a human brain. The same sulci and gyri can be identified, differing in details of their formation, yet recognizable as similar, and in all probability having the same rela-tions to function. The association areas of the cortex are much less ex-tensive; yet, for example, the great parietal association region can be demonstrated to be bounded by similar fissures. The fact that this parietal association region is so much more restricted in extent, that the "speech" areas are only feebly developed, and that the special sense areas for vision and for hearing are less well developed than in man empha-sizes the importance of these two senses in relation to attention and speech as human characteristics. A comparison of brains of anthropoid apes with those of Tarsius and the lemurs, and of these brains with those of tree shrews and jumping shrews, and of the latter with each other, quickly reveals elements of the natural history of gradual emanci-pation from the control of the senses of smell and touch, of the re-placement of this dual dominance by a combination of vision, touch, and hearing. We may be persuaded quickly too of the importance of the lengthy adoption of arboreal life, shared with us in their history by the pongids, in this emancipation from predominance of smelling. The increasing power and correlation of the newly dominant combination of senses of vision and hearing and touch, and the cooperation of them in influencing muscular activities, reach a climax in man, outstandingly in his speech.

As has already been noted here (p. 9), in the human brain there is a region in the posterior part of the left inferior frontal gyrus which when injured results in disturbance of the more motor aspects of speech

(Broca's area). It is this region which is among those feebly developed in the apes. Injury to an area around the posterior end of the left superior temporal gyrus (Wernicke's area) often produces a different type of aphasia, a difficulty in comprehending spoken speech. Adjacent to this area is the gyrus angularis, which is also included in Wernicke's area. This area is sometimes designated as the region of ideational speech, or the "word store" (Young 1970). It lies between the association areas connected with vision, hearing, and touch. Hence Wilder Penfield (1966) has dubbed it "the association area of association areas," and it is characteristically well developed in man.

In the second month of extrauterine life the human infant begins to be able to see someone approaching from a distance if at the time of the approach the infant is hungry. At this stage of elementary visual perception, observation leads to the inference that such perception is predicated upon tension generated by an ungratified drive. Spitz (1965) writes: "Two or three weeks later (about the eleventh week) we note a further progress: when the infant perceives a human face, he follows its movements with concentrated attention. No other 'thing' can elicit this behavior in the infant at this age level."

Nursing is not the only ministration of the mother during which the baby stares at her face; she offers her face for his inspection when she lifts him, washes him, changes his diaper, and so forth. At such times she often fixes her eyes on him, moves her head, and vocalizes. The face is indeed a frequently offered stimulus to a baby. In the first six weeks a mnemonic trace of the human face must be laid down for later the infant follows the face as the first distal signal of the presence of the need-gratifier. His own face later becomes, as the mother's face is, a superb instrument for affective expression, complementing the vocal apparatus.

According to Gesell and Amatruda (1947) premature infants, at a foetal age of 30 weeks, react to the sound of a tinkling bell by active movements or by cessation of movement. Normally anyway such responses to sound can be demonstrated at birth. These primitive responses become differentiated. Before six months, emotionally expressive vocal tones will elicit smiling and cooing responses or anxious cries. Thus if a mother is playing and talking with her baby until he is smiling and cooing and then another person interrupts with a harsh angry voice from a distance, his facial expression will instantly change to that of anxiety and he will start crying. After six months, the hearing child moves his eyes in the direction of sound, apparently trying to locate its source, especially if the sounds are of a familiar voice or a bell he has heard before. At about one year the sounds of speech are to some extent differentiated, and the child responds differentially to words he has heard frequently in connection with his experiences of pleasure and pain (e.g., *mama, bottle, bye-bye*). According to Jakobson's analysis (see Cherry 1966) twelve features are sufficient to describe all the phonemes of all languages, and nine are enough for the forty phonemes of English. This analysis conveys some idea of the number of binary selections accomplished gradually by the child's brain in his comprehension of spoken words as this progresses while he himself is babbling, lalling, and blathering without much mastery of consonants. It is these consonants which to a large extent will refine the information he will later offer; the vowel sounds are much closer to the open resonances that convey the nonlinguistic emotional signals of animals.

The differential responses to common words indicate coordinations between sight and hearing, and soon coordinations between hearing and the child's own vocalization occur too. According to Jean Piaget (1952) these coordinations are not simple associations but are reciprocal assimilations of one schema by another, a *schema* in Piaget's terminology being a cognitive structure, having reference to a class of similar action sequences. The activation of one schema (hearing or vision) excites others. For example, the child assimilates aural activity to the schema of looking, and visual imagery to the schema of hearing. Or, in Piaget's phrasing, the child tries to listen to the object seen, and look at the sound which the object produces. J. H. Flavell (1963) writes:

The same is true for vocalisation and hearing, and even more obviously so. The infant certainly assimilates his own sounds to the schema of hearing; the sounds he makes stimulate listening activity and are in part controlled by the latter. And the reverse is also true. Young infants show a kind of primitive imitation or contagion phenomenon wherein external sounds tend to stimulate vocalisation, especially if the sound and vocalisation in question are similar. Thus as with vision and hearing, the child assimilates sounds heard to his own vocalisation schemas as well as assimilating vocalisation to hearing.

From his own observations and experiments Piaget has achieved a special conceptual framework regarding cognitive growth which comprises older theories of association and gestalt notions and which resonates with the inferences that psychoanalysts have drawn of primitive kinds of identification in early life.

The enormous enhancement of the perceptual basis of orientation which visual imagery comes to provide has been previously sketched (see especially Section V). This perceptual elaboration provides the material for concrete thought, and when this elaboration is extensive it in time provides a sure foundation for abstract thinking. It has also been noted that excessive visual dominance may, on the other hand, impair the development of mastery of sound symbolism and of abstract thinking. As Allport (1924) has pointed out, vivid visual imagery in the earlier years of mental development enables a vast elaboration as well as preservation of sensory data, enhancing the meanings of the surroundings of the child and allowing him to perfect his adaptive responses. It is not surprising that the congenitally blind child often shows slower development of language and thought than the sighted child. Surprising, perhaps, is the finding that his development of logical thought is so often retarded as compared with that of the deaf child (Piaget and Inhelder 1969).

Studies of the deaf

Since usually language is acquired largely through hearing, when there is a hearing loss from birth or in early childhood and this loss is extensive enough to render the child incapable of adequate auditory contact with the environment, there is then a considerable increment of difficulty in the development of verbal symbolic thought. The situation of the child requires a sustained effort by those in his entourage to exploit kinaesthetic, tactile, and visual senses in order to interest the child in speech. Manual communication, lip reading, showing pictures and describing them, and writing may all be employed at different times appropriately, but even so the acquisition of language usually remains a slow process for the deaf child. This slowness is a major impediment to substantial educational achievement. If, however, the child is four years old or older at the time of hearing loss, since language patterns have already been securely laid down in memory, there is much less impediment.

Rainer and Altshuler (in press), working in a program for the deaf in New York State, found a twenty-point difference in I.Q. on language-dependent tests in a comparison of discordant twins, one of each pair being deaf. Interviews with a cross section of the deaf adults in the state depicted a group of people who were making slow progress toward educational and vocational opportunity, but who had generally a poor preparation for family living and underachieving patterns both in school and in work.

In the operation of a pilot clinic for the deaf these authors made note of common character difficulties which they designate as a lack of empathy, a diminished understanding and regard for the feelings of other people, a lessened awareness of the impact of the deaf person's own behavior on other people, and a tendency to impulsive behavior with limited control and constraint. It is evident that a vastly diminished contact with talking individuals takes its toll. Adequate experience of emotional closeness which language exchange helps so much to build is in many deaf people lacking. As Rainer and Altshuler note, "The soundless world of the deaf is unconsciously equated by many persons with lifelessness and impenetrability, and sometimes with hopelessness regarding vital human contacts." Often the response of those in the entourage of the deaf person has been one of avoidance rather than the increase in attempts at communication required for optimal possible development.

We are also reminded of Wegener's view (1885) that the logical predicate, the novel assertion, that is, the key element of a sentence, requires verbal exposition when this is not implicit in the immediate physical context, in order to secure the listener's understanding and thus a more adequate response to the talker's desire. In speaking, the child learns to develop skills in verbal exposition in order to resolve ambiguities; this development, as much as it is dependent on advances in object-relatedness which are preverbal, no doubt encourages through its success the attitude of trying to understand the listener. The great amount of time in such verbal practice found to be worthwhile by the hearing child is replaced in the deaf child by greater amounts of time which necessarily achieve much less. Moreover, Wegener (1885) depicts not only the advancement of cognitive structures through verbal dialogue but ethical advancement too in response to the increasing implicit demand to make concessions to the listener in order to be understood. In this respect he anticipated Balkányi (1968), who has more recently pointed out the enhancement of the inner "sense of rules" through the gradual learning of language as a system of conventionally related conventional signs. The fact that not only does phonetic symbolism crucially develop the organization of the ego but it enhances the differentiation of conscience, and of the superego has already been discussed (p. 50) only to consider the amount of vocal control and constraint normally exercised by parents over their children to realize that without this additional experience it would be difficult to internalize self-control and restraint more adequately than on the simple basis of sphincter control, which is enjoined before or at the time when speech usually begins. Rainer and Altshuler write:

One corollary of the latter trait (impulsivity) is that rage lies close to the surface rather than becoming internalised and indeed little or no retarded depressive symptomatology was noted (in the deaf patients). Paranoid symptoms and projective mechanisms were seen, but were not universal and basically were no more prevalent than among hearing groups. Organised obsessional mechanisms were rare. The most prevalent diagnosis among non-psychotic adult patients was passive-aggressive personality disorder.

Altshuler (in press) in another article notes that both the one deaf and contestably manic-depressive depression patient and the one deaf obsessional neurotic patient alluded to by Rainer and Altshuler had virtually no speech but a good command of language, as was evident from their excellent manual communication. Altshuler (in press) notes, "it should be emphasized that language is the prerequisite for such structuralisation (embedding of internalised constraints), not necessarily oral words."

The teaching of oral language to the deaf is very time consuming and tedious. Notable success can be attained only in about one case in four, and is usually belated. The assimilation of word symbolism is what is crucial for intellectual development, the detours in thought, the endopsychic displacements, which may diminish direct impulsive acting out; and it is word symbol formation which, in development, provides the adequate embedding of internalized constraints. Yet some mothers have been indoctrinated with the importance of using only the voice with the deaf child, and of eschewing communication by any other means available to the mother and child.

In one case a deaf boy 10 years old was brought to psychiatric consultation by his mother following scenes of uncontrollable rage against his older sister and attempts to poison her by use of his photo-chemicals. A change was suggested from exclusive training in an oral (lip-reading) method to instruction in manual language (including natural and conventionalized signs and finger spelling) as well as written communication. This resulted gradually in a substantial clinical improvement. Moreover the boy in later years achieved considerable educational success. It must be added, however, that in this case the new special teacher was exceptionally skilled, dedicated, and enthusiastic.

Orientation, laterality and speech development

Finally, we have to take into account that remarkable development which causes one side of the body to function differently from the other so that the phenomena of hand preference, often of foot preference, and even of ear and eye preference emerge in various activities during childhood. Although not invariable, one of the most constant phenomena of human cerebral physiology, associated with this general development of laterality, is the gradual dominance of one cerebral hemisphere, usually the left, in relation to speech. In his diagram of the structure of the differentiated mental apparatus (Figure 2), Freud

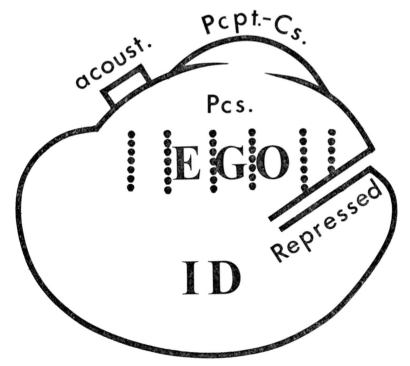

Figure 2. The differentiated mental apparatus as diagramed by Freud. Pcpt.-
Cs. = perceptual consciousness; Pcs. = preconscious; acoust. = special ac-
coustic sensory perceptual supply to Pcs. (Reprinted by permission from
The Complete Psychological Works of Sigmund Freud, ed. James Strachey,
XIX, 24, © 1961, by Hogarth Press and the Institute of Psychoanalysis.)

(1923) gave laterality appropriate expression. He added that the ego
wears a "cap of hearing" on one side—"It might," he wrote, "be said
to wear it awry."

Thus Freud embellished his sustained spatial metaphor of *the mental
apparatus* and emphasized his conclusion from the study of aphasia
(1891), namely, that verbal residues are primarily derived from auditory perceptions. In essence a word is centrally registered as a mnemic
residue of a word that has been *heard*, and this registration is eventually
unilateral in some of its features.*

It is certainly of interest in connection with the historical evolution
of scientific concepts of orientation that while Freud was investigating
aphasia, Breuer,† with whom Freud later collaborated in joint studies

---

* Secondarily, through reading there are visual components of word-presentations. There
are also, of course, important motor-sensory components which are auxiliary to the acoustic.
  † See Flugel, J. C. (1933).

of hysteria, was investigating the semicircular canals of the inner ear. He came to a theory of equilibrium (now attributed to him and Mach and Crum-Brown) on the basis of his discovery that changes in the position of the head cause, through inertia, currents in the endolymph, currents which bend the hairs on the ampullae of these canals and thus stimulate the passage of nerve impulses to centers in the brain. The three semicircular canals are placed roughly in the three planes of space and through the mechanism first investigated by Breuer make an important contribution to the orientation of the organism in space. Together with the effects of the otoliths in the respective utricles and saccules of the right and left labyrinths of the inner ears, the organism is partially enabled to achieve equilibrium reflexly. In concert with these reflexes, mediated through stimuli from the inner ear, are tonic muscular reflexes. All of these reflex activities in infancy underlie the development of an increasing awareness of orientation in the world developed in childhood. The asymmetric laterality of the body and of its functions gradually becomes more marked (by two years there is usually a clearly dominant hand) and aids in this orientation. Observation of the development of children's concepts of right and left clearly shows the association of the building of these concepts with increasing awareness of a differential, in sensations and skills, between the two sides of the body.

The study by L. S. Basser (1962) and by others quoted in his important article of hemiplegia of early onset in infancy and in childhood and of the effects of hemispherectomy indicates that one-sided cerebral dominance for speech usually develops in the following way: initially both cerebral hemispheres participate in subserving early speech development, and subsequently there is lateralization, most commonly left-sided, though sometimes right-sided. The evidence is primarily based on the relatively high incidence of speech impairment following right hemisphere lesions in children as compared with adults. Freud (1897) remarked upon the delay in the age of onset of speech in infantile hemiplegics, and it was later maintained that such delay and associated persistent defects were more marked in cases with left hemisphere lesions (Taylor 1905, Wallin 1949, Dunsdon 1952). When there is a unilateral cerebral lesion following the acquisition of speech but still early in life, the resulting speech disturbance is vastly different from that found in adults with unilateral cerebral disease. Sarah J. McNutt (1885) described a boy aged three years when he developed right hemiplegia and lost all speech. Six weeks after the catastrophe the child commenced to say single words "and then he had to be taught as when he commenced to talk." Freud (1897) remarked on the restricted vocabulary in such instances and on the transient nature of the disturbance. E.

Guttmann (1942) stated that "the clinical picture is uniformly that of diminished speech production, with dysarthria and telegraphic style in the recovery period," and he noted that recovery was often surprisingly rapid. Both Freud and Guttmann remarked that in early childhood the disturbance in speech occurred commonly also with lesions of the right hemisphere.

Such clinical studies provide convergent evidence that the outlook for recovery from aphasia is better the earlier its onset. In regard to this question of recoverability E. H. Lenneberg (1967) writes:

The chance for recovery has a natural history. This natural history is the same as the natural history of cerebral lateralisation of function.* Aphasia is the result of direct, structural and local interference with neurophysiological processes of language. In childhood such interference cannot be permanent because the two sides are not yet sufficiently specialised for function, even though the left hemisphere may already show signs of speech dominance. Damage to it will interfere with language; but the right hemisphere is *still* involved to some extent with language, and so there is a potential for language function that may be strengthened again. In the absence of pathology, a polarisation of function between right and left takes place during childhood, displacing language entirely to the left and certain other functions predominantly to the right.

As for those functions, primary among them is the ordering of spatial orientation which is to a large extent in right-sided people subserved by the right cerebral hemisphere.

Of course there is not only hemisphere difference but hemisphere interaction, as well as interaction between the hemispheres and other parts of the brain, so that we must beware of too simple views of localization of cortical functions. Nonetheless the development of lateralization of the cortical basis of more advanced speech function and, on the other hand, of more primitive orientation is sufficiently indicated by clinical studies. The possible biological significance of lateralization is a gain in adaptation beyond the gains already offered by deepening sulci among the convolutions to afford more room for cortical cells within the limits of the cranium, itself comparatively large. Specialization on both sides of the brain obviates the necessity of complete bilateral representation and avoids the redundancy evident in such organs as the kidneys. It became a factor advancing human development beyond that of the other primates. It is possible that cerebral laterality set the stage phylogenetically for an enhancement of the level of metaphoric symbolic achievement so important for evolved word language. Our orientation in our lifespace and in the cosmos is thus so much more finely

* Usually this process is completed by puberty.

achieved. On the other hand, the more concrete basis of spatial orienta-tion is safeguarded in the other hemisphere, and it is in the adequate interaction of the hemispheres that language bountifully flowers. In this connection it is noteworthy that Wegener shows that full-fledged word language depends on metaphor and on emendation, and the latter is particularly dependent on an orderly arrangement of the elements of speech in time.

X Conclusion

PHONETIC symbolic representation is an achievement which has a long phylogenetic history, though it takes a healthy infant only about 18 months to utter words like those uttered around him. It is, of course, by progressive increase in size and complexity of the brain that the primates emerge from among the mammalia and that man in turn transcends other primates. The power of phonetic symbolic representation with its special brain basis was somehow acquired by our primate ancestors, differentiating them as linguistic primates. Wegener suggests that two further principles of linguistic development, *emendation* and *metaphor*, followed that first step. We have tried to show how remarkably well an understanding of these principles clarifies some important clinical problems. It is evident, for example, that Kraepelin's categories of agrammatic disturbance and acataphasia in schizophrenic speech relate to these principles, and that both faulty emendation and disordered metaphoric symbolism contribute to semantic speech disfigurement in schizophrenia.

As we have also suggested, the original use of language in naming, fixing, and conceiving objects even away from immediate perception develops on a deep expressive level. This is a level which may sometimes be overlooked in the study of the definitively communicative use of words between individuals, especially because each child in his development is enveloped by, and interacts with, a purveyed language with its own social history. Wegener's principles of emendation and metaphor apply to both the individual and the sociohistorical development of language. We have indicated that the complex processes involved in the growth of the metaphor itself are rooted in a primitive symbolism to which Freud called attention; these roots of metaphor are uncovered sometimes in the ravages of disease. We thus learn that metaphor is an extension of primitive symbolism ultimately based on psychic representations of the forms and functions of the human body. Figure 1, page 22, attempts to take these relations into account.

It is beyond the scope of this book to evaluate upheavals in the current scene in terms of social pathology. However, when we understand how the sick individual, as exemplified in hysterical neurosis or in schizophrenic psychosis, departs from patterns of speech which Wegener shows to have been so neatly and so finely evolved for our use, it is tempting to speculate whether present problems in communication reflect more than the jamming of the airwaves and the oppressive immediacy of millions speaking at once.

Certain abbreviations of linguistic expression have in the past arisen from necessity, and inventive vernacular has frequently made the daily exchange more sprightly, even serving a warm social purpose in recognizing the vagaries of the common lot. Many healthy people, eagerly leading full lives, have managed handily to invest a mediocre speech with a highly adequate emotional particularity. Many well-educated persons continue to have reading understanding considerably more sophisticated than their speech, and leave the better part of a technical or professional verbal competence behind them when they leave the office.

Casually ordered ways of communicating can, however, only confuse in the absence of commonly perceived experience and shared anticipations. The vociferous rebels reject the very idea of a shared humanity on any all-inclusive scale and deny, in a schizoid way, that even—or most especially—the blood-tied members of the same household live within their own gestalt. Across the "generation gap" they cry "Hear us!" Across the "credibility gap" they jeer "Tell it like it is!" Uniquely able, in the physical sense, to disseminate words, they use language to separate themselves from those with longer memories, instead of using it for the traditional outreach of self to other.

On the other hand, as recent political campaigns with their accompanying propaganda of agitation have highlighted, words may become excessively persuasive definitions, narrowing their connotations and skewing denotation in the direction of evil. The word *permissiveness*, for example, no longer has a measure of precision shared by contending groups. To some it seems to mean "unpatriotic"—even to indicate the cause of unemployment or inflation. Yet, as a recent issue of *The New Yorker* (46:39:43-44) noted, many twist the word to show that it is being "permissive" to spend large sums of money on education, hospitals, and environmental protection, while it is not being "permissive" to spend them on military hardware of any kind.

Wegener patiently follows the finely dividing growth of human language, which continued through the years to branch from the large vessels of gross and general meaning to the capillaries of specific reference. Although at present countless new words are being added to the vocabularies of most languages—and even being exchanged among them —we hear over and over the special vocabulary of scorn and rebellion and see enormous public excitement being evoked by portmanteau slogans whose meaning depends more on the urgency and frequency of utterance than on any rational process of understanding.

Some who are most vocal today have little use for the shades of time discrimination so painstakingly developed. In the narcissistic "now" world, any present effort designed to bring delayed benefit is "irrelevant." Anything scorned is "sterile," although the ways in which it might be supposed to fructify remain mysterious.

Metonymy, metaphor, synecdoche, and all the other classic figures of speech continue to appear, and might encourage us to believe that language is still growing; however, they are not only "faded" but stretched badly out of shape, covering all sorts of lumpy puzzles. Confusion grows when we are admonished to "love" by people with faces full of malice and voices full of scorn. Their stereotypes fail to "chime" with what has gone before; they weaken the magic of "taming" a passion by naming it, or of awakening an aspiration by a noble word that might pierce the heart.

It is no longer only the mental patient who abandons those repressions which used to weave in and out of human communication, making it an artifact designed to reveal, conceal, and influence. Four-letter Anglo-Saxon words make a clear statement about our common humanity in its physical aspect but paradoxically speak louder of bondage than they do of freedom, in a world apparently putting so high a premium on individuation and "doing one's own thing." Further, they mask many variations of personal response which might be profitably communicated. The "Pygmalion" concept of language is anathema to an egalitarian society; nevertheless, persistence of an individual style of speech, with informatively balanced areas of reticence and disclosure, might contribute to the solution of the ubiquitous "crisis of identity."

Wegener wrote his history of language in a quieter day. One is obliged to wonder whether, like the other arts of man, language will take new directions rather than continuing to branch into ever greater specificity and refinement. Today, immediate sensory impact is favored over an elegant presentation for the gratification of mind and sense; perhaps this is consistent with the new technology. New directions need not be suspect, yet it may be possible to find a key with which to interpret the language of today's crowds by looking at patterns of language deviation in the mental illness of an individual.

THE LIFE OF SPEECH

Dr. Philipp Wegener

Translated from the German *Untersuchungen
ueber die Grundfragen des Sprachlebens*
(Halle: Max Niemayer, 1885)

Foreword

THE following studies are based upon two lectures given by the author at two conventions of philologists in Magdeburg (Autumn, 1883) and in Halberstadt (Spring, 1884). More comprehensive reports on the first of these lectures are contained in *Die Berliner Zeitschrift fuer Gymnasialwesen* [*The Berlin Journal for Secondary Schools*] (1884) and in the *Jahrbuecher fuer Philologie und Paedagogik* [*Annual Chronicles for Philology and Pedagogy*] of the same year. The content and scope of both papers, especially of the second, have been enlarged and deepened.

In both cases the content has been retained. The order, arrangement, selection, and limitation of the material has also remained the same. Had the author had at his disposal the necessary quiet and leisure, he would have attempted a systematic treatment of those areas mentioned, as well as of some related ones. But, under the present circumstances, he had to be satisfied with this loose form of investigation and relinquish a systematic arrangement until more propitious days appeared or his energies were less engaged.

PHILIPP WEGENER

Magdeburg, May 4, 1885

Contents

On the Life of Speech

I

I HAVE called the field from which I intend to present a few research results, the life of speech. This is a common expression which metaphorically describes language as a living organism—such as a plant. This is why one also speaks of the growth of language. The science of this life could be called the biology of language. Naturally that expression is a figure of speech, a metaphor with which one must not forget that language is not a being or an organism possessing spatial autonomy as is, for instance, self-determining man. Rather, it is a collective name, indeed an abstraction, for certain muscular movements of man which are connected with a definite sense for many persons of a social group; in psychological terms, which are associated by them with definite imagery. All this forms only a part of the entire psychical and physical life expression of man, a part which stands in closest connection and most active interrelation with the other processes in the human organism.

The physical muscular movements drive air streams out of the compressed lungs, modulate these through the changing positions of the vocal chords, the tongue, the teeth, the lips, and the uvula which locks the nose channel. The modified air streams become audible to the speaker as well as to other persons and call into the hearer's consciousness essentially the same sense which the speaker has connected with the muscular movements and the corresponding acoustic images.

Thus the word *language* is the abstract summary of all these human activities, which, characteristically, have two aspects, the physiological and the psychological. A division between their combined effect and the areas of each aspect or principle has been attempted (as Osthoff did in his report on the physiological and psychological principles in language); yet so far, in my opinion, such a division has been unsuccessful. Certainly, with regard to their origins, those cases of progressive assimilation (like the German umlaut, the German refraction, and the effects of the Greek *y* on preceding sounds) must not be considered as belonging only to the physiological manifestations of language. They belong to the psychological area. Furthermore, like the pianist's movement of fingers and hand or the technical movement of the woodcarver, potter and scribe, the production of the learned sounds in a man's mouth must not be attributed to purely physiological activities. What is often called physiological here is nothing more than an original spontaneous movement that has *become* mechanical or automatic. The physiological in this matter is only the nature of the organs, their position, and their form of movement. In contrast, the impulse and regulation of the movement of the organs has something to do with sound physiology only insofar as the nature of the organs opposes the intention of man with certain difficulties and inhibitions. The way in which complicated sound movements are produced is indeed to be judged exactly the same way in which the above mentioned technical movements develop; similarly with walking, running, dancing, and so on. If, on the grounds of mechanization, something should be said about the validity, invariability, and irrevocability of the sound laws, that is, the changes which occur during the course of time in the pronunciation of the sounds within greater sound series, then one cannot merely refer to the fact that one deals with a physical law. One also has to be aware at all times that one is in the area of automatic, mechanized, psychological processes. Everything remains to be done especially with regard to research in this psychical area. The second treatise will return to this subject for other questions concerning the life of speech.

So much, however, is clear: that the physiological as well as the psychological processes have to be viewed and examined in the observation of language itself.

The physiological conditions of speaking have been examined with care and some success in sound physiology, or phonetics, which has naturally taken living man as the object of examination. It seems certain to me that even this science is still in its beginnings. It obviously still separates the sound processes too much according to the sounds that have been dealt with in the old grammar. Since those were evidently very complicated systems, one wonders whether the media* is to be defined as a voiced plosive or as a lenis. Obviously the sounding, that is, the contraction of the glottis, is an articulation in itself, which can take place at the tenuis just as well. The sounding of the glottis could be defined very well as a kind of vowel, which continues at the locking of the soundbox, during the locking, and at the opening of it. Indeed, this pure sound can be found syllable-forming, while the locking is being produced (in Low German—at least west of Magdeburg—in proclitic forms *op mik, et iss, ik bin*). I have spelled the vowels in the pausa-form rather than in the mere sound, which is naturally not very exact. The contraction of the glottis must naturally slow down the expiration before the media as well as before the tenuis.

---

* *Editor's note:* In phonetics, the *mediae* are voiced stops (b, d, g) intermediate between the *tenues* (p, t, k) and the *aspirates* (ph, th, ch).

There remains much to be done for the sound physiology in its application to the history of language; indeed, it would be more appropriate to give this task to the history of language. Thus one can assume with certainty that sound changes occurred on account of a continuum of organ displacement from one point in a certain direction, until the historically confirmed place was reached; for example, with the transition of *s* to *r*. The knowledge of the starting point, the stages of this organ movement, and the end point belong to the complete understanding of such a transition.

The sound-physiological observation of the history of language has yet to discover the articulation of how *s* could become *r*. The transition happened in Latin and German, when *s* becomes voiced. The newly developed *r* had to be a tongue *r*, which could be formed on the alveoli or in front on the hard palate. The *s* sound, which arises at this articulation without vibration of the tip of the tongue, is not the so-called pure *s*, but *š*. From this observation follows the correct consideration for Latin, Greek, and German: whether the graphic sign *s* really was the so-called pure *s*-sound, or whether it was just in the place of *š*. The same transition from *š* to *s* is proved by the French *raison* from *rationem*. When *tj* became *t* with a hissing sound, then this could be no other than *ts*, as the Italian *ci*, is articulated *ce*. The same fact is to be considered for the Greek ζ meaning *dš*, e.g. in νομίζω (to own as settled, to deem, to suppose), for Greek ττ or σσ, thus πράττω (to do, act) was at least at a certain time pronounced like *pratso*. When in Greek σ becomes *h* between vowels, that is, voiced σ, then the tongue must be a little more distant from the palate. With this distance, a narrow space appears, which gives not the so-called pure *s* but *š*.

The knowledge of the psychological processes is still obscure, despite the excellent book by H. Paul, *Principles of the History of Language*, Halle, 1880.

The valuable articles of Steinthal and Lazarus also must be mentioned, as well as those of Whitney, who has judged many things in his sober manner. The slow advancement of this knowledge may be explained in two ways: First, the well-deserved discredit which the logical treatment of language has inflicted upon itself by regressing to the grossest empiricism; second, the one-sided inclination of modern language research to fix statistically the transmitted material of lost language epochs, or to consider only old language steps as worthy areas of research. With regard to the flaws of modern language research, a healthier direction can be noted in the work of the younger scholars of German. The physiological appearances can become clear only in the observation of living speech and, indeed, of the speech of the person himself. In becoming conscious of what we do daily, the living native language, which is understandable to the speaker in its finest subtleties, must also form the foundation and the orientation area of all psychological observations. Only these investigations can yield reliable speech laws from which we can, perhaps, draw significant conclusions about dead languages.

As the physiologist would not study or base his examinations on old Egyptian mummies or on petrifacts, but on the living body of animal or man, so we must learn to know the laws of the life and growth of language from the most apparent speech patterns of the living native language. From this perspective we may be able to interpret and understand the large rubble heap of materials transmitted from the dead languages.

II

THE distinct sets of sound which we call words, alone and in their connection or association with a definite meaning—that is, with a complex—must be learned, because the same set of sounds means something completely different in different languages. Thus LG *ssett*, meaning *sit*, is phonetically equivalent to the French *sept*, meaning *seven*. The accomplished speaker may therefore be compared with a skilled pianist who needs only to see a note, a complete chord, a complete measure or more on the music sheet in order to strike without thinking the appropriate keys on the piano. The accomplished speaker needs only to see a house or tree, to observe an action, to recall it without observation, or simply to feel a desire and, without conscious deliberation of the particular factors involved, he finds the suitable word and the logical sentence.

Indeed, it is actually impossible for the accomplished speaker to become conscious of the single impulses by which the muscles are stimulated to speech movement. It is equally difficult to be aware of the particular muscle processes themselves, or of the way in which this physiological activity is connected with the complexes in his mind. The same unconscious obscurity prevails in this case as in other mechanical processes of the body.

All of these movements are learned by man at a time in his life when everything is still veiled in unconscious darkness. It is even difficult to become conscious of single effects of these movements, for example, that the lips are rounded for the *u* sound, that we open the nasal canal for nasals, or whether we speak *r* with the uvula or in an alveolated position with the teeth. Certainly orthographic teachings demonstrate the difficulty of analyzing words by their sounds. Thus, the entire learning of the mother tongue, fully in the first years of life and also for the greater part of life in the later years, takes place in the obscurity of the unconscious. One no doubt perceives what a mistake in method it is to explain language phenomena as the distinctly reflective design of the speaker.

Of course, in the unconscious learning of language, it is possible that, at later stages of childhood, the adult comes to help correct the imperfect speaking of the child. But what means are used by the naive man, completely uneducated in phonetic physiology? He says to the child: "you must not say *l* but *r*, not *a* but *o*, etc. . . . ." Consequently, he does not give guidance as to the correct use of the organs: rather, he brings the child to awareness of the correct phonetic image. He works on the unconscious, nevertheless correct, supposition that all phonetic movements of the child consist of the imitation of such phonetic or sound images. Therefore, generally speaking, the child's learning of language consists of the following processes:

1. Sound or phonetic images are perceived. The muscles try to imitate them. Success comes gradually in reproducing the sounds of the original images.

2. These separate phonetic images, which are ultimately heard and reproduced, are perceived under two conditions: (a) when the child has certain sensations of pain, such as hunger or thirst; (b) when the child has certain optical sensations stimulated. Simultaneously with these sensations, or, more correctly, as a direct consequence, these phonetic images enter into the mind—that is, shortly after or before—and they form with them chronologically connected sets of ideas. The more frequently these sets appear in the mind, the stronger and more indestructible they become, and the more firmly the separate members of this set unite with each other.

Indeed, man never receives simply sensations of light or sound. Always directly connected with these are sensations of touch or pressure, conveyed by the finely organized nerve tissue of the fingertips or by other coarser and more callous parts of the epidermis, which are excited by the pressure of the position and attitude of the body. Added to these are the continuous sensations which the completion of metabolism entails. When the child hears the phonic image *milk*, he does so according to the described psychological conditions. He will often hear this word in association with the painful sensations of hunger and thirst. He will relate this word to the light sensations of the white fluid in the shiny bottle. He will finger the smooth, solid, heated bottle. He will suck and lose the discomfort of hunger. Very often this sensational course repeats itself with the words *milk*, *bottle*, and so on. According to the psychological rule, like images unite and reinforce each other and unlike images obstruct each other: that which as a complex is continually the same becomes permanently and indestructibly associated with the phonic image *milk*. Complexes formed in such a manner are called the meaning or sense of the phonic image, that is of the word.

Complexes, the phonic image and meaning which are associated with each other, can reciprocally recall one another. If the phonic image *milk* is heard, its meaning is recalled. Conversely, the recollection of meaning produces the phonic image. The phonic image is associated, through frequent utterance, with the sensations of muscle movements, which must necessarily take place with articulation of the word. Therefore, the muscle sensation is also associated, and the muscle movement which this sound image vocally generates is itself produced.

The words which children first learn are articulated very imperfectly. Sounds are not completely equivalent to those of the adult. Words, that is, sets of sounds, are incomplete. The reason for the latter phenomenon is threefold. First, certain sounds are particularly difficult to imitate, such as the *l* and *r* sounds. Very often in the first years children do not succeed in finding the appropriate muscle movements for these sounds, and hence they remain unarticulated. Second, not all parts of a word are exhaled with the same amount of energy by the accomplished speaker. One distinguishes between strongly and weakly stressed syllables, and these once again in various degrees. In sentences the stress relationship becomes more complex, since a gradation of the single words takes place before and after the stressed word. Certain words become unstressed, such as the enclitics and proclitics. The more weakly stressed syllables and words follow a familiar psychological law, *Weber's Law*: sensations increase like logarithms, when the stimuli increase like numbers.* Thus the sensations which the child receives when listening to the more weakly stressed syllables must be weaker in the given circumstances than the sensations received from the strongly stressed syllables. Hence, in the first years of the child's language, one finds the stressed syllables of the badly pronounced words relatively more correctly and precisely reproduced than the unstressed syllables. Finally, one often finds in children's speech the exchanging of sounds. I remember hearing from a child of about four years the sentence *sonne mân von dinne wette füttn* instead of *soll ich mal von diesen welche pflücken* [shall I pluck some of these]. Evidently the *l* sound was difficult for the child, and for that reason it was replaced by *n*, or left out in the difficult combination with

* Compare Wundt's *Lectures on the Mind of Man and Animal*. Volume I, page 108f.

f. The *k* sound was replaced by *t.* It is clear that the muscle sensation had coincided for the *k* and *t* sound in the mind of the child. A similarity of the acoustical sensation in association with this sound is certainly obvious, just as with *n* and *l.* Hence it follows, as with a set of other data, that the separate sounds can enter the mind by association because of the similarity of the acoustical sensation and muscle sensation. Similar sounds will be sensed and united as partially alike, or, through inexact observation, as completely alike. Such incorrect fusions of different sounds must be unraveled in the further development of the child's speech.

III

THE child does not hear merely single words. He hears most words in the context of a sentence. Nevertheless, unaided, he utters at first only single words. Thus the words he uses in the early stages of his speech development are first released from larger groups, the sentences. This process has already been described as unconscious abstraction, whereby like images unite and reinforce each other, while unlike ones obstruct each other. However, it still remains unclear why all words used with equal frequency will not be used simultaneously in the first stage of speech. The number of words actually used is very small. Among the words accumulated in the child's mind by that process of abstraction, there must therefore exist a difference between the psychic efficacy and intensity.

Such a difference is produced in two ways. First, the words of the same sentence have different stress strengths. Therefore, the sensations of the listening child must also be of different strength and must cause, as by the differently stressed syllables of the same word, a varying precision in their imitation and application. Since the stressed words are the most important components of the sense of the sentence, precisely because of their special strength, the child will first of all know and learn to use the words most important for his needs and his conceptual world. The observation leads to the second point of view by which the store of applicable words of the child is determined. The most important words are those associated with the appeasement of the strivings and needs of man, in this case, of the child. Words which are regularly associated with a strong sensation of pleasure or discomfort have an excessively

larger strength of sensation than other words. It is, therefore, the words
which, in the child's mind, are linked with sensations of pleasure or discomfort that far surpass other words in their strength of sensation and
their ability to be reproduced.

The psychological law expressed here is so well-known for its effects
that I need only think of days of joy or sorrow. We say that for us they
will be unforgettable. In accordance with this law, the child is soon in
the position to use word designations for his conditions of need and
striving. The earliest words of the child are therefore words like *Mommy*
[Mama], *bottle* [Fläschchen], *milk* [Milch], *Nana* [Babá], *light* [Kucke-
licht], *tick tock* [Ticktack], *doll* [Puppe], *up you go* (*onto my arm*),
[Oppa], and so on.

IV

A N IMPORTANT stage of the child's development begins during
his first two years, when he no longer simply cries out in discomfort, but also calls *Mommy* [Mama], *bottle* [Fläschchen], or similar
words. These words are firmly incorporated in his mind in the set of
sensations or pain—for example, the sensation of hunger until it is ap-
peased. And, what is more, the word enters this set at that position when
the sensation of pain is relieved. On the one hand, it is closely associated
with the sensation of discomfort; on the other, it is also associated with
the subsequent sensation of pleasure. In addition to this, we observe that
the production of this sound tends to eliminate existing sensations of discomfort, because the mother responds to the child's call and best knows
how to comfort him. The word, therefore, becomes a help or a means of
eliminating an existing sensation of discomfort.

This help will be employed when a sensation of pain is present; the
sensation of pain produces the reflex action of crying. The word thus
uttered during the crying is the means of demanding relief from the
pain. The child is, at the same time, trained by the parents. One tries at
every opportunity to break him of the habit. Although this training is
almost always successful, that is, the outbreak of crying will be suppressed, nevertheless, the crying muscles are regulated by pain. Even
when the crying is suppressed, therefore, one hears a whining sound.
This sound will be more and more relaxed in later life, but an echo
remains in the adult who knows how to control himself. I point out that

here an ethical factor enters into the development of speech and into the pattern of sound formation.

Thus the word which the child tearfully or whiningly speaks is a means of eliminating the sensation of discomfort for him. Yet for the listener and, above all, for the mother, it is a summons to bring help. This word is the imperative of the child, which no one misunderstands. However, the reason that this form of expression will be understood by the listener as an imperative is an ethical one, the feeling of obligation to help the needy or suffering, the feeling of sympathy. Later we will look into this point more closely.

In that this manner of the child's expression establishes a sensation of pain, it is an expression of the present. And if one remains indifferent during this expression of pain, if the listener remains merely an observer, then he will not sense the summons for help; he will not be hearing an imperative, but rather the simple fact that the child is sensing pain.

The doctor will face the suffering child in a manner similar to that of the physiologist facing the convulsions of a dog or rabbit. It should be evident by now that it is not the form of expression as such, but rather the way in which it is related to the mind of the listener which is decisive for the meaning and content of the words. But when pain indicates, by the use of a word, a means for its relief, this manner of expression becomes an expression of the future. The child shows simply the present when he cries out in pain or shouts with delight upon viewing a light or a shiny object, or in the joy of playing. When a change has taken place with these things, or when the child comes across these things unexpectedly, the exultant *light* [Kuckelicht], *tick tock* [Ticktack] or the astonished *my car* [mein Wagen], *my doll* [meine Puppe] are pure expressions of the present. However, if the child reaches for the lamp and can't grasp it, he experiences the painful sensation of obstructed striving and disappointed expectation. Now the whining sound *light* [Kuckelicht] is a pure expression of striving. The time which has control in the mind of the child and is revealed to the listener is the future. Similarly, when the child seeks an object but doesn't find it, he cries, perhaps, *my car* [mein Wagen], an expression which could be interpreted as an imperative, as a question, or as a pure expression of striving.

If the child has knocked against something, he runs crying to his mother, and tearfully or whiningly he calls *bump* [stossen], *door* [Thür], *stone* [Stein]; the mother concludes with certainty that the child has bruised himself. If the child has seen the lamp, he runs to his mother and calls *light* [Kuckelicht], and she knows that the child has seen the lamp. We have here the meaning of the present perfect tense, which reports the completion of an action and its continuation in the present. The precision of meaning of this tense becomes clear only in man's emotional life, where the action lingers on in the speaker as sensations of pleasure or pain.

If the father comes to a family scene after the passage of some time, and the child tells him *bump* with no traces of pain, with indifference, or even with cheerfulness, then the effects and continuation of the painful feelings have disappeared, the action is pure aorist. It is the same with sensations of pleasure. The fact itself lives on in memory, but joy and pain are now only faint points of the awareness, no longer living sensations. The grammatically skilled form of the aorist, not that of the perfect is, therefore, the correct tense for the cold recollection of the experience. This is the so-called aorist *gromicus* or *empiricus*.

Things exist for us only through our sensations of them. The first instances of which man becomes conscious are those which involve sensations of pleasure and pain. The faded, feelingless recollection of these give the most important components for the psychic stance which we call objective. Consequently, man does not need a vocal naming of the forms of being at that first stage of emotional speech. The forms of expression of being are the reflex motions, which the sensations bring forth in the voice organs of man.

Thus it may be proved that the child uses the word as a sentence. Indeed, these sentences exhibit the same temporal nuances which trained speech displays: present, future, perfect, and aorist (the form of desire, however, not the imperfect). The child intends the sentence in this temporal sense, as soon as he notices that it will be so understood. Thereby, the form of the sound becomes the means, the form of expression, and the mother actually understands the child so. Hence the child speaks a real and coherent sentence. All of these sentences, with the occasional exception of the pure aorist sentence, are accompanied by some kind of emotional excitement.

V

THE same word could be used for the various sentence forms and the various tenses.

It is thus not the word as such, not the body of the word alone which builds the sentence. Along with this is the tone or the manner of delivery, the *actio*, as the Roman rhetoricians called it, which is a second important element of this word-sentence. We have spoken of the crying or whining tone, by which the mother recognizes the intensity of the pain or the joy and desires of the child. The word is, for the listener, the explanation or illustration of the outbreak of feeling, in that it indicates the sphere of feelings, its object, or the aim of its desire.

Understanding of the subject, that is, of the person or thing about which the predicate is concerned, is not to be found in the word. Rather, it will be first indicated in the accompanying tone that it is the child which is happy, feels pain, or is filled with astonishment. Secondly, the apprehension of the subject will be gained by the unconscious, general assumption of the mother that the child is concerned only with his own sensations of pain or pleasure. Only with the intellectual advancement of the child, drawing the conclusion from his own utterances that other persons too have feelings, and only with the ethical advancement in sympathizing with others' utterances of feelings, only then will the child have risen above this stage of one-sided, elementary egotism.

Furthermore, the accomplished speaker, by controlling the tone, can make every word a command, or in grammatical terms, can make every word enter the imperative mood: *bread* [Brot], *cake* [Kuchen], *eat* [essen], *drink* [trinken], *away* [fort], *to/with me* [mir], *come here* [her, hierher, hier], *right now* [auf der Stelle], *more* [mehr], *something else* [was andres], *something more* [noch etwas], *forward* [vorwärts], *now* [nun], *quickly* [schnell], and so forth. This means of expression, so often used by children with a crying or whining tone—for example: *roll* [Butterbrot], *apple* [Apfel], *my hat* [mein Hut], *my boots* [meine Stiefeln] is under the circumstances not taken amiss. However, later in life it is considered ill-bred, and we forbid this form of request, since it does not respect the will and free initiative of the person addressed. But it is not the enunciation of the single word or phrase as such which will be tabooed. The supplicatory *a small piece of bread* [ein Stückchen Brot] of the beggar is, because of the submissiveness of tone, completely unassailable. This tone acknowledges the right and possibility that the request will be refused. With this tone the phrase enters the mood of supplication.

So it is shown what a mighty lever for communication the tone of delivery is. Its nuances and modifications are extraordinarily diverse. They are determined (1) by the order or sequence and distance of the musical tones, thus the melody of the sentence; (2) by the intensity, the form, and the tempo with which the airstream comes out of the lungs; and (3) by the position of the organs, how they are created by certain reflex movements, especially crying and laughing, and equally by the ethical reaction against these reflex movements, such as the swallowing of tears, the suppression of laughter, the restraint of the airstream with moaning.

Alongside the tone is the eloquent speech of the eye, the countenance and the gesture. The expression of feeling is really only a further continuation of the reflexes which modulate the tone of speech, and the arm and hand motions also.

The melody of the sentence and the reflexes differentiate the quality of the pain and pleasure sensations to be expressed, and thereby further the quality of the form of communication, order, request and wish, astonishment and question, assertion. The intensity and form of expiration modulates the degree of the passion or the feeling, such as the loud tone of voice, the haste, the stillness, the indolence with which it is spoken, and so forth. Naturally the three factors enumerated above always appear allied with each other in a sentence.

The lecturer, speaker, and actor know, at least unconsciously, the extraordinary diversity of the nuances in the human voice. Their success before the public is determined to a large degree by the correct choice and use of these means of tone. I can only advance a few cases of this modulation here, since no special research has yet been completed. With certainty we differentiate a flattering tone of the voice by moderate, retarded pressure of the muscles upon the lungs and a sentence melody which falls significantly after a high tone and rises again at the end. This tone in the sentence melody agrees with that of the question and statement of astonishment. It is differentiated, however, in the form and energy of the expiration. If a command is sung to this melody, the question will still be understood in the words beyond the summons, whether or not the person to whom it is addressed will comply with the request. This is the tone that we require of a well-bred child for a request, because we find in this tone the necessary respect for the self-will of the individual of whom something is requested. If we meet this tone in an assertive sentence of the accomplished speaker, we feel thereby the acknowledgement of the dignity of the addressed person, and consideration for him. From now on, the tone will be perceived by us as obligatory.

There is a great need in the science of speech for the study and exact statistical arrangement of these modulations. What has already been stated can be used to demonstrate what radical significance the fundamental ethical views of man have for the understanding of modulations of tone, both as a means of linguistic expression and for the application and working out of these means. Those forms of expression receive their conceptual content only with the recognition of an equal organization of humans, that is, with the desirability to work on the wills of others only with the acknowledgement of moral duties, to sympathize with the sufferer, and to help him. Methodical comparative philology here draws attention to one perspective of the comprehension of the human soul, which lies far above the sphere of the knowledge of languages in the usual sense.

The tone, first of all, provides the key for the understanding of words and sentences, and not only in the language of children. When we say in a shop or restaurant *may I please have the menu* [ich bitte um die Speisekarte], or one thing or another, the request will mostly be expressed with a certainty of tone, which no longer leaves any question as to whether it is convenient for the waiter, host, or salesman to give us what has been requested. The form is also similar to that which the more authoritative person uses with a subordinate. The superior says to his inferior *may I please have the papers finished within a week* [ich bitte die Acten in acht Tagen fertig zu stellen]. In spite of the linguistic form of the request, the tone tells us that we are dealing with a strict order. Evidently at one time the same ethical considerations prevailed as those mentioned in connection with the brusque demands and orders of the child. Thus, in business and official intercourse one wants to considerately and politely respect the free individuality of the other person. But as soon as the tone of the linguistic request becomes imperative, the word expression becomes an empty form, by which mainly an incongruity with the content is felt. This feeling ultimately disappears, however, and content and form appear harmonious. It is only when the form of rhetorical feeling is imprinted, that the request form is a finer or more noble form of expression for the command, as the language of intercourse of the higher society requires. We probably have a similar occurrence in the Latin prohibitive of the classic time, when the language of intercourse of the higher stations had tabooed the imperative and had replaced it with the perfect conjunctive of wish, or with the *noli cave*. Both the latter phrases express the prevention of an action, not in the interest of the speaker, but rather, in the interest of the addressed.

VI

AN ANNOUNCEMENT in the paper or an oral proclamation states *The Concordia Club is celebrating its Founder's Day on June 7, in the Club Meeting Hall in Berlin*. A young member of this club hears or reads the notice and calls cheerfully over to his friends *Founder's Day celebration at the Club Meeting Hall*. The members understand the young man or the young lady. Of course, they don't know of any other anniversary about which the young man could be interested. They know the day of the celebration and the city. Why then has the committee of the club issued an extensive notice when the young man's was shorter?

The newspaper in which the communication was made public addresses itself to many readers, including many who are not members of the Concordia, or who perhaps know nothing at all about this club. Furthermore, there are many other clubs besides the Concordia. The first words, therefore, serve to indicate to those addressed by the notice that it applies to them. The members perceive that a club notice has been made for them—concerning contributions, or a social evening? —no, concerning the anniversary festival, whose celebration on the seventh of June must be impressed on the forgetful. Now, what has actually been communicated? Hardly the anniversary festival and its celebration, rather, the place where it will be held, the hall of the club.

Everything, aside from the naming of the place, is completely uninteresting to the members. The rest serves only to make the central point comprehensible—comprehensible also for nonmembers, but for them the central point of the notice will hardly be interesting. Thus, the declarations, aside from the naming of the place, are like the exposition of a novel or drama, or as the relation of an anecdote is only preparation for the point. The central point of the notice is declared following that which was expressed as introduction and orientation, as in the following example: *The house on Wilhelm Street is finished* [das Hause in der Wilhelmstrasse ist fertig]. One is accustomed to indicating this relationship grammatically with the words subject and predicate. The group of ideas from which a declaration is made we call the subject, the declaration itself, the predicate. The subject is the uninteresting known, the declaration, the interesting and new. Of course, this relationship doesn't always take place between grammatical subject and grammatical predicate. With the stress on *your* in *your father said it* [dein Vater hat es gesagt] the grammatical subject is the new and interesting; thus, logically, it is the predicate. One may, therefore, call the exposition the logical subject, while the interesting and new may be called the logical predicate. Of course, the trouble with this is that the expression *logical subject* is a well-established technical term in grammar. One means the acting subject, especially when this doesn't have the form of the grammatical subject, the nominative, as in the sentence *The tree is seen by the boy* [der Baum ist vom Knaben gesehen]. Here, the logical subject is *by the boy* [vom Knaben]. For clarity it is, therefore, preferable to say *exposition* instead of *logical subject*.

The exposition serves to make the situation clear, in order that the logical predicate may become comprehensible. The situation is the basis, the environment, for the appearance of the fact, or thing. It is also the temporal precondition from which an activity originates. The activity we have designated as the predicate and the naming of the person to whom the notice is directed, are also part of the situation. In speech the situation is not determined merely by words, but more usually and extensively by the surrounding relationships themselves, by the immediately preceding facts, and by the presence of the person with whom we are speaking. The situation, given by the surrounding relationships and the presence of the addressed person, comes to consciousness through perception. Thus we call it the situation of perception.

If I am standing with someone in front of a tree, the word *Linden* is quite sufficient to stand for *This tree is a linden* [dieser Baum ist eine Linde]. The pronoun receives its content only by means of present perception. If I introduce someone at a party, it would be somewhat improper to say *This is Mr. Miller* [dies ist Herr Müller]. I simply point him out with my hand in order to differentiate him from the others present and say *Mr. Miller* [Herr Müller]. Vivid perception, made more precise by the gesture, is the situation and subject. It is clear that a present perception is not so simple that all of its parts could necessarily be the subject, nor the entire illustration. There is probably also an oak tree next to that linden in the park; many other things are visible, including the person addressed. The gesture and the direction of the eyes give clues for the separation of one part from this complicated mass; but also, of course, without this more specific illustration one can comprehend such a predicate. Actually, the gesture itself is an activity. The hand, the arm, a finger will thereby be shown. Why doesn't the listener mistakenly refer the predicate to this part of the perception?

In order to make the right connection, the listener must also draw a conclusion from the nature of the predicate as well as from the content of the perception. I am here only suggesting this question, which will be elucidated in the second discussion.

If someone takes a glass of wine away from his mouth and says *Excellent!* [vortrefflich!], I don't doubt for a second that he means the wine that he just enjoyed. From this exclamation I complete the sentence *The wine is excellent* [der Wein ist vortrefflich]. The situation is, thus, also determined by completed actions, which are still in the foreground of our consciousness. And the subject to be thought of is not merely the completed action. Rather, as in the case of drinking the wine, it is something affected in this action. Therefore, here also the perceptive person reaches a conclusion from part of the situation, of which more will be spoken later. This situation will be called in passing the situation of remembrance.

If the eyes of thousands of people are trained on a great spectacle such as a coronation, the exclamation *beautiful*! [schön!], *magnificent*! [herrlich!], is comprehensible while the crowd disperses, since one may assume that everyone in the audience remains concentrated on what he has just seen. Memory keeps alive what has just occurred, so that any linguistic utterance is related to it at once in the absence of further exposition. A difficulty can arise, however, when current perception competes with recent memory for the attention of the listener.

It is evident that any constellation of ideas of immediate interest permits communication to take place effectively with little or no exposition. There are also pervasive human concerns which permit the same ellipsis without loss of understanding.

With their high intensity, these interests are capable of so obscuring the immediately preceding ideas given by perception and remembrance, that they can cross the threshold of consciousness. They also have the greatest capability of being raised into consciousness by other ideas, even those ideas which admit only a distant connection. They form very important material from which other ideas will be supplemented. If someone says *The boards were freshly painted today* [die Bretter sind heute frisch gestrichen], the average person will think of some boards on a house or somewhere else. He will probably look around, if he hears this utterance suddenly, in order to see if the boards mentioned are within his view. An actor, on the other hand, could very easily think of "the boards" as signifying the world. If the hunter hears of *Loeffeln*, he is just as easily inclined to think of the ears of a rabbit as of the soupspoon at the table, even when he is holding the latter in his hand. In the same way, the military man has his special word connotations, as does the lawyer, the sailor, the philologist, the preacher, and so on. From this comes the charming anecdote related by Steinthal, in which a good judge of men undertakes to determine a man's station from the answers to a puzzling question given him by various people unknown to him. The many interest groups thus have their own ways of expressing themselves, the well-known *termini technici*, which complete their content from the situation of consciousness, that is, from the interests which have become established: thus *die Loeffel, der Lauf* of the rabbit,* *der*

---

* *Editor's note*: The German *Loeffel* normally means *spoon* but may mean *ear of a rabbit* in a particular context. *Lauf* normally means the *course* or *run* but may mean *foot of the rabbit*.

Schweiss of the deer,* the many legal terms, and the great number of trade terms. For the Romans, *testudo* could be a turtle, a military tortoise, or a lyre.

The types of situation named are the most important, but it must not be forgotten that all sensations and feelings which are present during the linguistic utterance can be important as measures of exposition. The feelings of joy and pain aroused by the perception momentarily present and the remembrance of facts shortly preceding, belong to the two categories of situation mentioned above, that of perception and that of remembrance. But just as the established interests proceed alongside those momentarily aroused, so will the momentary feelings be influenced by the total sensation and thought which the unshackled or easy course of the somatic functions of life bring with them. It is likewise with the feeling which usually *follows* a desired attainment or impeded course of life's goals. These established feelings are the dispositions of man, which as solid quantities in the spiritual life of man are also often called moods. These cheerful and lively dispositions or sad and melancholy feelings express themselves in the entire thought world of man and, therefore, also in his linguistic expressions. They color, happily or painfully, the complete tone of his voice, the *Actio*, and, thereby, bring a positive element of disposition into the utterances of the speaker. Feelings thus expressed should allow the listener to draw a conclusion concerning a preceding happy or sad event, or concerning a painful condition momentarily present. Such influences require such aid, as do the imperative and the question. However, when the listener sees that cheerfulness or depression is part of the general character or nature of the speaker, he can anticipate from this, as from every other peculiarity of character, the tenor of the communication. The effective significance of this mood upon the listener remains only a stylistic one. It is of great importance for poetry and literature to know the individual dispositions of the literary personality. Only from these sources can the value judgments of a man be understood and appreciated, because a melancholy man becomes very easily pessimistic in his judgments and sees bile where the cheerful one believes he is tasting honey. One sees decay where another perceives joyous, blossoming life. And thus from these established dispositions is derived significant material of expositive elements.

We spoke of the situation of interests which had become firmly established. However, not only separate classes within a community of

---

* *Editor's note*: *Schweiss* normally means *sweat*, but may mean the *falling blood* of a wounded deer in certain contexts.

people, nor only single families or groups have such collective interests. Whole peoples and whole cultural epochs have types of firmly-established collective interests. In this case one is accustomed to speaking of the prevailing ideas of a period. For example, it can be imagined that if in Berlin in the year 1809 one had shouted *freedom*, the people would have had different conceptions from those of the people of Paris during the years of the great revolution. A Prussian would have thought of liberation from foreign domination, a Frenchman of specific political freedom and equality in the domestic life of the state. In contemporary Paris the shout *revanche* would probably be clearly understood. What conceptual picture does the modern Frenchman associate with the word *Prussien* or the Prussian when he proudly asserts *I am a Prussian* [ich bin ein Preusse]. What concept did the Romans of the Golden Age have of *Graecus* or *Graeculus*, and what did the Persians who fought with Salamis think of in connection with this name?

Anent the linguistic and literary utterances of a period, the poetical and written works, we immediately note that a great many expositive elements that we would need remain unsaid. We think and feel differently from those men. It is all quite strange for us. The unexpressed expositive elements can also be called the prejudices of the period. When, in the Edda poems, Brunhild attempts to murder Sigurd as the result of her uncontrollable love for him, her assumption that she hopes to be united with him in the after life is not immediately clear to us. When the same mighty woman tries, through bribery, to persuade her servants to die voluntarily with her, it is incomprehensible to us. We are not familiar with the desire of the Old Germanic Period to enter the after life decorated and honored. The Edda poems give not a single word of exposition. Only in a subsequent presentation by Brunhild is this view revealed. Imagine that a modern writer wanted to revitalize these facts for the modern reader. He would surely strive either epically or dramatically to convey the leading ideas and decisive prejudices of that period. The period itself was of one mind about these views and wouldn't waste a single word on them since so much was implicitly understood.

Our whole conception of the world is determined by such value judgments, ordering the relationships of things among themselves, the relationship of man with God, views of life and world forces, and the duties of man to himself, to others, and to God; one calls this situation the view of life or of man. One may call part of this awareness of the world the religious and moral consciousness of the time. How much this view of life varies among different peoples and cultural epochs needs no discussion. The literary monuments of such periods and peoples actually become comprehensible to us only through extensive commentaries, that is, expositions of their utterances, which were comprehensible in those periods without expositions. Horace begins the eighth ode in the third book:

> *Martiis caelebs quid agam Kalendis,*
> *Quis velint flores et acerra turis*
> *Plena miraris positusque carbo in*
> *Cespite vivo.*

> [A bachelor, March calends see me fill
> My thurible with incense, pluck bouquets,
> And heap the living turf with coals, but still
> Thou standest in amaze.
> (Trans. C. J. Kraemer, Jr., N.Y., 1936)]

Thus, the festival of the matrons on the first of May was given meaning by the religious consciousness of that time. It was all comprehensible to Horace's contemporaries: the people which this festival celebrated, its ritual form, perhaps its deeper religious meaning, and the astonishment of Maecenas. But today we must laboriously try to bring these facts together from other sources in order to understand why Maecenas should be surprised about Horace's festival.

When the Roman said *pluit*, he gave no exposition of the situation. For him it was self-evident that Jupiter's rain god Pluvius brought rain. Does the expression *it is raining* [es regnet] without exposition mean the same thing to us?

It can be concluded without argument that the cultural differences of various peoples and places must produce significant differences in their exposition. We say today *He took the wood in order to make a fire* [er nahm das Holz um Feuer anzumachen] and everyone understands that wood is that which will be brought to flames by another fire or some other means of ignition. Would a man comprehend this idea if his culture knew only of lighting a fire by rubbing two sticks together? Would he understand the expression *steel and stone* [Stahl und Stein]? We call this situation the cultural situation.

Only by comparing our view of the world and the condition of our culture with others do we become conscious of what we assume and what we leave unexplained in speaking to our associates with the same view of the world and the same culture. The entire content of the words of all activities, forms of life, and tools—that is, the things which support this course of life—is determined by these assumptions based on our view of the world and our culture.

That should suffice to give an idea of the conceptual material which I have called the cultural situation.

VII

THE clearer and more complete the situation becomes through perception, the less it needs linguistic means. Thus the linguistic expression which is directed at an actual perception may be kept as short as possible. Among the various kinds of poetry, drama played on the stage needs the least words; pantomime manages without linguistic means. In the presentation of pantomime all remarks are omitted because the ensemble of the scene depicts those needed facts and relationships directly and bodily. How simple the understanding of the words becomes by means of this ensemble on the stage. For example, at the beginning of Egmont: *Now go on and shoot so that you all have taken part. You still won't take it [victory] away from me! In all your born days you haven't shot three black rings. And I would therefore become this year's champion.* [Nun schiesst nur hin, dass es alle wird! Ihr nehmt mir's doch nicht! Drei Ringe schwarz, die habt ihr eure Tage nicht geschossen. Und so wär' ich für diess Jahr Meister.] Without the perception of the group on stage, would one be in a position to reveal that a firing of crossbows is taking place, that Soest is a shopkeeper or at least a burgher, that Jetter, to whom he directs those words, is likewise a burgher? Who would know that during this speech soldiers are also present? Who could even approximately guess the time of the action, or the place, whether the action is taking place in the woods, in the village, in the city? The dramatist, therefore, is using lively, actual perception as a very important element of exposition. How much longer the exposition would have to be for a novel choosing the same mentioned situation! The novel and, even more so, the tale need the most words of all, because they have the most expositive information to give.

The situation becomes less apparent the farther apart and more diverse the number of the surrounding persons and objects becomes. To a great degree the indication with the hand can still be helpful here. But the single occurrences of the single persons can no longer be observed with the same thoroughness. In a large and crowded wine cellar it would be difficult to tell whether the shout *excellent!* [vortrefflich!] referred to the wine, to the meal, to an anecdote, to a suggestion, or to something else.

The determination of meaning is more difficult when speaker and listener are at a distance one from another, or when the subject being discussed is not close at hand. Face-to-face conversation is often clearer and less complicated than an exchange of information by means of a letter, and a description of an Indian landscape by a man in Paris will be less readily grasped than if it were being offered in Agra. The discussion of something distant in time may be even harder to understand than the description of something far away in space. This is the case in the excerpt from Egmont. If the author of a novel leads us back to ancient times—for example, to that of Egyptian or Greek history—he senses a much greater difficulty in exposition than Spielhagen who places us in the modern life of a German city.

Finally, the larger the circle of people addressed, the more difficult exposition becomes. An author who addresses himself to a whole nation, or to all of the educated world, cannot rely on a single-minded and uniform understanding of his message, nor on the ready understanding furnished by local or family reference. The more widely diverse the interests of his audience, the greater will be the demands on his ability to explain himself clearly in words. One must be aware of the difference between a community of thousands of well-educated individuals, the tiny world of the child with his imperfect but adequate speech and the small tribal community in which the daily activity is so predictable and repetitive as to require little sophistication in language. Recognition of these differences demonstrates the law that not only the phonetic form of language but the manner of expression of groups originally within the same language community will change with spatial separation or alterations in the mode of life.

VIII

IN CONTRAST to the exposition is the logical predicate. As has already been indicated above, this is not the same as the grammatical predicate, although there is naturally a close connection. That member of the sentence which carries the tone, the stressed part of the sentence, is the logical predicate. According to the grammatical form, this can be a subject, a designation of time or place, or any other grammatical category. The following sentence can thus be variously stressed: *The battle of Leipzig was fought on the eighteenth of October. The battle of* Leipzig—*was fought on the* eighteenth *of October—was fought on the eighteenth of* October [die Schlacht bei Leipzig ist am 18. October geschlagen. Die Schlacht bei *Leipzig*—, ist am *achtzehnten* October

—, ist am 18. *October*—geschlagen]. One immediately senses the difference in meaning of the sentence in conjunction with the difference in stress. If *Leipzig* is stressed, it is thereby stated, *this* battle took place on October eighteenth; to be sure, another one occurred on a different day. From the confirmed fact that on October the eighteenth a battle took place, the declaration is predicated which one this was. If the number *eighteenth* is stressed, an assumption is thereby contradicted—the assumption, let us say, that this had occurred on October the twenty-fifth. From the confirmed fact that in October there was a battle near Leipzig, the correct predicate is expressed. Consequently, with the different stress there arises each time a different meaning, because each time the logical predicate and the situation, or the logical subject, are different. It is worthy of notice that in our sentence it is precisely the *grammatical* predicate which cannot be stressed.

From this example also emerges what had already been mentioned above, that the predicate always contains the new and interesting segment of the communication, or, to express it more precisely, the more valuable element. We will hear more about this point when we face the question concerning the purposes of speech.

From this it is even now obvious that only those words which are in a position to communicate something valuable to the listener can be the logical predicate. As far as I can see, this is possible only with a relative pronoun. Otherwise, all the so-called form words could be the stressed parts of the sentence, for example, the prepositions: *that's right* next to *the house, but not* in *the house* [ja *neben* dem Haus aber nicht *in* dem Haus]; and the other adverbs: very *beautiful, you say?* [*sehr* schön, sagst du?], he *makes it* much *too hard* [er macht es *gar* zu arg] *your brother* also *came* [dein Bruder kam *auch*]. On the other hand, the relative pronoun *who, which* [der, welcher] cannot easily be stressed; except perhaps in contrast to the correction of an assumption: *I only went to him* when *I heard it* (*not beforehand*) [ich ging zu ihm erst, *als* ich es hörte (nicht bevor)]; *I have written* because *I love you* (*not although*) [ich habe geschrieben, *weil* ich dich liebe (nicht obgleich)]; *That will happen* if he *comes* (*as you maintain, but it is doubtful whether you are right*) [das wird geschehen *wenn* er kommt (wie du behauptest, aber es ist zweifelhaft, ob du Recht hast)].

The means by which the speaker distinguishes both highly differentiated classes of sentence elements from one another is the higher or lower intensity of the tone. I am here disregarding the fact that, in the languages with a musical accent, a simultaneous musical raising of the tone in pitch takes place. The importance of the accent for understanding the sentence and its meaning is demonstrated by comparing a clumsy and monotonous reading with a well-accented delivery.

The means are fully sufficient to allow the logical predicate to become prominent. One even finds in modern languages, especially French and German, the endeavor to allow the stressed part of the sentence to come to prominence, also by means of grammatical construction. One becomes especially conscious of this endeavor if one compares these languages with Latin and Greek. We frequently translate sentences such as *primus Caesar hoc fecit* as *Caesar was the first who did this* [Cäsar war der erste, der dies that]; and, likewise, with the stress *Caesar hoc Fecit, it was Caesar who* [Cäsar war es, der]. In such cases, French uses the expression *c'est que* so much that examples are unnecessary. One can say that especially stressed secondary determining factors are in this manner frequently advanced to the foreground in modern languages, for example: *it was his brother with whom he came* [sein Bruder war es, mit dem er kam]; Latin, *cum fratre venit*; *it was night when he returned, it has been a long time since* [es war Nacht, als er zurückkehrte, es ist lange her, seit]; and many other examples.

One gets the impression that this shows a contradiction in language feeling, bringing the stressed part of the sentence into a syntactical relationship which in general serves as an expression of secondary determination. One also needs to advance the most important member of the communication to the front, which is not always easy because of the fixed arrangement of words in modern languages. Characteristic of this is the fact that one makes the logical predicate also the grammatical predicate in such cases. At this opportunity, I would like to indicate that (1) there are endeavors to put the logical predicate at the front and to make the logical predicate the grammatical predicate, and (2) the unusual position of the grammatical predicate in modern languages is behind the subject. This is obviously a logical contradiction to which we must return.

IX

THIS question now arises: how does language actually satisfy this need for a logical predicate and exposition; which forms will be used for this; and how does the grammatical form pertain to the established relationships of closed sentence structure just described? The following sentence is very illustrative: *Themistocles, a Grecian from Athens, a contemporary of Aristides, at Salamis defeated the Persians, who had come to Greece in order to subjugate this country, in a sea battle.* [Themistokles, ein Grieche aus Athen, ein Zeitgenosse des Aristides, schlug bei Salamis die Perser, welche nach Griechenland gezogen waren, um dieses Land zu unterwerfen, in einer Seeschlacht].

Let us follow the courses of this presentation: first, a personal noun as subject—for one versed in history it suffices to indicate the native country and lifetime, because there is only one Themosticles of historical significance. For the unlearned, an elucidation of time and place is required. This is contained in the double appositive. Evidently the narrator has been moved in his representation by the consideration of the level of knowledge of his listener and which expositive elements he must give to him. The elucidating appositive comes after the subject needing explanation; one would expect from a well-arranged presentation, that the exposition would precede those words needing such an exposition. Therefore, *Themistocles* is here related to his appositives, as the logical predicate of the sentence is related to its expositive factors, to its exposition, or to its logical subject. A clear and simple narration would say: *At the same time as Aristides, there lived in Athens a man named Themistocles* [es lebte zur Zeit des Aristides ein Mann in Athen mit Namen Themistokles].

The presence of the Persians at Salamis is explained by the relative clause. This is the exposition to the logical predicate: *The Persians were defeated at Salamis* [die Perser wurden bei Salamis geschlagen]. Both types of exposition—apposition and relative sentence—always stand behind their logical predicate. And thus these simple, familiar forms of exposition are logically in the wrong position.

For an explanation of this surprising fact it need only be reflected how the speaker generally becomes aware that his presentation needs some exposition. In general, man, especially one who is naive, assumes that his fellow human beings are so organized and internally determined, that they think and know the same things as he. If he begins his presentation with this presumption, he must very often realize its invalidity from the unresponsive expression in the face of the addressed or, even more directly, from the questions, what are you talking about, when was that, where did that happen? Thus, the speaker will notice that he must add certain particulars as an explanation. It is easy for the speaker to misjudge the amount to be communicated in the exposition. If he gives too much he will become boring or will appear a cautious pedant. If he gives too little he will be unintelligible. He is advised about this from the facial expressions of the person he is addressing. If these expressions are absent-minded and disinterested during the presentation, the speaker can conclude that he is being verbose. If he can read on the face of the addressed person expressions of surprise or lack of understanding, or if he hears a direct question, then he knows that he must explain more thoroughly what he has just stated.

Moreover, it is precisely the logical predicate which interests the speaker most of all. It is, for the moment, his main thought. It is completely at the foreground of his consciousness, and, because of this, it is the strongest force to be communicated. This mechanical dominance of the logical predicate in the mind is accompanied by the awareness that an exposition is necessary for understanding, and this is required to maintain equilibrium. How often, nevertheless, this awareness succumbs to the overpowering force of the psychological powers of feeling and striving has been demonstrated by moral science everywhere.

The natural dominance of interest is further reinforced by the increased animation carried along with it. This may be contrasted to the tranquility of writing and also by the elementary striving of man to be interesting. It is for this reason, psychologically only natural, that a naive man expresses the expositive elements only after he has spoken the predicate. The speaking form, once created and firmly established, is also retained by the artistically-minded creative poet and author. The appositive and the relative sentence are therefore supplementary corrections of our imperfect presentations.

X

IT IS interesting that the grammatical form of subordinate clauses gives us insight into the creation of expositive form, somewhat in the manner that petrifacts reveal to us the forms of ancient life. In the Indo-Germanic languages, two classes of stems are most often employed to form the subordinate clauses: demonstrative stems and stems of the interrogative pronoun. In Greek, Latin, and German we have for this (1) the demonstrative stem *ta-* Greek *το-*, German *tha, da*, NHG *der die das*; (2) in Latin the interrogative stems *qui* and *quo-*, German *hwa-*, from which comes NHG *wer, was, welcher*, with their derivatives. It is from these stems that most of the important conjunctions of these three languages are derived. However, since these languages do not agree in the choice of stems, it is therein proven that the development of the subordinate clause was first executed within the individual languages. It is even more noticeable and interesting then, that there is an agreement about the inherent principle used in forming these sentences.

The origin of the relative sentence from the demonstrative is very clear: *The Greeks defeated the Persians, which was a nation from Asia —they came from Asia—at that time Xerxes was king* [die Griechen schlugen die Perser, das war ein Volk aus Asien—die waren aus Asien gekommen—damals war Xerxes König]. As demonstrative sentences, they are similar to the parenthetical expressions of former times and are still used today. They are related also to the functional sentence appositives, thus the supplementary corrections of presentation.

The sentence appositive is, of course, to be found in all three languages, but it is not in every case the established form of the subordinate clause. It has neither become nor remained even that of the relative clause. In German it hasn't remained so, in that the relative clauses have adopted a different word arrangement from that of the parenthetical appositive clauses. This word arrangement is also common to all subordinate clauses which have arisen in other ways; for example, the directive sentence formed with the noun *while* [Weile]: *while I was watching him* [weil ich ihn sah]; those sentences formed with a participle: *during the time I received the letter* [Während ich den Brief erhielt]; the indirect interrogative sentence: *I asked him whether he had seen him* [ich fragte ihn, ob er ihn gesehen hätte]; and, likewise, the subordinate clauses formed from interrogatives. The demonstrative sentences have subscribed to the usual word arrangement of the subordinate clause, and, thus, have submitted to the constraint of a system. In the Greek language and its varying dialects, the relative form ὅς with time seems to have made headway against the forms of the stem το-.

However, not all German subordinate clauses formed with the demonstrative can be explained in this manner. In a sentence *he left after the sun had risen* [er reiste ab, nachdem die Sonne aufgegangen war], the demonstrative expression *after* [nach dem] can etymologically only be related to the main clause, *he left after a time; this time was: when the sun rose* [er reiste ab nach der Zeit, diese Zeit war: die Sonne war aufgegangen]. Likewise, *since* [da] must be counted etymologically with the main clause: *we are so happy since you are coming* [wir freuen uns, da du kommst]. Also in sentences with *because* [indem]: *because I am waiting here, he is already planning murder* [indem ich hier verweile, dingt er schon Mörder]; sentences with *according to which, so that* [je nachdem, auf dass]: *you should honor father and mother, so that it will go well for you* [du sollst Vater und Mutter ehren, auf dass dirs wohl gehe].

If we have been etymologically connecting and constructing correctly, the demonstrative is shown to have the same function in principle as the appositive. The clause *he left after* [er reiste ab, nach dem] is spoken as if the demonstrative expression could be understood by itself. The speaker himself attaches a certain content to the demonstration. The following clause *the sun had risen* [die Sonne war aufgegangen] is attached as a correction, as a supplementary exposition. In the same manner are those sentences to be understood, from whose example the many German connections with *that* have been formed; for example, *I think that he is coming* [ich glaube dass er kommt]. First of all, the neutral *that* [dass] was the object of the verb *I think* [ich glaube], and if it was incomprehensible, one added parenthetically or appositively *he is coming* [er kommt]. The use of the sentences with *that* [dass] was most certainly originally confined to its relation with transitive verbs. However, as soon as one no longer sensed the pronoun merely as pronoun, but related it to the following sentence, the gate was opened wide for the expansion of ways of construction.

That a simple main clause can serve as a supplementary explanation of an incomprehensible word can be completely understood from the free use of parenthetical sentences, for example: *He visited the other brother (he was a farmer)* [er besuchte den anderen Bruder (er war ein Farmer)]. It may also be used as a formula of the personal pronoun in the relative sense, for example: *with you, who are the crown of all virtues* [mit dir, du ein krône bist aller êren]; further in sentences with *now* [nun], in actuality, *at present* [jetzt], for example: *I can die in peace, knowing that I have now recommended her to you* [ich sterbe ruhig, nun ich sie dir empfehle]; likewise with *eh* [before], MHG *ê*, *eh* corresponding to the etymological relation of *nu* [now] and *ê* with in MHG *daz* [that] will also be added; likewise *weil* [while], MHG *die wîle* [while that] and *die wîle daz, die wîle und* [while that and while]. Also the MHG *doch* [yet] in the sense of *obgleich* [although] is also in this category. The original participle *während* [while, during] can equally be construed etymologically as part of the main clause.

It cannot be doubted then that a special method used in forming German expositive subordinate clauses accompanies the demonstrative in cases when it is not comprehensible to the listener, and, therefore, in need of supplementary elucidation. It is the method of correction. In discussing this phenomenon we have found other forms alike in principle; only in these forms, the correction accompanied a different word in need of correction. This phenomenon is interesting for the history of language in that the part of the main clause which was kept too general gradually became part of the explanatory subordinate clause. We will encounter this phenomenon even more often.

XI

IT MAY remain undecided whether the stem of the Greek relative pronoun ὅς and the relative forms of the το- stem should be regarded as interrogative or demonstrative. However, since the demonstrative meaning has definitely been certified for the Greek language, and since the relative sentence has developed without a doubt in the country of this single language, I can then see no reason to deny the origin of these secondary sentences from the demonstrative pronouns.

Indeed, one might explain these Greek sentences in the same manner as the German or Latin relative sentences, but the results of our investigation, in search of the linguistic means which characterize the exposition, would not thereby be altered. Most certainly the Latin relative sentence, with its pronoun *qui* and its derivatives, has developed itself from the interrogative sentence. The fact is that the relative clause has, as its introductory word, a form of the interrogative pronoun; for example: *Themistocles, qui Athenis natus est, vicit Persas* [Themistocles, who was born in Athens, conquered the Persians]. The relative clause contains the explanation of the name by naming the place of birth. The speaker could not ask the person he is addressing who was born in Athens, since he has just given this information as a fact to explain the name. The interrogative sentence cannot come from what the person being addressed is thinking either, because, up to now, nothing was said to him about anyone born in Athens.

But, of course, the interrogative pronoun is derived from what the listener is thinking. What *will* he ask when something seems questionable about the name Themistocles? Obviously, who Themistocles was. The old construction was: A says *Themistocles*, B: *Who?* A: *He was born in Athens.*

Latin *quianum* means *why?* or *wherefore*; *quia* means *while*. The old construction was: *The Persians traveled to Greece. Why? They wanted to subjugate* [die Perser zogen nach Grieschenland.—Warum? —Sie wollten unterwerfen].

Quippini means *why not* [warum denn nicht]; *quippe* means *because* [denn]. The sentence introduced with *quia* and *quippe* contains the answer to the question *why* [warum]. It would be impossible to introduce the answer itself, clearly and consciously from the basic meaning of the words *quia* and *quippe*, with such an expression as *why* [warum].

We construe, chiefly from the sentence form, that the exposition will be given subsequently. Furthermore, it will be given in the form in which it usually first becomes clear to a speaker that it is his responsibility to give such an exposition. This form is also used frequently enough, not merely in naive speech, but also in educated language; for example: *I want to move away. Why? (Well,) I don't like it here* [ich will fortziehen. Warum? (Nun) es gefällt mir hier nicht].

We will later discuss how it is conceivable by itself that the interrogative meaning of these stems *qui* and *quo* has developed from the demonstrative. I do not want to deny the possibility that the single languages could have had an interrogative originally. However, it is just as probable from the comparison of the Greek stem πο-, the Latin *quo* and the Germanic *hwa*, that before the separation of languages took place, this stem had obtained its interrogative meaning.

The explanation given above, which appears to me to be the only possible one, is therefore also valid for the others of these stems and the derivatives formed from them, thus for: *quod* [because], *ubi* [when], *unde* [whence], *ut* [that], *quam* [than, as] *quom* [when, since], *cum* [when, since], *quando* [when, at what time].

We find here further, a very interesting fact for the history of the language: two sentences (1) an interrogative sentence, whose predicate was to be completed from the preceding information, and (2) the answers to this question; both are fused into one continuous organically complete sentence.

In this fusion process, one must answer the question of how it is possible that an interrogative sentence forfeits its interrogative tone, because only when the following tone of the interrogative word is softened can it be fused with the assertion sentence of the answer. It must first of all be ascertained that the interrogative *who, how* [wer, wie] and so on, will be spoken by the same person who also gives the answer. Thus it follows that the speaker is able to deduce the question by watching the person he is addressing: *"How," you ask* ["wie" fragst du].

Cases such as these, in which a direct utterance is reported by another person and taken over, are extraordinarily frequent; for example: someone has spoken to a person with *thou* [du]. The latter answers *"Thou," I forbid* [du, das verbitte ich mir] or *I forbid the use of "thou"* [das du verbitte ich mir], or in connection with a preposition *You spoke to me with the "thou" form* [du hast mich mit du angeredet], or with a verb derivative using *thou* [duzen] or *ye* [ihrzen]. The address of the first person—that is, as a direct oral utterance—thus becomes the object of the other person and, thereby, adopts completely the character of an appellative noun. The tone of the word *thou* [du] can be lost in the address and it will naturally be regularly lost when the borrowed word is declined or receives derivative suffixes. Likewise we say *the how* [das wie], *the where* [das wo], *the when* [das wenn], Greek τό πῶς [the how], τό ποῦ [the where], τό ποῖον [the what], the *Lord's Prayer* [das Vaterunser], and declined, [des Vaterunsers], Greek ἀλαλά and ἀλαλάζω [alala (a war cry), to raise a war cry]. *Hoorah, hoorah!* [Hussah, hussah!] we shout, or adverbially *da geht es hurra hopsassa.* The Greek ἦ μήν [Editor's note: not translated, only used to indicate an oath] is an affirmative participle and is, therefore, quite appropriate in oaths and solemn pledges. But it is also given its authority by an infinitive, which is dependent on a verb of swearing or pledging. From Tacitus, in the classical period, *an* has come to forfeit its interrogative tone. For example: *finem vitae sponte an fato implevit,* but the expression was probably developed from the direct question: *Did he die of his own accord—or of a natural death?*

This appropriating of a direct utterance of another person in a reporting statement, whereby the original tone of sensation is lost, makes it even possible to build actual linguistic words with fully developed natural form from interjectional sounds. And so it was possible from the interjection *ach: das Ach und Weh* [alas! the Oh and Woe] to build the verb *ächzen* [to lament] or perhaps even the Greek ἄχος [ache], or οἰμώζω, στενάζω [to wail, to groan, etc.] Only the complete loss of the tone of sensation allows words of sensation to take part in the developments and changes in the sounds of the language, such as sound shifts. The interjectional sound itself may stay outside of such changes and along with it every word which is *clearly* dependent for its linguistic consciousness on that interjection.

But here I should interrupt this stream of thought. Those relative clauses formed from the interrogative pronoun may be illustrated by the German sentences *er ist gestorben. Wie—das will ich dir erzählen* [He has died. How? That's what I'm going to tell you] or *das wie will ich dir ererzählen* [I'm going to tell you how]. When the interrogative pronoun has become an integral part of the relative clause, then it is self-evident that the grammatical purpose of the pronoun must be determined by the verb of the original sentence of reply. For example: *ab urbe profectus est, quem vidisti* [he has left the city, I saw him], etymologically the construction was *ab urbe profectus est. Quis? vidisti (eum)* [He has left the city. Who? I saw (him)].

XII

THUS all forms of the pronoun subordinate clause are a result of the supplementary correction of a presentation with insufficient exposition. Only when the language has been cultivated with fine arts and education must one meet the obligation of placing the exposition in front of the logical predicate. It is this striving for a preceding exposition which accounts in enlightened times, for example, in the classical Latin period, for the relative expositive sentence being placed in front of the main clause. Thus, with the feeling that the logical predicate should be the verb (of course, often the case), the verb came at the end of the sentence—that is, behind all the determining factors, which appear as exposition.

A study of the verbal declension of the Indo-Germanic language leads to the same result. The pronoun suffix which characterizes the person is placed after the word stem; and, in contrast with the verbal stem, it is so weakly stressed that it joins it enclitically, thus completely forfeiting its independence as a word. Since the logical predicate carries the stress, the form of the verb declension decidedly arises from those cases of the usage of language in which it is not the person characterized by the pronoun which contains the logical predicate, but the stem of the verb. This formation is somewhat similar to the German form *kommt'r* [he's coming], a frequently used contraction of the proper form *kommt er* [he is coming].

Since the verb form constructed with the enclitic pronoun provided the model for all verb forms, then the most frequent case of all must have been the one in which the verbal stem contained the logical predicate. Therefore, the expositive subject must have come right after the predicate. The pronoun suffix was so firmly fused with the stem, that it was even retained when a special subject word was used with the verb; thus *I I-say, you you-say, Carl he-loves* [ich sag' ich, du sagstu, Karl liebt'r] form the patterns for this.

Even in the period when the value of the suffix as a pronoun was clearly perceived, it was not unusual for the third person that a new exposition would be affixed to the indefinite exposition with the pronoun *he*, as in the pattern *Carl (he) is coming* [Kommt er Karl]. This form, completely analogous to the appositive, is very often heard in

actual conversation and, likewise, in the category of corrections of expositions. Following are several examples of this manner of correction
from artificial speech—from Goethe's songs, for example:

*Of course he is to be praised, the man. . . . And who is to tell about it, the
most manifold misery? . . . It was sad to see, the various belongings, etc.
—Goetz: Dogs, the cavalry! It becomes sour for one, the little bit of life and
freedom.* [Freilich ist er zu preisen, der Mann. . . . Und wer erzählet es wohl,
das mannigfaltigste Elend? . . . Traurig war es zu sehen, die mannigfaltige
Habe, etc—Goetz: Lumpenhunde, die Reiter! Es wird einem sauer gemacht,
das Bisschen Leben und Freiheit.]

> *I can hardly wait for it,*
> *The first flower in the garden.*
> *The first bloom on the tree.*
>
> [Ich kann sie kaum erwarten,
> Die erste Blum' im Garten.
> Die erste Blüth' am Baum.]

Or from the songs of Eckhard:

> *They are coming, the nocturnal horror is already coming.*
> *They are the hostile sisters.*
> *They drink what was fetched with difficulty, the beer,*
> *Then they are gracious to you, the ungracious ones.*
>
> [Sie kommen, da kommt schon der nächtliche Graus.
> Sie sinds die unholdigen Schwestern.
> Sie trinken das mühsam geholte, das Bier,
> Dann sind sie Euch hold, die Unholden.]

These examples, which are abundant in Goethe, demonstrate the extent of this form of correction in the language. Here it has even become
a popular and decidedly effective stylistic tool.

XIII

WHILE the actual meaning of the noun suffixes in ancient languages is unknown to us, it is clear that (with the exception of
the vocative, theoretically a pure stem) the modulation of relationship
of the stem, i.e., the function of case, is given in the suffix. We derive
this fact from studying the few remaining suffixes such as the Greek
-θεν, -δε, -σε, -θι, the Latin -tus. These suffixes are absorbed by the

tone of the stem, the model for the formation of the noun being created by the most frequent instance in which the stem contains the logical predicate. The structure of the elements thus has exactly the same arrangements with nouns as with verbs. Also the form of declension of nouns has its origins in the supplementary correction of insufficient exposition. This manner of formation is similar to the German slang form: *wo er draus erkannte* [from which he recognized], *wo er rein ging* [where he entered], *da hat er sich dran gemacht* [he set to work there]. Quite commonly in everyday speech we use a noun quite out of all context and only later do we add required relationships: *das Haus, da bin ich rein gegangen* [the house, I went in there], *dein Buch, da habe ich viel drin gelesen* [your book, I read a lot in it], and so on.

It appears worthy of notice that modern languages misplace the succession of elements in their new formations. The Romance and German languages actually inflict the personal pronoun of the verb for the second time, but put forward: *j'ai, tu as, I have, you have.* Likewise the newly-formed helping morphemes are placed in front of the verbal stem, while in the older Indo-Germanic formation, the help stood behind it; Greek ἔλυσα [loosened], λύσω [loosen], ἐλύθην [was loosened], Latin: *amabam, amabo, amavi*, Germanic: *suohta*. The case functions of the genitive, dative, locative, ablative, and instrumental—frequently in the Germanic languages, regularly in the Romanic—will be rendered by the preceeding prepositions. In several cases, the Romanic languages will even lead the way for Latin and Greek.

In these new formations, most of the sentence elements used as exposition stand in their logically valid positions. It is certain that here, also, the case formed the model by which these elements of purpose stood as unstressed or expositive. This is proved by the proclitic form of the prepositions, by which they are differentiated in many ways from the older adverbial forms. It is further proven by the proclitically originated form of some personal pronouns, such as the French *je* and LG *'k* meaning *ich* [I]. Also, the word arrangement of the modern sentence, generally with the subject in front of the verb, belongs here; likewise does the proclitical position of the conjoint pronoun in the Romance languages. Although, of course, the grammatical and logical predicates are not identical.

One may certainly say hereafter that the history of language unveils a picture of the general advance of man's mind: sober, reasonable reflection and calculation of the comprehensive ability of the fellow human being who is addressed wins the upper hand over the primitive power of feeling and striving.

However, before I leave this point, I must mention several interesting relics of this phenomenon of supplementary exposition, firmly established grammatical forms, such as the Greek ἄλλος τε καὶ ἐκεῖνος [besides others, that], Latin *cum alii tum ille, cum ceteris rebus tum hac re* and the German *ausser anderen dieser* [this in addition to the others], ἄλλος τε καὶ = *präsertim cum* [and another besides = particularly because]. The expression *other* indicates the remains of a subtraction process. One speaks of a number of men, then separates from these, several or one. Those who remain are the remainder, the others. The extent of the remainder and, along with it, in the expression *the others* [die Anderen], *others* [Andere], is first comprehensible when one is given the minuend and the subtrahend. In the above expressions, however, the minuend is assumed to be known, then follows *cum alii, ceteri.* Thus the remainder is given, and only after this, the subtrahend *ille.* This is obviously a process against which the mathematician would raise a very energetic protest. This order of the elements is possible in that the speaker has already completed the subtraction in his mind when he begins his sentence, and he doesn't concern himself with whether the listener knows the elements necessary for the subtraction. The situation is stated incompletely and therefore needs a correction; this correction is *tum ille.*

The same neglect of the exposition is also demonstrated in the corresponding particles: τε—καί, καί—καί [both—and] οὔτε—οὔτε [neither—nor], *et—et, que—et* [both—and], *nec—nec, nec—et* [neither—nor], *aut—aut* [either—or], *sive—sive* [either—or]. One can proceed from *et—et* with the meaning *also* or *and.* In both cases it signifies, for example in the clause *et Caesar et Pompeius,* that the predicate also stands for Caesar. Thus, Caesar is placed on a level with a person who has not yet been named. The listener does not know the assumed person, but the speaker does, of course. It is Pompeius, who will only be named supplementarily. Caesar and Pompeius are augends; by means of the first *et* the addition is completed. First *one* augend is named, the other follows only after the addition. We had in the first case the succession: minuend, remainder, subtrahend; here we have the completely corresponding sequence: first augend, sum total, second augend.

It is exactly the same in the form of the alternative in ἤ—ἤ, *aut—aut* [either—or], likewise in the double question with *utrum—an,* πότερον ἤ, *neither—nor*: both elements which are indicated with *utrum,* πότερον, *weder* [neither], are really not given to the listener. They must therefore be supplemented in the form of an appositive clause: *utrum abis an manes*—actually *which one of the two?* [was von beiden?]—assumes the knowledge of an alternative between two cases. Since this is not present, it is given supplementarily: *are you going or are you staying?* [gehst du oder bleibst du?].

The same process of supplementary exposition is valid for comparison. The comparative *larger* [grösser] already contains the results of the comparison. If I say *he is larger than you* [er ist grösser als du], I have thus given with *he is larger* [er ist grösser], the facsimile of a comparison between two people, thus the facsimile of a calculation. It is in reality only *one* person, the member of the proportion first named. I must therefore put up with the question thrown in: in relation to what (Latin *quam*)? This I must answer by supplying supplementary information about the as yet unnamed person, thus, by presenting the second member of the proportion.

Also belonging to this category are the expressions *so* and the formations made in this sense, such as *tantus, talis,* τόσος, τοῖος, *such a,* and so on. These expressions are only then immediately comprehensible from the situation when the compared objects are in front of our eyes and ears as a perceptual quantity, or if they have just been named, for example *and it happened so* [so kam es]—that is, as it has just been stated. But if the speaker has in mind only the object to be judged, he doesn't put the listener in a position to understand the comparison. Therefore, a supplementary correction is necessary with *than* [als], *like* [wie], *that* [quam, ut, dass], *what sort of* [οῖος, quantus], and so on.

It is self-evident that one's language feeling at the more developed stages of speaking does not sense the least trace of defect with these sentence forms, once they have become firmly established. Moreover, they appear to be the really logically adequate and congruent expression of thought. Nevertheless these sentence forms have arisen from the naive assumption of the speaker that the listener must be aware of the same thoughts and be able to compare, as if the criterion of the speaker were a generally known and absolute one. Thus the child uses unsuspectingly *so schön* [so beautiful], *so gross* [so large]. The more developed German language has the comparative form *so* without an exposition, even in the most sublime stylistic nuances; for example, *es wär' so schön gewesen, es hat nicht sollen sein* [it would have been so beautiful, it should not have happened] (Scheffel). Without an exposition is the Latin *haud ita multo post,* Tacitus' *non perinde,* (meaning *not as it should be*), and the comparitive in the sense of *too* [zu], *all too* [allzu].

However if the speaker has one time cleared up the situation, the predicates which follow no longer need the expositive elements anew. For example, *Scipio went to Africa; he made a camp* [Scipio ging nach Africa, er schlug ein Lager]. It would be quite offensive to repeat the exposition *Scipio*. The elevated Latin language even has the capability to express the new predicates after the exposition without any reference to the subject by the infinitive, that is, by a nominative noun form: *Caesar cum Rubiconem transiisset, obsider oppida, vincere exercitus.* We can also say in the same manner: *When Caesar had crossed the Rubicon,* (*there were*) *sieges of cities, victories over armies* [Als Cäsar den Rubico überschritten hatte, (da) Belagerung von Städten, Sieg über Heere]. This form of expression, stemming from the language of emotion, has preserved the stylistic character, vitality, and descriptiveness of emotional speech.

Just as every object of an actual perception can form the exposition to a predicate, in the same way every group of thoughts of which the listener becomes conscious can be the exposition for the utterances which will later join them. Only with this principle is it possible to join a long series of predicates and sentences in a unified presentation. This is because the linguistic series would become infinite if the whole exposition had to be repeated for each new logical predicate. To demonstrate the relationships of the members of the presentation mentioned above, the same means may be used as those employed in indicating the actual perception, the demonstrative pronouns. In this demonstration of an element of remembrance, instead of an element of perception, the meaning of the demonstratives would naturally be changed a great deal, as in the *Casus obliqui* of the Latin *is*, of the Greek αὐτός [he, the one], and of the German *er* [he].

Simply by means of retentive remembrance are such sentence forms possible as *Cäsar ḳam, sah, siegte* [Caesar came, saw, conquered], or with the objects of Greek and Latin sentences like *Caesarem vidit et amavit*, where German would need a demonstrative with *ihn* [him], *er sah den Cäsar und liebte ihn* [he saw Caesar and loved him]. The nominative connections are made possible in the same manner: *Caesaris frater et filius, mein Sohn und Bruder* [my son and brother], the supplementation of a common verb: *vidit Caesarem et Ciceronem*, and so on. A glance in any story followed by simple reflection would show that every past utterance of the narrator forms the exposition for all following predicates. We need follow this path no longer, since we will later come back to related and supplementary questions.

XIV

PEOPLE have long disputed whether or not a word can have several meanings. The word *lion* [Löwe] has, to all appearances, only one meaning. As with all words, this meaning is the sum of all thoughts which will be connected with its combination of sounds. But for whom will these sounds be connected? If one shows a picture of the animal to the zoologist and the child, will they really associate the same thoughts with this word? Will not the African traveler or the animal trainer, who have more than once come into contact with the lion, have different thoughts about this name than the more detached reader of animal stories?

The zoologist has more, clearer, and better classified thoughts about this word than does the child. The lion hunter probably has incomplete and unclassified thoughts about the anatomical structure of the animal, but perhaps he knows the character of the animal better. With the name of the beast he associates all the feelings of fear and horror which he felt when he encountered him. Thus the substance of words is differentiated (1) according to the point of view of the completeness of the associated thoughts, (2) according to the arrangement of the actually associated thoughts, and (3) according to the type and intensity of the feelings which memory has accumulated from the associated thoughts. The first two points together can be called the point of view of comprehension, the third one is ethical and aesthetic. It is thus obvious that a given word will not have the same meaning to all people in the same language community, in spite of the fact that its phonetic form undergoes no change.

From the points of view indicated, it appears that a group of thoughts evoked by a word, for example, *lion* (Löwe), will link itself by association with other groups of thoughts in the mind of the listener, and that these associations differ from one person to another. Because of his training the zoologist thinks of the criteria for classifying an animal as a lion. The child and the non-scientist, only incidentally alike in this respect, relate the lion to other golden creatures with manes. The kind of feeling each has about such animals will lead to an ethical and/or aesthetic value judgment, and determine whether the beast is conceived of as beautiful, noble, good, and useful, or simply terrifying.

Such value judgments are conditioned by whether or not the constellation of thoughts evoked by a word is part of everyday thought or whether, rarely impinging on the consciousness, such thought maintains the attraction and interest of novelty. The man who sees a mountain for the first time has feelings about it which are different from those of the man who has always made his home on it. The more frequently a combination of thought and sound is encountered, the blunter the attendant feelings become; the listener is indifferent toward the familiar. The modification of word meaning in accordance with the accompanying feelings and value judgments is obviously significant.

Thus a word is not uniformly understood either in relation to mental or emotional processes. Persons within the same language community will differ in understanding precisely what it represents in reality and in what style of utterance its meaning will be clear to others.

We can conclude also that the meaning of a word is likely to undergo change during a human lifetime. Many constellations of ideas gain significance and wider application with time, and some are refined into discrete categories, gradually detaching themselves from the more general concepts with which they were once connected by reason of superficial likeness.

With advancing years many people lose the freshness of the feelings with which they responded so readily during childhood and adolescence. The old man is apt to reflect sadly upon the vanished joyous effervescence of youth evoked by the very word; he is equally apt to have a stronger ethical objection than when he was young to words representing ugly and coarse aspects of life. He refrains from the use of many of the coarse words which the child inadvertently employs and which indecent young men use to sound forceful.

Thus anyone who believes that the meaning of a word is fixed and uniform must see only that an identical group of thoughts and feelings are evoked in a listener throughout a given interval of time. Measurement of this interval presents a problem and invites disagreement. No agreement that could come into consideration with the *ratio ruentis acervi* will persuade the student who understands the lightning-fast changes which occur not only in the content of a verbal utterance but in its relationship to other thought patterns.*

And there is another point of radical significance for the study of language. Let us stick with our example *Löwe* [lion]; it is by all means clear that in the sentence, *der Löwe kann die stärksten Knochen zermalmen* [the lion can crush the strongest bones], different characteristics of the animal are brought to consciousness from those in the sentence, *der Löwe ist ein edles königliches Tier* [the lion is a noble, royal animal]. In the first sentence we are conscious of the animal's powerful jaws, the power of his muscles, and of their application. Thus, we are conscious of their ability to devour a cow. In the second sentence we think of the animal's bearing and his physiognomy as an expression of his ethical

---

* *Editor's note*: Here Wegener anticipates the modern studies of affective connotative meaning. For example, the Semantic Differential is a technique, devised by Osgood, Luci, and Tannenbaum, which utilizes a set of seven-point scales, anchored by pairs of contrasting adjectives: good and bad; kind and cruel; active and passive; strong and weak; beautiful and ugly; and so forth. The task presented to the subject is to define the meaning of, say, a key word he himself uses repeatedly, by placing a check mark on each scale, thus building for a particular word a semantic profile. This may resemble or be in marked contrast to other words he also uses repeatedly, or neither of these alternatives may obtain. Models of connotative meaning may thus be utilized in the analysis of language, as was accomplished by R. L. Johnson and H. S. Gross in the case of an extravagantly and floridly deluded individual.

character; perhaps we also imagine certain magnanimous acts. How is the understanding of these sentences realized? The lion is noble, that is, the thoughts which we associate with the notion of the word *noble* [edel] may be connected with the *lion* group of thoughts. Evidently, it will not be connected with every thought in this group, rather only with a few of them. If we are successful in discovering from which of these few thoughts *noble* may be predicated, we can thereby amplify the predicate. If we are not successful, then the speaker must tell us with which thoughts this connection is possible. The speaker will then explain how the animal looks, how it behaves in the presence of human beings, and so forth. This exploration is nothing more than a selection of the available thoughts with which the predicate, by the addition of missing ideas, could be connected. And the speaker? All he is doing is stating what is presently in the foreground of his consciousness, the nobility, not the strength or the digestion. In the fact that it will always only be parts of a group of thoughts of which one is conscious (unless one is thinking reflectively) is to be found the reason for the very common phenomenon that the presentation of a subject is distorted, that is, too broad or too narrow.

We must therewith reject the assumption of the uniformity of word meaning.

The disadvantages of such an assumption are shown even more distinctly in another employment of the word: *He is the lion of the day* [er ist der Löwe des Tages]. The expression in this case positively excludes thinking about the yellow color of the lion, of his anatomical structure, or of his residence on the African plain. In such an expression, I personally can only think of the prominent role which a person so characterized must play.

Therefore, if we use a word within the complex of a sentence, its connection with the other words allows only one part of the group of thoughts which are connected to the word to become conscious. The others remain under the threshold of consciousness. And with regard to the logical subject of the sentence, only those parts of the groups of thoughts will become conscious which serve as exposition of the predicate.

XV

BUT even more important for the development of language is the question of how the logical predicate behaves in such connection. If I form the sentence: *Carthage was extinguished by Scipio the Younger* [Karthage wurde vom jüngeren Scipio ausgelöscht], I would perhaps only be fully understood by those who know that the relations of Scipio the Younger to Carthage consisted of his destruction of the city. This brings another significant fact to my exposition, namely, that Carthage is to be thought of in this example in the figure of a light. Others will say that the sentence makes no sense, but surely *Carthago exstincta est* must have been comprehensible to every Roman. Were the Romans psychically differently organized that we are? Most certainly not.

The German sentence would be more easily understood if I wanted to say: *Das Licht Karthagos wurde vom jüngeren Scipio ausgelöscht* [Carthage's light was extinguished by Scipio the Younger]; then I would add the elucidatory exposition to the logical predicate, that Carthage is to be thought of as a light. The Romans needed this exposition with *exstinguo* no more that we need one for the expression *der Krieg entbrennt* [war breaks out].

Actually we don't think any more about *entbrennen* [to be ignited] in this connection than we do about *ausbrechen* [to break out] when speaking about war, although if we thought about it for a while we could say that the expression *entbrennen* [to be ignited] presents war with the figure of a fire. But with *ausbrechen* [to break out], which is also a figurative expression with respect to its origin, it is impossible to discover certainly its original perceptual meaning any other way than with historical research. In the course of the development of language, the recollection of the original perceptual content from which one part of a group of thoughts receives its predication can be completely extinguished from linguistic consciousness.

Thus is shown to us a developmental series of metaphorical usage. It begins hypothetically with the requirement that in order to understand the metaphorical predicate, the exposition must indicate that the subject is to be thought of in terms of this object. It concludes with the situation when one no longer even senses the object from which the metaphorical expression was contrived.

Having given the above comments on the linguistic forms of the exposition, the naive man will quite often have added the exposition in a merely supplementary manner upon the demand of the listener. It is further evident that often this will not be required, if the whole situation is so transparent that the listener also understands the sense of the metaphor without an explanation.

The metaphor is based upon the association of groups of thoughts of partial similarity and, therefore, will always be individual. If a single individual has used an appropriate and felicitous metaphor, it will be applauded and copied, just as it is with fashion, and the metaphor will perhaps become part of current linguistic usage. An event of recent times might elucidate this process. Herbart compared the processes of the mind with mechanical movement: as physical bodies retarded each other the psychic ideas inhibited each other too. This conception gradually found approval, or at least the figure of speech was regarded as felicitous. Today every liberally educated man understands the expression *inhibition of ideas* [Hemmung der Vorstellungen]. One no longer needs the troublesome exposition *one must think of an idea as a mechanical quantity* [man hat sich die Vorstellung als mechanische Grösse zu denken].

In our example of the war it thus becomes evident within the sentences: *der Krieg entbrennt, der Krieg bricht aus* [war takes fire, war breaks out], that the only sense derived is that required of the situation. The thoughts which would otherwise be connected with the word *entbrennen* [to be ignited] are completely forgotten in this connection.

In this series of development there are three stages to be differentiated:

1. *War blazes up like a fire* [Der Krieg lodert auf wie ein Feuer]— one thus adds an expositive comment to the figurative idea. In this case, along with the beginning of the war, the moment of the fire's ignition is also conceived. Thus the substance of this expression is graphic and picturesque.

2. *War blazes up* [Der Krieg lodert auf]—one senses that the predicate is taken from the fire. However, one no longer contemplates the similarity of the two groups, because the comparison has already been made and is familiar; the comparison is shortened or compromised.

3. *War breaks out* [Der Krieg bricht aus]—we are now only aware of the ideas contained in the group war, no longer of those in the original simile.

This process is the same as that which has been called the wearing out and reduction of words. It is not by chance that I have described the process of reduction with figurative expressions. The necessary prerequisite for all reduction is that the logical subject and the logical predicate do not completely agree with each other, that the predicate does not completely coincide with its function. The reduction consists

precisely in the fact that the predicate loses all ideas which do not correspond to the situation determined by the subject, and that it assimilates all those ideas which are required by that situation.

This reduction can only take place with a logical predicate, because
the logical subject must correctly present the situation in its simple
reality. Therefore, it is not permitted to arouse any ideas which are not
found in the situation. Thus I can surely say *die Lohe des Kriegs ist
ausgebrochen* [the blaze of the war has broken out], but certainly in
speaking about the war, not simply *die Lohe ist ausgebrochen* [the blaze
has broken out]. However, if by reduction in the predication of *blazing*,
it had coincided with war, then it too could be the logical subject. The
interpreters of Horace thus rightfully objected to one segment where
Tiberius says:

> *impiger hostium*
> *Vexare turmas et frementem*
> *Mittere equum medios per ignes.*
> *(Odes* 4. 14. 22)

> [with warlike ire
> Their squads to vex, and through the fire
> To hurl his snorting steed.
> (Trans. by Dr. John Marshall)]

If *ignes* is related to the battle as the context demands, then this
figurative expression is used in the exposition where a simultaneous
correction and rectification is not possible. However, since it is very
improbable that *ignes* was reduced to the meaning of battle, we must
either reject this relationship to the battle, or here observe one of those
not isolated cases in which those rhetorical-poetical rules, upon which
the Romans educated themselves, led to affectation.

XVI

THE law discovered here is of the greatest significance for the development of word meaning and for the whole history of language.
If *dens*, ὀδούς, means *that which chews*, then in relation to a tooth, it
could only be a predicate, because in addition to the tooth there are many
other things which could be called *that which chews*. It would only be
able to be used as a logical subject after it had become congruent in the

extent and content of the thoughts given by the conception of the group of thoughts embodied in *tooth*. Thus, without exception, all words which could be logical subjects, that is, could form an exposition, first attain this capability by their reduction in use as a predicate. Before language possessed this reduced word for a logical subject, it was incapable of characterizing the situation any other way than by referring to a perceptual situation.

We want to clarify the particulars of this process, and the following discussion will give the basic reasons for this phenomenon. In our previous discussions we have dealt with the realization of congruity (1) of verbs like *ausbrechen* [to break out], *entbrennen* [to take fire] in relation to war, (2) of nouns like *dens* in relation to a tooth. Obviously the expression congruity must stand for something different in each case. In the first case, *der Krieg entbrennt* [war breaks out], the verb becomes congruent with the activity or with the condition which appeared as the beginning condition of the war. In the second case, *dens* becomes congruent with the group of thoughts which we indicate by the word *tooth*. However, in both cases it was the intention of the speaker to characterize that which was concerned, *thus beginning of the war* [Anfang des Krieges] and *tooth* [Zahn]. To arouse these respective thoughts was thus the task or function of the verb and of the noun. More keenly formulated, the predicate becomes congruent with its particular function.

The situation as a memory or as a perception always contains a noun element. If we say that the logical subject was developed from the logical predicate, we can only relate this to the word which characterizes the substance and such words we call nouns. We are now concerned with the question, how is it possible that predicate nouns can become logical subjects which congruently characterize the situation and which are always prepared to call a certain group of thoughts into the consciousness of all people involved? The expression *he who eats* [der Essende] calls a decidedly different group to consciousness than the expression *tooth* [Zahn].

Let us say that we are standing in front of a building, for which the congruent designation would be *castle* [Schloss]. Perhaps we are mainly astonished by its size and shout *an immense structure, a mighty work* [ein gewaltiges Bauwerk, ein mächtiger Bau]. We survey the lines and the groupings of the parts and call it a *beautiful, a noble, a magnificent work* [einen schönen, einen edlen, einen herrlichen Bau]. We observe the ornamentation and the foundation, and finding agreement with a certain historical form of architecture, we call the castle *a Renaissance building, a Gothic building, a Romanesque house* [ein Renaissancegebäude, einen gothischen Bau, ein romanisches Haus]. We become conscious of the human activity in it, as opposed to the works of nature, and we call it *a work* [ein Werk], *a structure* [ein Bauwerk]. Or, if this consciousness is associated with the feeling of human weakness in the face of God's omnipotence, we speak of *a work of man* [Menschenwerk]. If the purpose which the building served comes to mind, we say a *dwelling* [ein Wohnhaus], a *palace* [ein Palast], *a residential palace* [ein Residenzschloss]. Further designations would depend on the various connections made: *practical, comfortable building* [praktisches, wohnliches Gebäude], *castle* [Castell], *fortress* [Festung], and so on. Similarly, if a man named Müller stood before us, he could be a *wise, clever man* [ein weiser, kluger Mensch], *a fool* [ein Narr], *a scoundrel* [ein Schurke], *an ass* [ein Esel], and so forth.

All of these designations are judgments, and the names themselves are the predicates of the present perceptual picture. And with every predicate we are conscious that the perceptual picture is being further described for us. Of course, it is not designated immediately with its fully congruent name, rather the name of the perceptual picture is assigned to a certain category of ideas in our mind. This class or category, however, is not that type which would fully embrace the perceptual picture by its significant characteristics. Thus it could be Gothic buildings, churches, private homes, city halls, company houses, etc. The real category, whose significant characteristics are also the significant characteristics of the observed individual object, we designate as *castle* [Schloss]. Nevertheless, we attach the perceptive picture immediately to the category *castle* [Schloss], with the predicate *Gothic* [gothisch] as opposed to that designation *Gothic building* [gothisches Gebäude]. And from this we have the sensation of having heard a secure designation, which is only somewhat more copious than the pallid *castle* [Schloss]. Thus as opposed to the perceptual picture or, on the ground of the perceptual situation, the designation which is not sufficient or congruent to its function is completed to a congruent designation. But we must add that in this situation the designation is always completed as an individual designation, because the group of thoughts sensed with this designation is identical with the perceptual picture, and the perceptual picture is always individual. The castle under consideration is thus either Gothic, Romanesque, or something else. The designation itself, however, is general.

One asset of the imaginative writer is his ability to vary the names of the objects or persons of whom he is speaking. In various places where a noun designation is necessary he varies the designations, and they will be formed in the same manner as we have just discussed with the perceptual pictures. They are predicates of that object in its most diverse relationships. So if Rome is spoken of, it will later be indicated by *the city* [die Stadt], *the sink of iniquity (of the Roman empire or the Italian)* [das Babel (des römischen Reichs oder Italiens)], *the capital* [die Hauptstadt], *the city of seven hills* [die Siebenhügelstadt], *the city of the Tiber* [die Tiberstadt], and so forth. If Goethe is spoken of, instead of repeating the name, the author later says *the poet* [der Dichter], *the lyricist* [der Lyriker], *Karl August's friend* [der Freund Karl Augusts], *the man of genius* [der geniale Mann], *the noble spirit* [der edel Geist], *the son of the burgher from Frankfurt* [der Frankfurter Bürgersohn], and so on. If in a general presentation the four cardinal virtues are named, instead of the cardinal virtues they will be called *virtue* [Tugend], *moral character* [sittlicher Zustand], *morality* [sittlicher Character], *noble meaning* [Sittlichkeit, edler Sinn], and so forth.

In this case, the later designations are neither complete nor congruent with their function, but they will, nevertheless, be made so by remembrance of the former expositions. Thus the incomplete designations, which I will characterize as free designations, will become complete and congruent designations through the situation of remembrance. According to whether the once-created situation is individual or general, the free designations will thus be sensed as individual or general.

In villages situated near a certain city, for example, near Berlin, this is a common expression *to go to the city* [nach Stadt gehen] or *to the city* [in die Stadt]. No one thinks of any other city but Berlin. Thus the city of which one is most conscious, and the city most probably referred to by the activity expressed in the verb, will be understood by the listener from this free designation. It is obvious that *city* is not a sufficient expression for Berlin. Yet, within the narrowly limited horizons of the listener as well as those of the speaker, only this city is thought of, and therefore the appropriate group of thoughts can be associated most easily. Thus the free designation will be sensed as congruent on the ground of the situation of consciousness, as we have already called this type of situation. The group of thoughts with the designation is individual. Likewise, in all expressions within a limited circle, as in *to go to the castle* [aufs Schloss gehen], *the church (local church)* [die Kirche (Ortskirche)], *to the ale-house* [in den Krug], *to the pub and to the school* [auf die Kneipe und in die Schule], the speaker will be thinking of a certain school, church, and so on.

Within a certain house *the closet* [der Schrank], *the suitcase* [der Koffer], *the kitchen* [die Küche], *the piano* [das Clavier], *the bookcase* [der Bücherschrank] are quite definite particular items. If one imagines that next to the first city a second one arose at the same distance from the village, this one would perhaps be called the new city [Neustadt or neue Stadt]. Thus these are nothing but individual characterizations which sometimes are the same as the actual names which originated in this manner, whence come so many names with *houses, house, burg,* and the like. Similarly, personal names like *Karl or August* within a small community designate a very definite person.

But we find within a small community not only the supplementation of a general expression with an individual one through the power of the situation of consciousness and without the necessity of further words, but equally so the supplementation of a genre with a type. The miner thinks of *Todliegend* [lying dead] as a certain type of stone; the student thinks of *Rein* [clean] and *Unrein* [dirty] as fair copy and outline respectively; *der Erste* [first] and *Letzte* [last] in student circles, is he who occupies the first or last place in the class. For the foot soldier *mit vollem Gepäck* [with complete luggage] means with satchel, coat, and haversack; for the Roman, *insigne* means insignia, *bonum* good, *mortales* the concept of man. We have here basically the same phenomenon as in the process of development of the general expression to the individual one. The difference is here only to be found in the consciousness of the speaker and the listener, otherwise the expression could be related to many individual things. The student thus attaches a particular meaning to the word when he says he has finished his *Unreine,* that is, his outline.

It is equally possible to understand type or individual designations as general, if the situation of consciousness gives supplementary help. The well-known verse *sint Maecenates, non derunt, Flacce, Marones* shows us the way in which the Roman *Palatium* could provide the source for the naming of *emperor's palaces, palace, palatinate.* People and individual perceptual pictures have their unique character, that is, the sum of their individual qualities. According to these, the genres can be characterized. These designations will be sensed as complete by the situation of consciousness.

The really important type of situation in the transformation of the logical predicate to the logical subject is, therefore, the situation of consciousness. The situation of perception and of remembrance vanish again after a short time. But the situation of consciousness, of the most easily associated groups of thoughts, can originate only when the situation of perception and of remembrance become fixed in our mind by frequency and interest. To this degree, both of those types of momentary situations are significant for the development of word meaning.

The multiplicity of denominations is especially conspicuous in the names and designations of the gods. Both Zeus and Odin are polyonymous. Some points of view from which dead objects can be named were mentioned above. These same points of view naturally come into consideration with people and gods also. Here, however, the ethical designations, as well as deeds attached to these people play a large part, thus the historical consciousness. Such surnames as *Numantinus, Afri-*

canus, Asiaticus of the Scipios are well known; frequently enough these surnames must designate the person himself without the addition of an exposition. Prevalent among the gods are such surnames as *Delius, Pythius, Cypria,* and so on.

With *Delius, Cypria* and other denotations based on extraction, a misunderstanding would be very easily possible, but here the predicate is added as elucidation. Thus *Africanus Carthaginem delevit* distinctly means the younger Scipio, because this fact makes no sense with anyone else. This is the exposition of the logical subject by means of the logical predicate, a means of exposition which empowers the listener to differentiate which one contains the name of the logical subject as a congruent designation, from the types or individuals of a group. We will bring the particulars of this process into the following investigation.

It is self-evident that in this development from free naming to a concrete, congruent name, we are concerned not only with the simple words but also with words which, as compounds, are under an accent like *Bettelmann* [beggar man], *Rathaus* [city hall] and other compounds such as *Edelmann* [nobleman], *Rotkehlchen* [robin redbreast], *Gelbschnabel* [greenhorn] which have arisen from an attributive connection of adjective and noun. Their original meaning was attached to the group from which they were predicated. However, they were only sensed as complete if the exposition was given by perception, remembrance, or consciousness. It is the same with certain connections of adjective and noun which haven't developed to a complete compound: *the gray lion* [der graue Löwe], *the speckled, the striped hyena* [die gefleckte, die gestreifte Hyäne], *the yellow fever* [das gelbe Fieber], *the black death* [der schwarze Tod], *Asiatic cholera* [die asiatische Cholera], *gray salve* [graue Salbe], *the guilty part* [der schuldige Teil], *malicious abandonment* [böswillige Verlassung], *negligent killing* [fahrlässige Tötung], *sulphurous acid* [schweflige Säure]. All of these denominations as fixed names designate certain categories or groups in which not only the linguistically named characteristics are contained, but also many others. These denominations have become congruent with the thoughts connected with such categories.

Thus the child's and primitive man's need for communication led to sentences composed of single words. These no longer suffice for a complicated situation. Man needs more copious means of exposition; the material for these means is supplied by the words which as predicates of the primitive sentence have been reduced, and whose groups of related perceptions and thoughts have become congruent. With the help of these means the speaker supplements the insufficiencies of the exposition which were disclosed to him by the interrupting question and the unresponsive facial features of the listener. These corrective forms become established forms of speech, whose origin the consciousness of language has completely forgotten. Originally sketches, by which the distorted picture was improved by supplementation, they become the established and basic contours whereby a later consciousness of language can have the logically pleasing feeling of clarity, and the aesthetic-ethical sensation of beauty and nobility.

One will perceive how the basic ideas of the investigations presented here point further in all directions, how they are of significance as aspects of the history of knowledge, ethics, and aesthetics. This is because all phenomena of human mentality form a self-contained living organism, and the stimulation of one single unit of this organism thereafter causes vibrations in the other units, and the results of this, poetry and art, nobility of mind and ethical grace, developed on the twigs and branches of this organism. From this woody edifice several fibers and cells came under closer consideration here.

Understanding Speech

ALL known human language is articulated. It is not a sum or aggregate of natural tones and sounds. All sounds truly related in a language are formed by a great number of individuals guided by a general norm. From living with other individuals, the accomplished speaker has learned the way in which to form these sounds and how to connect groups of them to form a definite meaning. However, we learn a language by becoming accustomed to associating a certain sound image with a certain meaning, and by comprehending the association of these sound images together to form a definite sense. But who has told us what meaning should be associated with those groups of sounds? No one; because no one can tell us unless he first understands the language himself. It is quite clear that linguistic understanding is not dependent solely on the knowledge of the words and their meanings, nor on the knowledge of syntactical forms and their meanings. Otherwise, we would never understand language nor learn how to use it independently. *It is thus important for the understanding of the existence and development of language to state clearly which factors and processes make it possible for us to understand language at all, and to investigate in what way these factors gain significance for the formation of language.*

The Cause and Purpose of Speaking

I

OUR first question concerns the cause and the purpose of speaking, a more difficult question than it might at first appear. All speaking has a cause, but not all speaking has a social purpose. Aimless

speaking is monologue, primarily at the same level of involuntary reflex sounds as coughing, clearing the throat, sneezing, smacking one's
tongue, audible breathing, wheezing, groaning, moaning, crying,
laughing and cries of pain. These inarticulate, natural sounds cannot
be considered as actual speech. For, although moral and aesthetic regard for beauty and education plays a large part in transforming the
form of such outbursts of feeling and brings about the wide range of
diversity in their articulation, these emotional exclamations lack the
makeup of the established sound system of language. On the other
hand, these interjections are part of speech: *o, ach, weh, na nu, ach
Herrje, brr, äks, pfui, ei, Donnerwetter, tausend, potztausend, Gott,
Christes ne* [oh, ah, woe, well, oh, my goodness, burr, hey, fie, indeed,
damn it, great Scott, God, good Christ, no] and many others. They too,
will be aimlessly uttered in certain emotional situations.

These exclamations are not merely naturally formed sounds, but in
many cases are engendered by words of speech, like *God* [Gott] *damn
it* [Donnerwetter]. The invocation, *God*, and the curse, *damn it*, are
actually forms of prayer, presume an addressed person, the diety, and
thus originate in purposeful dialogic speaking. Thus also, dialogic words
are so firmly interwoven with certain processes of sensation that they
too will sometimes be spoken involuntarily—that is, without a definite
conscious purpose.

Indeed, there may be no substantial difference between the interjection and the syntactically structured exclamatory sentence. The shouts
oh, how beautiful that is [ach wie schön ist das], *how magnificant* [wie
herrlich], *how ghastly* [wie grässlich], *too beautiful* [zu schön], are
sometimes clauses not meant to be heard. They are, rather, the involuntary outbursts of our emotions. The form of the sentence with the interrogative *how* [wie] is borrowed from dialogic speech, where the
question is asked with the intention of receiving an answer.

We thereby observe the well-known transition from arbitrary to automatic movements. This is understandable enough, since speech is actually a movement. For the listener these monologic sounds and groups
of sounds are signs of certain mental processes that he must understand,
because they engender the same sounds in himself as well as in others.

Without further ado, we might here consider monologic speech as it
is employed in drama. Here the transition is even more extensive, because the customary sentences consist of expositive elements which were
chosen originally only with regard to the addressed person. An interesting and important question is: to what extent does the monologue
come under the influence of strong emotion in real life? I can offer very
little as a solution; but I would like to call attention to the fact that with
strong emotion, probably always but certainly often, a disturbance of the

situation of consciousness enters—that is, the illusion that we are facing some person with feelings of hate or love, pain or joy, fear or hope. The dramatic monologue is also very often clearly within the power of this illusion. Let us take, for example, the closing monologue in Egmont. Here Egmont is primarily addressing Alba: *Malevolent man! You didn't believe you would confer such kindness upon me by means of your son* [Feindseliger Mann! Du glaubtest nicht mir diese Wohltthat durch deinen Sohn zu erzeigen']. Then apart from the addresses, *Sweet sleep* [süsser Schlaf], *you beautiful picture* [du schönes Bild], *daylight has scared you away!* [das Licht des Tages hat dich verscheucht!] He turns to the people of the Netherlands, *Stride on! Good People! The goddess of victory is leading you!* [Schreitet durch! Braves Volk! Die Siegesgöttin führt dich an!]

Lady Macbeth converses similarly with her husband in the monologue (act I, scene 5):

> *Glamis and Cawdor art thou, and wilt become*
> *What is prophesied to these.*
>
> [Glamis und Cawdor bist du, und sollst werden
> Was dir verheissen ist!]

Likewise, Banquo (act III, scene 1):

> *Thou hast it now: King, Cawdor, Glamis, everything.*
> *According to the prophesy.*
>
> [Da hast's nun: König, Cawdor, Glamis, Alles,
> Nach der Verheissung]

It can be observed from one's own experience that at times one imagines oneself in a situation of a conversation, an argument, a speech, or the proposal of a motion, and that one then forms words and sentences which could perhaps be used in such situations. Yet these forms may actually never be uttered audibly. One can't dismiss the possibility that in developing the dramatic dialogue, this artificial means may have sprung from a mistake of the dramatist, who had to communicate certain of his characters' thoughts to the listener and who let the characters themselves relate these thoughts, thereby unconsciously exceeding the limits of his artificial means and slipping back into the epic situation. The approach to many lyric situations is also closely related to this question, since true lyric poetry is an outburst of emotion which, according to the whole situation involved, is not affected by the addressed person. Even if the lyric poet thinks also of his reading audience, as in the literary times of today, still, this thought is meaningless for the lyrical situation itself. Nevertheless, a lyrical work of art must contain those elements of exposition from which the atmosphere is to be made intelligible to the reader, because the communication of these elements must appear to be completely purposeful. Thus the question as to what extent expressive lyric poetry is the artificial cultivation of the natural human artless outburst of emotion can only be answered through an exhaustive treatment of the extent and the nature of monologic speech.

II

THE foremost purpose and intention of dialogue is to influence the listener in a specific way. The groups of sounds here are thus means of speech.

The view that the purpose of all speech is the communication of ideas certainly contains an element of truth if one limits this definition to the dialogue; but which ideas do we communicate, and why? The definition is also too narrow in that all influencing of the mind in its various forms in language (such as the imperative, the request, the challenge) does not appear to us as communication of ideas. Moreover, that which is actually stated is not always the purpose of our speech.

The purpose of speech is always to influence the mind or judgment of a person in a way that seems valuable to the speaker. Thus, in forms of commanding and wishing, the mind of the addressed person is to be primed for action; in the question, it is to be primed for an explanation about groups of thoughts valuable to the speaker. The demanded action and requested answer are no more a purpose in themselves than the food which we require; they are merely a means to a higher purpose. The imperative phrases *just consider* [überlege mal, ob], *just think* [denk dir mal]; Latin *recognosce mecum, iam intelleges*, contain the rhetorical question (represented by the conditional clause in German), which is not the main purpose of the linguistic utterance, rather only an aid, a means. These phrases, in their subordinate significance, are partly distinguished because they have become subordinate clauses used to satisfy one's feeling for language.

The purposes are arranged like the feelings of value in an infinitely graduated system. The world of values begins with the elementary sensual desire-stimulation, continues through the whole series of sensations of desire to the purest desire of all, inner ethical gratification. This world of values includes the feeling of desire for satisfied curiosity, and of proud accomplishment with which we are filled, for example, on having solved a difficult scientific problem.

These values are the aims of the linguistic means. With them, the speaker tries to influence the mind of the addressed person either to gratify his own selfish desires, to urge him toward selfless ethical action, or to reveal to him through advice and teaching the good things in life. With these means he tries with selfish conviction to convince the listener of the justification of his views, as well as to lead an ill-bred and poorly educated person to good human judgment, and to disclose to him the ideals of his own view of life. Further discussion of such purposes belongs to the sphere of ethics.

Both light small-talk and the strait-laced fulfillment of an obligation in a conversation are always designed for one purpose, the realization of something valuable. Either the speaker may want to arouse enthusiasm for his own interests, or he may try to refresh some cherished memories. He might even wish to appear brilliant and, thereby, win respect or he might be trying to satisfy etiquette, thus avoiding the contempt of society.

All the purposes of the speaker can be placed in two main classes, which are both ethically and psychically related to each other: (1) to arouse sympathy or interest for one's own ideas or value judgments, and (2) to show sympathy and interest for the ideas and values of others.

The first category contains the selfish purposes, the second contains the selfless. It is quite apparent that *a selfish purpose can become the means to a selfless purpose*, and vice versa, because all inferior purposes are means to higher ones. In this way the acquisition of money can become the means to charity and humanitarianism. Conversely, the support of a needy person can become the means to one's own advance. The forms of selfish purposes can equally be the means to selfless purposes, as orders and demands are means of education. Conversely, the use of flattery as proof of sympathy for unfamiliar ideas is really a means for selfish purposes.

In the same way that society would deteriorate if its members were ruled purely by selfish purposes, so too would the speech dependent upon society deteriorate. This is because *sympathy is the most fundamental prerequisite for all understanding of speech*. Without it, no mother would understand the crying of her child as a summons for help; no one would understand the tearfully spoken *roll* [Butterbrot], *my boots* [meine Stiefeln] as an imperative. No one would understand the pointing at an object within view as a request to look at the man, house, animal or room. Indeed, no one would even listen to a speaker, or follow the antics of a dumb person, if this basic ethical element were lacking in man.

The importance of sympathy for the most basic of all human activity, that is, speech, clearly demonstrates that man, in living with his fellow human beings, must cultivate his sympathetic instincts and, thereby, attain a basis for all morality. This is a development in man which adapts itself with the same certainty and necessity in society as does the development of temporal and spatial perception.

But the understanding of speech would be equally impossible if the selfish instinct were lacking in us, if we didn't ask about the purpose of every linguistic utterance of another person. We would not be in a position to recognize the means to a purpose in this linguistic utterance if we didn't assume from our own example that every man undertakes certain action only when he wants to attain something.

The selfish instinct thus causes us to regard another's speech as purposeful, whereas sympathy causes us to pay attention to another's speech and to interpret it. The criteria and the patterns by which both take place are founded upon our own states of desire and emotional excitement. We unconsciously assume that the speaker has the same psychic processes and the same psychic organism as we ourselves. The sympathetic frame of mind is really the state of sensibility which even provides the possibility of the interpretation of unfamiliar ideas.

The Influencing of the Mind

III

IF WE construe those whining cries of roll [Butterbrot], *bottle* [Fläschchen], *my boots* [meine Stiefeln], *in the sense of an imperative,* we have then concluded, following the example of our own mental processes, that the reason for the crying is condition of pain. According to the course of our own sensations, we conclude further that *roll* [Butterbrot] must be related to the feelings of pain. Since a roll by itself usually causes a child no pain, we conclude further—again following our own example, also because we can see no roll in the child's hand—that he is without a roll, and, therefore, desires one. From this is derived the further conclusion that this feeling of pain is hunger. We now feel in us the ethical voice of sympathy, which summons us to help the suffering child. With this originates the idea of the imperative meaning of that form of speech.

Had the child had the roll in his hand when he cried, it would have led to completely different findings, namely, that the child didn't want to eat the roll. Thus the interpretation of the cry of pain, along with the thought content of the word and the perceptual situation, leads to understanding.

Had the child eaten the roll and cried out *roll* [Butterbrot] in the same way, the interpretations could be (1) another roll, or (2) the roll has caused the child pain. In this case the memory of the listener must intervene in the interpretation of the actual situation. Thus the external elements from which the interpretation is derived are in themselves by no means such that they must give a suitable conclusion; there may be ambiguity.

The same reasoning applies to the question as it does to the imperative. We hear the astonished exclamation *table* [Stuhl], *chair* [Tisch], and see the eye of the speaker directed at us, and we conclude that he expects something from us. We know the discomforting feeling of confusion, which comes from the inability to recognize something, or from the inability to find a relationship among certain thoughts. Using our knowledge of the speaker's awareness and frame of mind and, further, of the peculiarity of the situation, we can tell from the astonished cry *chair* [Stuhl], whether the distressed person is unable to recognize the chair as a perceptual picture; whether he is looking for a chair which he expects to find here; or whether he cannot grasp the relationship of the chair to his present situation. If we have deduced all of this, we are sympathetic to the uneasy emotions of the speaker, and we respond to the ethical demand to help him and to give him information.

We feel this sympathetic demand to bring help in the face of another's suffering, even when he does not employ linguistic means. *A means, however, is anything whose effect we ourselves have experienced, and only this. Means are not invented, but discovered.* If we have experienced the sympathetic effect of another person's expressions of suffering (for example, crying), then these expressions will seem to us well-suited to obtain the same sympathetic effect with other people. And so the *purposeless monologic utterances* and all other reflex utterances whose effect we have experienced will become *means for our purposes.* Therefore, the child cries in order to influence his mother, as soon as he notices the effect of his tears upon her. Therefore, one can only break the child's crying habit if one does not allow the intended effect to materialize.

Thus is proven *a double transfer of monologic speech and dialogue.*

The purposeless utterances become purposeful utterances because of the effect they have; on the other hand, through the mechanization of movement, the meaningful utterances may change themselves into purposeless monologic outbursts of noise again. Through this process, the dialogue receives phonetic signs from the multitude of reflex sounds, and the reflex sounds become more and more incorporated into the system of sound and word formation created by the dialogue. As a result of an evolution, neither the sensation sounds nor the tones of a speaking man, nor even the sentence melody, are to be regarded as natural sounds. The melodic succession of tones within a word and within sentences is very diverse. Even though no one hears fully the melody in the dialect which he himself speaks, he hears it all the better in the dialects of the other language communities. The silent pointing with the hand and directing with the eyes are also seemingly purposeless, but as a consequence of their effectiveness they become purposeful means.

From what we have just said, one can easily see how a vocable, a word which was previously unknown, is revealed from the other perceptions from which we obtain our understanding of speech. One can see, too, how in this connection such a word must gradually be sensed as an effective means, and how it gradually attains its meaning and substance from the ensemble of elements which forces the listener to those conclusions which we call the understanding of speech. I am only indicating this process here, because I do not plan to lead the investigation into these primitive stages of vocabulary learning, but rather into the developed stages, where the vocabulary has become well-known and fluent to the speaker and listener. At this time I would like to point out, however, that *words, above all, are not first learned as containers of sounds with specific substance, but as means to definite purposes.* What we are accustomed to calling the content of words is the most faded abstraction in which the use of a word for the most varied purposes gradually divests the word of its character as a means. This character remains only with those words which always have one and the same or only a few functions—those words with a one-sided formal function, such as conjunctions, articles, pronouns, and prepositions. It would be just the same for *roll* [Butterbrot], *bottle* [Fläschchen], *my boots* [meine Stiefeln], if, in speech, these words served only the purpose of quieting hunger or protecting bare feet.

IV

I T MIGHT appear that the ethical and psychic facts obtained above by dissection and analysis are of importance during the first stages of speaking and understanding, but lose their effectiveness very quickly. This impression is incorrect; the same factors remain continually active in the life of speech. However, with the traditional imperative form of the verb and the grammatically firmly established forms of the question, we no longer sense these rather complicated conclusions. *But it is a general psychic law that complicated series of conclusions through frequency and habituation disappear so quickly that consciousness of the individual intermediate conclusions becomes completely lost,* and that the components of the conclusion can only be found again with reflective analysis. It is the same with the formation of space perception, with the illusive movements of facile piano playing, with reading, and with all technical dexterity. These intermediate conclusions should therefore be executed more slowly and more clumsily by a child than by an adult; that is, in fact, the case.

Equally valid is the law that originally spontaneous and conscious means will gradually be used automatically and unconsciously. Just as, therefore, the speaker in the end, conscious of his purpose and without consideration, purely mechanically reaches for the imperative and question forms, so also the means must summon the purpose mechanically into the consciousness of the accomplished listener. This mechanization of the means of speech is a necessary prerequisite for the cultivation of speech to its higher and highest tasks. In the same manner, the mechanization of the technical movements first guarantees the craftsman or artist the complete success of his creative activity, or the mechanization of the muscle activity in walking and the difficult performances of the tightrope walker or bareback rider brings assurance and complete self-control.

Forms of speech which in a language community have become the automatic and mechanical means of their purposes, merely summon this purpose into the consciousness of the listener. Thus, one can also call them *congruent speech signals from the standpoint of the understanding of speech*. They are congruent in that the thought content which was really consciously accomplished by them is the same as the thought content which they sought.

The *Indo-Germanic imperative form* was naturally not immediately mechanized. The second person singular was the pure stem, and, as long as the verb was not actually declined, these stems were used in all other syntactical connections. They were thus kept alive for the later stages of speech in the vocative of the singular (later in the first components of many compounds, such as *parricida* [patricide], ἀνδροκτόνος [man-slaughter], *Wohnhaus* [apartment-house], and so on, the really genuine Indo-Germanic compounds) where they perform the same function as the limitative genitive. In the stage of the Indo-Germanic language before declension, an assumption was necessary in every instance in order to understand the meaning or function of the stem for each individual case.

Modern languages have never had a special word arrangement *for the question*, and even now the interrogative word arrangement is not peculiar to interrogative sentences alone. The same arrangement is used in interpolated clauses. Thus the determination of the syntactical purpose is still only possible with assumptions, even though these may disappear very swiftly. Certain types of *Greek questions* clearly demonstrate the way in which an inference is drawn. The basic pattern for this usage is in the forms of οὐ in a sentence like: *Then he hasn't come* [also er ist nicht gekommen], or in the forms with μή: *May he be prevented from coming* [behüte dass er gekommen ist]. I do not want to inquire at this time to what extent the named connections can be regarded as sufficient interrogative introductions, and whether or not the etymological consciousness has been preserved in one or another of these connections. These questions have not yet been fully answered.

Such sentences implying a conclusion spoken in a tone of astonishment frequently serve as a question in German too, but in our language this form is not mechanized, as it is in Greek. However, in Greek the form with οὔκουν [indeed not] is only used in cases where the speaker in the situation could find no definitive inducement for that type of conclusion.

The mechanization of the means of speech is precisely the reason why the chosen form is no longer understood according to its original meaning, but only in its function for a purpose; this is *the obscuration of the etymological consciousness.*

The original Greek interrogative form contains, aside from the tone of astonishment, no indication of the request for information. It is nothing more than an astonished assertion; it is equally so in the interrogative sentences with μή, meaning *by no means* [behüte], or *hopefully, that isn't the case* [hoffentlich ist das nicht der Fall]. The mechanization is clearly shown here by the use of μή in an indicative main clause. The request for information can only be inferred by the listener from the uncertainty with which the speaker states his assertion. The Latin interrogative sentences with *ne* and *num* are also negative assertions of this type, as is shown by the meaning of *ne* in *ne-que, ne-cessarius,* and so on; furthermore the meaning of *num* in *num-quam* along with *um-quam* are merely mechanized assertions.

The astonished assertion is, however, not always mechanized. It lives freely in the language, of course not using *ne* and *num.* These little words can only eke out their livelihood in mechanized usage.

The tone of astonishment can also be designated as a *mechanized means of speech.* It too can be replaced by words which express the lack of understanding in a freer manner. Instead of saying in astonishment *There is a chair missing here* [hier fehlt ein Stuhl], we can also say *There is a chair missing here, I don't understand that* [hier fehlt ein Stuhl, das verstehe ich nicht], or *I cannot understand why there is a chair missing here* [ich verstehe nicht, dass hier ein Stuhl fehlt]. The tone of astonishment indicates the uneasy feeling of not understanding and thus has an effect upon the sympathy of the listener. The sentence *That I don't understand* [das verstehe ich nicht] reports the fact of lack of comprehension and, from this, allows the uneasy feeling to be inferred. At the same time it could be understood as a request to have information given; not necessarily, of course, but in certain situations.

Therefore one can say that *before speech has obtained mechanized means through habituation the question can only be indicated by astonished intimation.* We now differentiate *two categories of the question*: (1) *the question of substantiation,* for example, *Has A gone away?* [ist A forgegangen?], in which the speaker requests information as to whether a supposition of his is correct; and (2) *the question of supplementation,* for example, *Who did that?* [wer hat das gethan?], *Whom did you see?* [wen hast du gesehen?], *how, where, why* [wie, wo, warum], and so forth, in which there is an inquiry about an unknown part of the thought relationship, although the fact itself is certain and known.

The Indo-Germanic languages have developed certain *pronouns* for this second class which have *interrogative* as well as *indefinite* meaning: Latin *quis, qui, ubi* (from *cubi*), *unde* (*cunde*), *quo; OHG hwer, NHG wer, was, wo, wie, warum* [who, what, where, how, why]. These questions have also emerged from assertions in the tone of astonishment; *quis (who) fecit?* actually means *someone has done it* [irgend einer hat es gethan]. To this type of assertion the listener feels himself obligated to give an answer.

This form of the question of supplementation is alive even today.

Someone searching for something can thus say: *somewhere I have laid the book down* [irgendwo habe ich das Buch hingelegt], and since this indefinite *somewhere, some, who* [irgendwo, irgend, wer] is itself a mechanized means of expressing ignorance, even the expression *I don't know the man who did that* [ich kenne den Mann nicht, der gas gethan hat] could in certain circumstances be construed as a question.

V

SINCE we are continually making the observation, on the one hand, that certain expressions influence us in a definite way and, on the other hand, that unintentional expressions of our own have an effect upon others, then *new means of speech must be continually created.* Since effectiveness always obeys the same psychic-ethical laws, the newly created means must always be *formed according to the same laws. The actual field of observation* for the effectiveness of the means of speech is therefore *the freely executed presentation, not the mechanized syntactical forms,* in which the succession of conclusions is shortened. The syntactical mechanizations are, like fossils, only intelligible from freely executed speech.

The painful tone of the imperative which arouses sympathy can, as in the case of the question, be replaced by the actual communication of pain. One who goes to the doctor says: *my arm hurts, my eye is paining me* [mir thut der Arm weh, das Auge schmerzt mich], and thinks thereby that he has requested the doctor to come to his aid; the latter understands him in this sense. In order to obtain food or drink the child says *I am so hungry, I am thirsty* [ich bin so hungrig, ich habe Durst]; the child who wants to be taken to bed complains: *I am so tired* [ich bin so müde]. Thus mere arousal of sympathy through communication of suffering serves as an imperative influencing of the mind.

In order to be an effective imperative, the suffering person's expressions of pain must immediately show his wish or will. The actual communication of what our wish or will is, may, of course, be equally effective as an imperative. If we enter a book store and say *I wish to have the Lessing, I would like the Goethe, I would very much like to have an Atlas* [ich wünsche den Lessing, ich möchte den Goethe, ich hätte gern einen Atlas], and the salesman senses in this communication of desire the demand to bring the appropriate book, he might even answer *At your service* [zu Befehl]. The Romans use the form *hoc factum volo* for a "measured command." From the given examples, the importance of the assumption of a definite purpose or an intention of the speaker for comprehension again becomes clear. Had the book salesman not assumed that the speaker wished to obtain something through communication, then his interpretation would not have recognized the imperative.

Wish or will is aroused by the idea or thought of something good or valuable. Children who see cake on the table want to have it; the gourmet salivates at the mention of oysters and champagne. In most cases it therefore suffices to excite the mind of the addressed person merely by naming a valuable object or by indicating its value. If the child sees someone eating cake and says *cake sure tastes great* [ja Kuchen schmeckt schön] or *cake is my favorite food* [Kuchen ist mein Lieblingsessen], the listener concludes from this that he should share some of the cake. Since the child connects his intention with the words, that is, to receive some of the cake, and since the listener has the fulfillment of this desire in his hand, the words will be sensed as a demand of the will.

A wish can only become will if we believe that it can be fulfilled. In the described situation, the child must regard the wish's capability of being fulfilled as dependent upon the will of the listener. Such influencing of the mind is called *dropping a broad hint*, that which allows no misunderstanding. This probability of understanding proves the following *important psychic fact: we apply indefinitely made expressions of speech in which something general is comprehended as something specific in the view or consciousness of the given case. It is as if one were speaking not of a general, but of a concrete case.* Thus, through perception, a general sentence is made into a concrete group of ideas. For the most part this fact is the same as the one we discussed in the giving of names and in predication. For example, the words *man, closet* [Mensch, Schrank], in a present perceptual picture, or in an individual picture held in memory, in spite of their general meaning, will be sensed as congruent as an individual picture. However, in the first case we were concerned with the predicate, here we are concerned with a complete sentence.

The same process is frequently found in moral admonitions in general sentences. These sentences will be sensed as predicates of one's own ethical frame of mind and must appear individually. If we say to a dissatisfied person, for example: *only the satisfied one is happy* [nur der Zufriedene ist glücklich], he feels that the statement is a judgment of his dissatisfaction. The same thing happens with teasing; with ironic statements, the spoken thoughts will be given a new interpretation consciously or perceptively.

We do not need a special presentation to demonstrate that the same relationships which play a part in the positive influencing of the mind are also shown on the negative side, in the *prohibition*. The only new factor is that with prohibition, the speaker makes the assumption each time that the addressed person intends or desires to do something specific. The speaker wants to prevent just this assumed and feared action.

It is well-known that in such a case a mere disapproving wave of the hand (evidently a shortened and mechanized gesture to defend against the approach of something evil), a threatening or warning raised finger, or a *no, don't* [nicht, nicht, doch] is sufficient. The relation of the defense to excitement of the will consciously present, or to the action about whose execution we are anxious, is easy to draw; but this does not mean that we have given it the correct interpretation. If a servant is passing food around the table, and the hostess makes a defensive motion, it could be interpreted according to the circumstances as: *don't pass it around* [nicht herumreichen], or *don't present it to the people in question* [nicht den betreffenden Personen präsentieren], or *not from that side* [nicht von der Seite], or *not in that fashion* [nicht in der Form]. If the person addressed correctly understands the motion, comprehension can only be won by reflection: what could be forbidden in the prevailing circumstances? The conclusion can only be drawn from a comparison of the actual event with the consciousness of what is due and the normal awareness of what is correct. *But the conclusion is never inevitable, only probable. Consequently the understanding of linguistic expression depends upon the possibility of relating thoughts to each other*, an important psychic law.

Disapproving motion and the prohibitive negation are mechanized means; the free means of speech which serve this purpose are based upon the same mental processes as the means of the imperative.

Among the means of influencing the mind are also found *the threat and the promise*. Here also the listener must first deduce the intention of the influence. One says: *It will be bad for you if you do that, you will get hit if . . .* [es wird dir schlecht gehen, wenn du das thust, du erhältst Schläge, wenn . . .]. This sentence is of a very general type; it means *Every time you do that, you will get hit* [in jedem Falle, wenn du das thust, erhältst du Schläge]. Thus, this general sentence must be related by the listener to its specific intention. It is also not stated from whom the addressed will receive the blows. This will all be inferred from the relation of the general sentence to the specific intention. With mechanized forms of the threat, in which aposiopesis is frequently found, it will no longer be sensed at all that the speaker is speaking generally, for example, *too bad if you do that; well if you do that, you'll really do it* [wehe dir, wenn du das thust; na, wenn du das thust, thust du das]. The threatening tone, which has many degrees of intensity and severity, makes comprehension easier.

The promise must be likewise deduced, for example, *a gulden for a glass of water, a kingdom for a horse!* [einen Gulden für ein Glas Wasser, ein Königreich für ein Pferd!]. This threat is incapable of being misunderstood. *Take a look at the whip* [Sieh dir mal die Peitsche an] or *Do you know the switch?* [Kennst du die Rute?]. In this case, however, only the idea of something bad is brought to mind. The connection of this with the intention meant by bringing this to mind must be inferred by the listener himself, today as it was in ancient times. It therefore suffices to point out the whip, or to indicate the switch, or to say *For nice children I have something nice* [Für artige Kinder habe ich etwas Schönes].

There are even more forms of the influencing of the mind which can be observed, such as the *question as inquiry*. For example, if one inquires of a salesman whether he carries a certain item the intention of buying the item is immediately inferred. Because the knowledge of this fact must be valuable to the person inquiring, the salesman thus concludes from the most obvious thought complex that the inquirer wants to buy the item. This is only *one* of many interpretations, however, because the statistician can use the same question for completely different purposes.

Especially common is the question *why not* [warum nicht], for example, *Why don't you go* [warum gehst du nicht]; in Latin the corresponding interrogative form is completely mechanized with *quin*. This question has retained its etymologically justified construction with the indicative *quin conscendimus equos* [Why don't we mount up?]. If *quin conscendite, quin conscendamus* [why not mount, why don't we mount?] is also said, however, a construction appears which is appropriate for the whole purpose of the expression, thus for the function of the whole question, but not for its etymological form.

Since the established speech forms of influencing the mind are also based upon such possible interpretations, then in the time of their free usage, that is, before they become mechanized, they must have allowed other interpretations. But as soon as they become mechanically active their meaning appears fixed. They become congruent with their purpose.

The artificially fashioned public speech pursues the purpose of persuading a number of individuals to perform a certain action, or of dissuading them from a definite plan, or both simultaneously, as for example, in Cicero's speech *de imperie Gnaei Pompei*. This too is an *imperative or prohibitive speech form of influencing the mind*. A legal speech tries to persuade the judge to acquit or convict; the preacher attempts to move the listener to a definite manner of religious and moral conduct. They are all nothing more than the influencing of the mind, using linguistic means. And for all these speakers, there are no other means at their disposal than those which have been shown as imperative or prohibitive.

In addition to the multitude of free means of speech, they must also use, as a matter of course, the mechanized means of influencing the mind. The lawyer tries to arouse the judge's sympathy for the accused. His suffering condition will be very effectively *miseratio* and elaborated in great detail. This sympathy for the suffering and unhappiness of one's fellow man will also be used in political and moral speeches as a means of inducing the listener to help. The requested action is presented as a good, as something worthwhile; the opposite action is suggested as something bad. The path which should be taken is described as possible and quite achievable.

These are exactly the same points of view which we found with the imperative forms. It is only that in this case the means are multiplied, because the listener is to be persuaded. The individual psychic passages and phrases are not condensed but spread out. *The speech is an imperative*, in which is present the exact opposite of the mechanization of the speech means found in the syntactical imperative. The means themselves are created, however, from the same source. We can call these forms *disjoined*, but we call the established syntactical forms *condensed or compressed*. In the latter forms, only the result of the train of thought will be sensed; however, in the former, the individual parts are clearly and effectively sensed. For this reason the content of the disjoined form appears much richer than that of the compressed form, and from this comes the completely different artistic taste of each form. *The differences in artistic taste are decided by the quantity and quality of the sensations from which we become conscious of the linguistic purpose of the speaker.*

The more often a language community has cause to influence the mind, the larger the number of mechanized means must become, because frequent usage mechanizes. The more difficult and complex the relationships are in which this influencing takes place, the greater the need becomes for new and fresh formations which permit the psychic-ethical course of thought to enter the consciousness unabridged. The wealth of the language thereby is enriched with stylistic nuances. The more often the listener himself has had to produce larger groups of thoughts directed at a purpose and related to that purpose, the greater will be his capability to master more expansive quantities of speech. Characteristic of this is the example of the Spartans who maintained that at the end of an Attic speech they had forgotten how it had started. *The connection of grammar, rhetoric, and style is therein intimated.*

The Substance and the Sentence

VI

LET us resume a former discussion, namely, the fact that all label-ling of objects and people occurs through predication of their acts or attributes, as *dens*, meaning that which eats, has assumed the mean-ing of *tooth*. Apparently such a predicate designation is not the same as a definition, and only a definition should be in a position to summon an object or person clearly to consciousness. But we have demonstrated before that the predicate can become congruent with its subject by mechanization. However, this fact requires more exact presentation.

We are in the fortunate position of being able to understand more exactly single noun formations; these are *the adjectives serving as nouns*, for example, *the noble* [der Adlige], *the civilian* [der Bürger-liche], *the black* [der Schwarze], *the Negro* [der Neger], *the red* [der Rote], etc. *It is plain that the adjective designates the quality, and the article the substance.** The designation of the substance here contains the reference to a person of masculine sex and is no different from the expression *the man*. The whole noun *the black one* [der Schwarze] is, however, not the same as every black person of masculine sex; one thinks also of the African race with certain mental and physical quali-ties. The designation is for a generality; like every linguistic naming, it refers to a definite class, excluded from the whole of humanity. If all individuals of a language community have excluded this class, and if for this class *the black one* is the generally understood designation, then a habituation, thus a mechanization, must have preceded it. With this mechanization, the inferred ideas contained in the content of the desig-nation must also be considered.

---

* *Editor's note*: Unlike English, the German article *der, die* and *das, die* also indicates sex and number.

Along with these, we have the same type of formations which are not mechanized by usage, for example, *the good one* [der Gute], i.e., the man whose single differentiating characteristic is morality; *das Schöne, das Grüne, das Warme,* i.e., everything which is beautiful, green, and warm. In these examples, no other attribute will be associated with the given characteristic. This contrasts with *the black* [der Schwarze], *the Negro* [der Neger], and *the red* [der Rote]. *The associated attributes can only be matched with the content of the designation by supplementation. But supplementation can only ensue from those thoughts which possess the highest degree of associability.* We have seen above that the advantage of associability is in its possesion of those thoughts (1) given by perception, (2) retained by memory, which were just or recently brought to consciousness, or (3) contained in the situation of consciousness. The supplementation must, therefore, be created from these. This supplementation remains necessary for each individual instance in which the word is also possible in other contexts; and, with most words, this is the case. *The black one* [der Schwarze] can also be said of the chimney sweep, the devil, or a man dressed in black clothing. Which meaning is intended should be inferred from the circumstances, that is, from just those thoughts of perception and remembrance which possess the greatest associability.

The black one will unhesitatingly be understood by *supplementation of perception* as the African, if such a person is standing in front of the speaker and listener. Likewise the designation will be surely related to the Negro if we are reading a chapter whose title is *Africa* and which begins *The blacks are a powerful and impressionable race* [die Schwarzen sind ein Kräftiger und bildsamer Stamm]. In this case we have the *supplementation of remembrance* in relation to the continent of Africa. Without any such indication that *Africa* and *the black one* could be related we exclude the possibility of relating them to each other.

This type of supplementation is of the greatest importance for coherent speech. Africa is logically the subject because it is the exposition for *the blacks* [die Schwarzen]; nevertheless, it would be impossible to connect both concepts grammatically as subject and predicate. Such a connection would be something like *the blacks in Africa* [die Schwarzen in Africa]. Yet the given relationship is logically present because it is possible, even necessary, for us to sense, along with the idea of the continent, the idea of its inhabitants. To be precise, the group of thoughts associated with Africa and embodied in *African inhabitant* [Bewohner Africas], is the logical subject. *In this way thoughts closely associated with a designated group, even though they are not named themselves, are active factors in the understanding and formation of speech.*

This fact is so important that I cannot completely ignore it in passing. We say, for example, *The fire in the oven isn't burning* [das Feuer im Ofen brennt nicht]. In this case we do not think of the subject as the warming flame; on the contrary, the fuel in the oven is not burning. Actually, that expression is a self-contradiction; only from a certain category associated with the fire, i.e., fuel, is the connection given some sense. Equally misleading in the literal sense are the expressions *to light the lamp* [die Lampe anzünden], *to read Cicero* [den Cicero lesen], *a whole city in mourning* [die ganze Stadt trauert], *to eat a cup of ice cream or to eat a bowl of soup* [ein Glas Eis essen, einen Teller Suppe essen]. If we say *to guild a house* [ein Haus vergolden], we mean only those parts where such a thing is usually done. On the other hand, *noon bread* [Mittagbrot], or *evening bread* [Abendbrot] connote not simply the bread, but all the other types of food we eat at those times. If we invite someone for a cup of tea he knows for certain that many other things will be offered. With *puppis* the Roman associates the whole ship, as with *keel* [Kiel], or *rudder* [Steuer]. We can thus see that the poetical forms of the *pars pro toto* and *totum pro parte* are connected with the fact *that we never think of well-known groups individually, but rather in connection with a series of associated groups.* These suggestions may suffice to present the importance of *thought complications* for the understanding of speech.

We now return to our interrupted main stream of thought. If I have spoken of Rome the sentence *The city was situated on the Tiber* [die Stadt lag am Tiber] will surely be understood as Rome; the indication of the genus city is supplemented by the remembrance of the individual thought, *Rome*. This is only possible when I relate the new designation *city* as a predicate to the previously indicated thought. In the example *Caesar was murdered on the Ides of March; he had gone into the Curia* [Cäsar wurde an den Iden des März ermordert, er war in die Curie gegangen], *he* is a predicate to the Caesar present in memory. This relationship to Caesar would also be drawn if the second sentence began *this man* [dieser Mann], even if there were another man perceptually present besides the speaker and the listener.

Nevertheless, if Caesar had not been previously mentioned, the expression would necessarily have to be related to the third person present. Thus an impulse of remembrance actually here prevails over an impulse of present perception. Why? Because if the speaker makes a communication about Caesar it must be of value for him. So we conclude that this person connected with a feeling of value must stand in the foreground of the speaker's consciousness. Without this relationship and the supplementation following therefrom, we would not be in a position

to understand the relationship of the two sentences. It must be remembered, however, that *this relationship, even if not expressed, is nothing
more than an associated predication of the second expression from the
first, thus, for example: the blacks of Africa* [die Schwarzen von Africa].

VII

*A THIRD type of supplementation ensues only subsequently. Thus,
it is indicated at first only generally and imprecisely through a following correction or limitation of a group of thoughts.* We hear the
sentence *The blacks live in Africa* [die Schwarzen wohnen in Africa].
The ambiguous designation *the blacks* [die Schwarzen] is made un-
equivocal by the addition *live in Africa* [wohnen in Africa]. The psychic
process passes so swiftly and so mechanically that we are not at all
conscious of the change in the group first brought to mind by the subject. But just imagine the following very slowly spoken: *the reds—have
—again—executed a putsch in Paris* [Die Roten—haben—wider—einen
Putsch in Paris gemacht]. There we sense the tension and expectation of
what will be understood by the *reds* [Roten]. That is, we anticipate that
a definite species of humans, all of whom could be called red, are referred to by the speaker; but we don't know which one. If we have
heard the predicate, and if we are familiar with the political jargon,
the necessary supplementations will be immediately deduced, and the
limited perceptual picture will be in our minds. This is the process intimated in the first discussion and called the exposition of the logical
subject by the logical predicate. We remarked above that this process
appears, when, from a plurality of possible meanings, a specific one is
to be chosen.

   Let us follow this process a little further. In the case of the phrase
the reds [die Roten], we search in our treasury of thoughts for one
group to which we can relate the expression—that is, from which we
can predicate the expression *such a class of humans are the red ones.*
The required group is the logical subject of the expressed predicate. Our
mind would have formulated the question *what is that, the reds?* [Was
ist das, die Roten?]. However, if this were followed by the predicate
have executed a putsch in Paris [haben in Paris einen Putsch gemacht]
immediately after that grammatical subject, then we would be conscious of neither our question, nor the corresponding answer, because

the understanding of the sentence would pass mechanically for us as a consequence of habituation. It would be different if we first confronted a Kantian deduction with Kantian terminology. There we ask ourselves *What is the transcendental?* [Was ist das transcendental?]. We think about it and give ourselves an answer. However, if we have read up on it, the *transcendence* [Transcendenz], *aesthetics* [Aesthetik], *apriority* [Apriorität], and so on, officiate with mechanical assurance. It is exactly the same for us in interpreting a sentence of a foreign language if we are not mechanically fluent in the language.

We thus search for the group of thoughts which is to be connected with the spoken word, and we do that because the speaker is talking to us. Therefore, our mind must certainly feel stimulated to produce the groups of thoughts corresponding to the words; otherwise the sounds of the speaker would dash past us without leaving an impression, just as do the multitude of thoughts which simultaneously enter the mind. *In this way we sense the words of the speaker as an imperative*: in order to be heard, the speaker makes use of such imperative forms as *just think, just imagine, just consider* [denke dir mal, stelle dir einmal vor, überlege einmal], or the vocative *take notice, listen* [merke auf, höre zu]. He uses the demonstrative, that is, an audible signal demanding one to turn one's attention to an object or person. In addition, he makes the gesture of looking at or listening to the perceptual picture, for example, *this picture!* [dieses Bild!]. Right after this he might say *beautiful, magnificent!* [schön, herrlich!]. The listener looks, sees the picture, and understands *beautiful* [schön] as the predicate to *this picture* [dieses Bild].

If one imagines this series of words as mechanized then we have the simple sentence: *This picture (is) beautiful* [dieses Bild (ist) schön]. The Romance languages illustrate very clearly that the demonstrative was originally an imperative which became part of the sentence in mechanized speech. For example, French *ce livre est beau, ce* is derived from Latin *ecce* or *ecce id*; thus *ecce id, liber, bellus est*. And what is the relationship of *ecce* and *id* to each other? Each one is actually an independent sentence by itself (*just look, this*), that is, two imperative sentences. From *id* the term *liber* will now be expressed again as a predicate in an independent sentence, *It is a book* [es ist ein Buch]. From the perceptual picture thus provided with a predicate a new predicate will be expressed, *bellus est*.

This is exactly the same procedure as in elementary instruction in perception. A child describes an object, for example, a tree as *That is a tree, it is green, apples are on it, they will be picked* [das ist ein Baum, der ist grün, darauf sind Äpfel, die werden abgenommen], and so forth. The adult who recognizes with mechanical assurance the graphic and coloration signs of the artist would say concisely *The apples of this green tree will be picked* [Die Äpfel dieses grünen Baumes werden abgenommen]. The predicates have become attributes.

Consequently, there is nothing in spoken words and signs which can basically describe the true nature of a substance. The word with which we associate the spoken understanding of the substance, however, is an imperative which demands attention and observation from us; this attentive observation of the eye or ear builds a perceptual picture into consciousness. This perceptual picture is the substance.

This psychic process of understanding occurs actually so quickly that in the end we no longer sense the factors, but rather the demonstration of the perception appears to us as a congruent designation of the substance.

With this is concluded a very important problem of the history of language. For a long time we have known that the masculine and feminine -*s* in the nominative singular of the Indo-Germanic languages (for example, in *magnu-s*, ἀγαθό-s, Gothic *fisk-s*) is nothing more than the demonstrative *sa*, which still lives in Gothic *sa*. The meaning may have corresponded to our NHG *he* [*der*]; ἀγαθός would thus have been *good he* [gut der], that is, the same as the sentence: *he is good* [der ist gut].

The neutral *t* in *illud* or *illut, quod, quid, id, hod-ce hoc,* or Gothic *thata* is likewise a demonstrative stem and, as the article in Gothic and Greek shows, was not in usage for the personally acting subject. Thus an *illud* would likewise have been a sentence: *that, it,* meaning *that is it.* The -*n* of the weak German adjectives is probably also a demonstrative stem, which can still be recognized in the Latin *an*. Moreover, a number of suffixes such as the Greek -θεν, -θι, -δε, -σε can be traced with certainty back to demonstrative pronouns.

Speech thus proves to us from the manner of its formation, still retained in the mechanized remains of older stages of speech, that *the word was once a sentence whose meaningful element, the predicate, is retained in its stem and whose substance will be indicated in the endings by demonstration.* Following this, we must also conclude that the adjective, which was provided with the same substance designations as the noun, was likewise originally a sentence, condensed or compressed into a noun. The transition from noun to adjective is executed then in the same way as it is with the *victor exercitus* [victorious].

VIII

*T*HERE *is only one difference between those old Indo-Germanic noun foundations like:* ἄνθρωπο-s [man] *and the modern ones like: the good one.* In the old formations the demonstrative imperative, which indicates the substance, follows; in the newer formations it precedes. This is the same contrast we found between the formation of logical subject, the supplementary correction, since the logical subject τίθη-μι and *I place.* We called the type of formation with a following logical subject, the supplementary correction, since the logical subject is only given subsequently, out of consideration for the comprehension of the listener.

We find in the Indo-Germanic language two large classes of nouns (1) *The personal* (2) *the impersonal.* The personal nouns are naturally divided again between masculine and feminine nouns. Thus the sensation one has with the personal substance is approximately the same as with the nouns *person* [Person], *man* [Mensch]; with the impersonal, it is the same as with the noun *thing* [Ding]. The personal substantive aspects are classified gradually, again according to the most varied points of view, into a great number of classes and groups, which at the same time can be called substances. This is because when we are dealing with a purely psychological concept of substance, we should not think of the logical-metaphysical valueless concept of substance, otherwise even the masculine-personal and the feminine-personal substances would fail to contain numerous qualities. *The psychological substances are always associated with qualities,* even the completely indefinite neuter. For example, in cases in which we see something in the distance which we cannot yet recognize, it is for us a *something* [etwas]. We ask *What is that* [was ist das]; thus it is neuter. This appearance has qualities, as do all appearances. Corresponding to these are the sub-substances, the noun, generic, and special designations, for example, *Mensch* [human being], *Mann* [man], *Tier* [animal], *Löwe* [lion], *Ding* [thing], *Baum* [tree], *Haus* [house], *Berg* [mountain].

If speech has obtained its substance designation by supplementation, and thus obtained nouns from mechanized sentences, then by demonstration these nouns themselves can appear as representatives for the most general of substance designations. In this way are formed *der Gute* [the good one], *der gute Mensch* [the good man], *das schwarze Tier* [the black animal], *die grosse Stadt* [the large city].

The position of the substance designation behind the adjective appears to be very old, if one compares Greek and German; and thus it is the same position which the demonstrative occupies in ἀγαθός [good]. The phrase *die grosse Stadt* [the large city] originally also had the meaning of a sentence, formed according to the pattern of the supplementary correction, with the adjective originally as predicate, and the noun as subject. The process corresponds to the Indo-Germanic compound, with the substantive concept following and the predicate preceding: *Ratmann, Hausthür, parricida, Edelmann, Grossvater, magnannimus* [councilman, housedoor, one who commits patricide, nobleman, grandfather, high-minded]. The preceding always contains the limiting attribute, modifying the subsequent generic determination. The first component corresponds to the logical *differentia specifica*, and the second component corresponds to the logical *genus proximum*.

This old form of sentence construction, also seen in the appositive, is engendered by the lively interest of the speaker in expressing the really important and valuable things, and it takes little heed of the possibility of comprehension. The smoother and more advanced the entire thinking and ethical forms of intercourse become, the greater will be the consideration given to the listener. For this reason, the following sentence pattern became widely accepted: first subject, then predicate. The old word arrangement was, of course, mechanized, and thus retained. Then, however, it was only sensed as a congruent means of designating a limited substantive group, no longer as a means of designating the developing group of thoughts in a sentence. In this function, as an attributive connection, the form has been retained.

The mechanization could, of course, after ascertaining the word order, embrace the predicative sentence connection in the same manner as before. In this way the Greek οὗτος ὁ ἀνήρ [this man] is mechanized with an attribute to an expression of substance, after Greek had already established its differentiation between predicate and attribute. The article shows in this connection as in that with ἐκεῖνος, ὅδε, πᾶς, (*completely* [ganz] *all* [all]) *that* ὁ ἀνήρ was the subject, and that the pronoun was the predicate. The same thing happened to the adjective πολύς [many], which admittedly had the position of a predicate, but was apparently also sensed as an attribute.

If this mechanism went further and also embraced the connections of the adjective with the noun (which, according to the established word order, should be a predicate), then, according to the pattern of supplementary correction, this form could take its place alongside the old one. And both types of position could be used together for the attribute, as in German *der Ritter gut* [the good knight], and as in the apparently arbitrary positioning of the attributive adjective in Latin.

If the presentation above is basically correct, then *the psychic result of a larger group of predicative judgments about a substance*, for example, about a person, an animal, or a house, must always be the same for the listener. *All of these predications*, which are issued by extended series of thoughts, *are condensed in consciousness to a composed picture; they are compressed to a group of thoughts* in which all of these predicates are now incorporated as inherent attributes. And this is actually the case. Imagine, for example, that we are reading the description of an animal, listening to a story about an historical person, or developing the characterization of a poetical hero: What picture do we have in our minds at the end of the story or passage? We no longer have the original series of predications, but rather a solid group in which all features and all predicates are assimilated as inherent characteristics, thus as attributes. It is just the same in the predicate sentences, for example, *the man is good* [der Mensch ist gut]; the psychic result of this series for the listener is the group *the good man* [der gute Mensch]. The speech groups of a thorough characterization are, however, too long to be mechanized, although this is very easy with the smaller sentence groups, especially if they renounce a specific verb form. They will then only stimulate the group of which we are conscious, and will be sensed as equivalent means of expressing a substance provided with an attribute.

The entire discussion above is based upon the demonstration of a present perceptual picture; but the nouns *the good one* [der Gut], *the black one* [der Schwarze] are not limited to the present perception. We saw at the end of the first discussion that, as a matter of fact, the picture of remembrance has the same significance for the supplementation of a predicate as the perceptual picture. For example, if a bird has just flown by and is no longer visible, or if the bird has just been named, the indication *this, the, he* [dieser, der, er] is related to the group *bird* with the same amount of assurance as if it were perceptually present. We observed further at that time that an established conscious picture also has the same force as the supplementation, and that this configuration of consciousness can be general or individual. If the conscious picture is common to a larger class of individuals, it will have become conscious along with so many individual differences that these will inhibit each other, and only an abstract will be active in consciousness. This abstract, however, is the general configuration of consciousness. If I were to say, *the dead one* [der Tote], a small circle, for example a family, would very probably think of a specific deceased individual, whereas a larger language community would think of deceased man in general.

Also in this general case the demonstrative *the* [der] has the function of an imperative, causing the listener to become conscious of a configuration. In this case, it surely lives as a solid picture of remembrance in him, but momentarily not in the foreground of his consciousness. This picture thus made conscious can naturally be no different from the abstract generic configuration. In contrast to the indication of a perceptual picture, in which the individual peculiarity can be new, the indication itself can give nothing new. Thus this indicaton alone can no longer be sensed as a predicate.

The indication of an established conscious configuration is possible, as long as this group is something familiar like *the good one* [der Gute], that is, the group which all the listeners would select with this name. But the indication in itself is not in a position to make this group conscious. The mere *der* [the one] is not in a position to reproduce the group *good man* [guter Mensch], if it has not already been named immediately before. With the present pictures of perception and remembrance, this possibility is extant, of course, as we have seen; because if a black person is standing in front of us, the indication *der* [the one] can make us conscious of this picture. If we hear *der Gute* [the good one] without a picture of perception or remembrance, we can think of nothing specific with the article. Clarity is first delivered by *Gute* [good], and this *good* must now appear far more important to us than the article. The article thus guides our consciousness by pointing forward to *good*; pointing forward obviously in the sense that, as our expectation is aroused, *der* [the one] is to be explained or further illustrated. Thus it is conceivable that a series of thoughts *der—gute—ist gestorben* [the —good one—has died] can be combined on the basis of the situation of consciousness. This would hardly have been possible with the perceptual picture, since, in that case, the visualized picture itself would have provided the illustration for *der* [the one].

Upon the basis of the situation of consciousness, the demonstrative pronoun, because of its inferior value for illustrating, was subordinated to the following predicate word, and the pronoun had to become proclitic, that is, to change itself to an article. On the other hand, if the pronoun followed, the first word must have had the decisive meaning for understanding. *In this case the pronoun became enclitic.* In this way the stress was developed *der Ménsch, des* [the man, of the] or *Menschen* [of the man].

Thus the way in which we understand linguistic utterances is decisive for the illustration value of the individual parts of the sentence, and along with this, for the intensity of tone and tempo with which we pronounce these parts, and therefore, *for the sound structure of the*

word. We observed this same process of leaning forward in the formation of the relative sentence: *Caesar venit,—qui?—Rubicon transierat.*
The original interrogative word has no illustration value at all; it does,
however, arouse the expectation for an illustration. The consequence
is the proclitic leaning on the actual illustration, the subsequent answer
sentence *I believe that,—he is coming.* [ich glaube das,—er kömmt].
The *das* [that], which has become useless for the illustration, leans forward on the illustration *he is coming* [er kömmt]. In this case it will be
written *dass.*

IX

TO COMPLETE what had been said it is necessary to look at still
another class of noun formations whose nature is equally clear. *Like
the Greek language, modern languages can make a noun out of every
single word, by placing the neutral article in front of the word: the alas*
[das Ach], *the ding-dong* [das Klingling], *the ugh* [das Pfui], *the when*
[das Wenn], *the but* [das Aber], *the coming* [das Kommen].
 Ugh [Pfui] is the emotional sound of disgust; *the ugh* [das Pfui] indicates the fact that *ugh* [Pfui] is said. Likewise *the alas* [das Ach] indicates the fact of saying *alas* [Ach], and it can be said *there was much oh
and woo* [da war viel Ach und Weh]. *The where, when, how, but* [Das
Wo, Wenn, Wie, Aber], indicates the *saying of the when, where* [das
Wenn, Wo sagen], or the situation and its relationships in which one
uses *where, how, but* [wo, wie, aber]. *The tomorrow* [Das Morgen],
the today [das Heute], *the yesterday* [das Gestern] are all unspecific
substances, although they are known to the listener and may be stated
tomorrow, today, yesterday [morgen, heute, gestern].
 If someone has said *höre ich etwas, so werde ich es dir schreiben* [If I
hear something, I will write you about it], he can be answered *höre ich
etwas, das ist ein schlechter Trost* [If I hear something, it will be poor
comfort]. If someone is called by another person *mein lieber Freund*
[my dear friend], he can answer him *mein lieber Freund das verbitte
ich mir* [My dear friend, I object to that] or *das, dein, (jenes, dieses)
mein lieber Freund verbitte ich mir* [the, thou (that, this) my dear
friend I object], or *ach was! mein lieber Freund* [certainly not! my dear
friend]. He who used the expression the first time recognizes his own

words again in the answer and thereby understands *wenn du mich mein lieber Freund nennst, so verbitte ich mir das* [When you call me my dear friend, I object to that].

In this manner every linguistic utterance can be used as a signal to help recall the situation in which this utterance was made. If many people use the same sounds in definite situations, these sounds become the signal which naturally reminds one of that situation in which many people or everyone uses these sounds. Common to many people are also the reflex sounds at the most primitive stage of development, such as crying and laughing. These reflex sounds can thus become a means of summoning to the consciousness of the listener the situation of laughing, crying, groaning, and so on.

The listener must be able to recognize that these reflex expressions are not the actual emotional reflexes of the speaker, but are rather a signal and means of expressing a strange sensation. The use of reflex sounds as an imitation of the sounds of another person can best be understood when the other signals for the emotional state of the speaker point to a completely different sensation from that of the reflex sound. This can be shown, for example, when one laughs with a wrinkled forehead, hostile look, or threatening fist, or when crying is imitated with a happy face. When this reflex imitation occurs in the middle of a conversation, which itself offers no motivation for a corresponding change in humor, the imitation will also be obvious in every case.

Nevertheless, even in these cases the listener will find it very difficult to recognize, within the laughing or crying of the speaker, the imitation of another's laughing or crying. Daily speech gives us a very significant clue as to how we should *discern a reflex utterance as imitation*. If someone has shouted *oh my God* [ach mein Gott], and another mockingly reproduces this expression, he intentionally exaggerates the passionate tone with which the words were spoken. In such a fashion children try to anger each other by exaggerating and distorting the passion, the crying, and the astonishment of other children. In doing this they create a difference between the original and the imitation, from which the listener immediately infers the derision. The intentional distortion of the original sounds is, in this case, the means of (1) presenting those sounds as another's sounds, and (2) making a judgment about them, thus expressing a predicate about them.

Next to this we have another case. Someone has shouted *ach mein Gott* [oh, my God], another person has answered *ja, ach mein Gott— das kann gar nichts helfen* [Sure, oh my God—that can't help anything at all]. The speaker in most cases or certainly very often, as has been mentioned already, will not in any way reproduce the emotional tone with which the original shout was spoken. As we have seen, the exclamation *alas* as a noun is likewise completely without emotional tone, just as *das Vaterunser* [the Lord's Prayer] is completely without vocative tone.

It is further conceivable enough that, if the speaker himself does not have the corresponding emotions, the emotional tones can only be imprecisely reproduced. And there is nothing more natural in this case than that the imitated emotional tone will be replaced by the tone which is in accordance with the actual emotion of the speaker. We are evidently dealing here with the substitution of one emotional situation for another.

This phenomenon is extraordinarily important for the life of speech and needs a little clarification. A is happy, and B reports the fact. There are two personal situations of feeling and consciousness present, of A and B. If A has spoken words in his happy mood, they are engendered from his emotional and conscious situation. The report from B, on the other hand, is derived from A's words. An exact reproduction of that first situation and the utterance which occurred in it would require that B be completely transplanted into the situation of A, which would be very difficult. It would also require that B repeat exactly the corresponding form of the utterance with the specific individuality of A, for example, the pitch of the voice, the tempo of speaking, and so forth; this is even more difficult. The demands made on B's report are thus exactly the same as those made on an author who wants to delineate an action completely objectively, and, moreover, the same as those made on an actor who wants to give a true imitation of an historical figure like Frederick the Great. The latter is completely impossible, and the difficulty of the former is proven by the course of literature. The portrayal of the conduct of other persons, as it really is and without the garnishing of the author's own individuality, has been approximately successful only in the most recent times. Earlier stages of all branches of literature demonstrate that the situation which is being reported becomes blended with the situation of the reporter. The Homeric poems give a picture of the historical and cultural situation in which they flowered, not the time in which the related actions took place. The heroes of the Lucretia tale in the *Emperor's Chronicle* are people of the twelfth century, the people of the *Song of the Nibelungen* are from the turn of the thirteenth century, and so it continues to the Greek heroes in wigs. Such anachronisms are also found in Shakespeare and Goethe.

The same principle can be observed in the simple reproductions of one person's linguistic utterances by another person. The difference can be seen most distinctly in those great deviations; but the result of this simple repetition shows clearly enough the intensity of distortion to which the report can lead. The result is indirect speech. This was not accomplished all at once, but rather its forms have developed gradually.

The designations are changed according to the position of the reporting person, for example, the second person singular to the first, or the first to the second or third, as the tense and mood shift.

Through such a distortion, basically similar to a reproduced sound, a reflex sound of one person can become the way by which another person indicates a condition, situation, or emotion and for which indication the reflex sound will be chiefly used.

A very similar occurrence is demonstrated in the onomatopoetic means of speech. That these are present in speech is certain. To what extent will always be very hard to determine. In any case we do not want to investigate this question. Indubitably onomatopoetic in the child's speech are *Muh* [moo] or *Muhkuh, Wauwau, Haufhauf* [moo-cow, bow-wow, mutt-mutt] or *Haufhund, Pilepile, Tucktuck* [mutt-dog, roly-poly, chuck-chuck]. These are word formations which imitate the sounds of animals. In addition to these are numerous imitations of mechanical noises and sounds: *batzen, klatschen, bauzen, baffen, knat-tern* [blot, clap, smash, knock, crackle]. But these imitations likewise dispense with an exact reproduction of the actual tone, as does *Schnet-terenteng* for the tone of the trumpet. Thus here too the situation of the reporter, namely the peculiarity of his sound organs, has assimilated the situation in which these noises and tones were formed. These speech formations have become mere suggestions.

Likewise those *expletives* which a man uses in a humorous manner or too frequently become characteristic signs of that person. Well-known is *Jasomirgott, Marschall Vorwärts* [Oh my God, Marshal Forward]; I know the nicknames *Eben* [Exactly] and *Wie* [And How] for persons who use these words constantly.

All tone, noise, or sound aspects of a living thing or of an inanimate object can thus be used as a means to summon the object itself into consciousness. *Even today these phonetic signs need no grammatical form in order to fulfill the grammatic function* of representing sentences. For example, if someone has fallen, we say *smash! bang!* [bauz! bums], or with an additional sentence of explanation *Bang, smash, there he lies* [bums, baus, da liegt er]. The psychic law discussed above stated that those parts of the sentence which were actually illustrative appositives because of their greater intelligibility for the listener, or because of their illustrative value, also function as the main thought. Thus, according to this law, one senses mainly *bang, smash* [bums, bauz], with *there he lies* [da liegt er] substantially as a descriptive adverbial addition. It is similar to the sentence *lickety split* [nun huldrdebuldr], with the addition *it went* [ging es] or *Then it went lickety split* [nun ging es hul-drdebuldr]. The usage of words as nouns has already been treated.

As a means of summoning the appropriate situation to consciousness, these words are the linguistic predicates of the situation. We can say that all predicates are ways of indicating or remembering a situation. At first they must be sensed as a demand to imagine the appropriate situation or to bring it to view; they must be sensed as an *imperative of remembrance. Thus the means of speech for the substance (demonstrative pronoun) is the imperative, or the demand to see or hear something present; the means of speech for the predicate is the demand to remember a situation.*

X

I N THE presence of a perceptual picture, a mere pointing of the finger and the direction of the eyes are usually sufficient for the demonstration. When the words of speech suited for this situation are used, the so-called demonstratives, it is obvious that these words must have the same relationship to the indicating and emphasizing of the situation as have *Wauwau, Pfui* [bow-wow, ugh], and so on to the situation itself. This should be remembered on hearing such words. *Thus the demonstrative stems are also predicates of the situation-of-indication.* As means of speech, they must originally have served the purpose of calling the situation-of-indication to remembrance. The meaning must have been something like *siehe hin* [look here] or *hier gibt es etwas zu sehen* [there is something to see here].

From this can be discerned that originally there were no phonetic means of speech to indicate a substance. Rather, all means of speech were predicates, that is, means of remembrance by which the familiar situations could be indicated. These situations were of a complicated type in which inanimate bodies, spatial relationships, people, and sensual qualities were all contained. Because of the function of these predicates for a definite purpose, they became indications of certain parts, attributes, or relations of this situation picture.

The simplest linguistic utterance begins as an imperative, the command to the listener to remember a situation, with each new word an imperative. Through habituation, fluency, and mechanization of the course of comprehension, these imperative sentences are sensed no longer as sentences, but only in their results as groups of thoughts. Through the conclusion of the listener about the purpose of the speaker, the words attached in a row are formed into a sentence in which the

individual parts have different values for the purpose. Such rows or
sentences can be mechanized again into simple words of speech.

One must imagine that originally speech related individual sounds as
predicates of perception. Sounds were connected with other sounds to
form new sentences; these were then again mechanized to roots. A root
predicated by a root was mechanized to a stem; a stem predicated by a
stem was mechanized to a declined word, word sentences again to
larger whole words, thus to compounds. As in a simple sentence, these
words which originally were sentences by themselves behave the same
way in relation to the whole sentence and its predicates as do the sentences of a paragraph towards the predicates of that paragraph, and
again as the paragraphs behave within a given speech in relation to its
purpose or theme.

This is the picture then of a continual atrophy and a continual rebirth
and strengthening of the simple cellular structure of the mighty tree of
developed speech.

Before I leave this area and the verification that the word in speech
was developed from the sentence, let me *conclude by compiling a group*
of clear and illustrative examples in which the individual sentence com-
ponents which have been mechanized into words are still perceptible.

Latin *quamvis* has become a particle, although it was originally a
sentence, meaning *as much as you want* [wie sehr du willst]; it must
have been a pure particle in the indicative, at the very latest then with
the Augustinian poets.

Greek εἰ δὲ μή, with continual omission of the verb, is the same as
the adverb *otherwise* [sonst].

Greek οὐ μὴν ἀλλά, originally meaning *however this didn't happen,*
but [doch dies geschah nicht sondern], receives the meaning *disregard-*
ing that, nevertheless [dem ungeachtet, dennoch].

Greek οἶδ' ὅτι, δῆλον ὅτι are pure adverbs.

Greek ἄλλως τε καί means simply *especially* [besonders].

Latin *sine* is actually *if not* [wenn nicht]; the character of the word is
clearly shown as an ablative preposition.

Latin *quisquis, quicunque* were, during the Livian period, simple
pronouns with the meaning *each* [jeder], as in the classical period in
connection with *modo* and *ratione* [by the means].

Latin *forsitan, forsan* and also simply *fors* mean *perhaps* [vielleicht].

Latin *ideo* is certainly nothing more than *id eo* (*that is therefore the*
case) [das ist darum der Fall].

French *peut-être* means *perhaps* [vielleicht].

Latin *quasi, as it were* [gleichsam] from the meaning *as when* [wie
wenn]; compare ὡς ὅτε in Homeric similies.

Italian *è un anno, un anno fa,* meaning *one year ago* [vor einem

Jahre], French *il-y-a quelque jours*, meaning *since* [seit]; Italian *tempo fa, a short time ago* [vor kurzem], *tre mesi fa*, and so on.

Italian *poffare (puo fare)* meaning *the thousand!* [der Tausend!]

Latin Terence uses *id propterea*, meaning *therefore* [darum].

Latin *scilicet, videlicet, nimirum* with the meaning *obviously* [selbstverständlich].

The application of such sentences as subordinate clauses is an intermediate stage between their importance as main clauses and their importance as words. As subordinate clauses, they will then be of inferior importance and meaning to the main thought, to the purpose of the speaker, or to his main predicate. In the etymologically transparent forms, a complete mechanization also appears; that is, all of these expressions only permit consciousness of the purpose which they are serving and their function in attaining this purpose, and no longer the original sentence meaning from which the function was inferred. *There are even stages in this decline to a subordinate clause*, as in the Latin imperative or conditional sentence: *raise up this opinion, you will support it* [tolle hanc opinionem, sustuleris]. According to its form this is probably still sensed as a main clause, but the function is the same as that of the subordinate clause with *si*, and therefore always the asyndeton. On the other hand, no one senses the German interrogative conditional clause as a main clause, for example *hast du das gesagt so wirst du* [If you said that, then you will]. The logical main clause is introduced, therefore, with the subordinate clause particle *so* [then], and the interrogative melody has completely disappeared. Closely related to the form of the main clauses are probably the Latin concessive clauses in the subjunctive. On the other hand, the prohibitive clauses with *ne and* μή, for example, after the verbs of fear, have become pure subordinate clauses. In Greek, therefore, the optative can also appear, that is, the form of indirect speech in the subordinate clause. Clauses at the beginning of a story, *A man had worked his whole life long, but only earned a little; then one day came...* [Ein Mann hatte sein Leben lang gearbeitet, aber nur wenig verdient, da kam eines Tages. ..], or the corresponding Latin forms, for example, *Forte per angustam tenuis volpecula rimam Repserat in cumeram* (Horace *Epistles* 1. 7. 29) [A lean little fox squeezed through a narrow crack in the basket] will be treated later. These clauses are main clauses according to the form; nevertheless, their function is that of subordinate clauses as the pluperfect demonstrates, *as a man had worked* [als ein Mann gearbeitet hatte].

The logical meaning, the function, is the same in both sentences, but the stylistic feelings of the listener are different, because the slower the supplementary conclusions are drawn, the larger is the sum of the conscious thoughts which convey the speaker's purpose to the listener.

Through mechanization, however, this feeling of the great number of thoughts can disappear, and the expression can appear harmonious with its purpose, as in the case of numbers, which were actually nouns; for example, *mille*, which through its function became an adjective, and ἐξεπλάγην [was amazed] through its function, which was basically the same as ἐφοβήθην [feared], also offered the possibility of assuming the construction φοβεῖσθαι [to fear]. Indeed, this same development was undergone by φοβεῖσθαι itself. In this way the Italian *si* with the active verb in the sense of our *one* takes on this function in the vernacular, for example, in an expression like *quando si è constretti*. In the same manner as the partitive genitive in the Romance languages, which takes on the functions of the subject and the object, the sign of the genitive is simply sensed as an article of separation.

The individual clauses and periods in a larger linguistic whole are grouped exactly in the same manner as those clauses in short expressions. The most important part is the predicate of the whole; all other clauses are graduated according to their value and their importance for the predicate. The predicate in this case can be the point of an anecdote, a general sentence in a fable or parable, a fact which should be proven, or the idea of the whole. But the words themselves and the linguistic form are not in a position to even approximately make clear the balanced relationship of the individual sentences, which in the simpler expressions will be approximately determined by the forms of the main clause, subordinate clause, and the word. The less developed a language is, the fewer means it has to do this.

The arrangement and grouping of the individual members in their relations to the idea of the whole must, to a certain degree, be left to the listener's ability to combine and construe. In actual speech, thus also in declamations, the manner of stress and the tempo are important expedients for the listener. For this purpose writing has devised several signals known as punctuation.

We have seen then, that the main clause is mechanized in a series of stages to the subordinate clause and to the word. The opposite is naturally not to be excluded, that subordinate clauses can contain the Predicate; this occurs often enough. Nor is it so seldom that certain clauses, which according to their form are subordinate clauses, often or regularly indicate the main predicate. Certainly such a case occurs in the main clauses with εἴθε, εἰ γάρ [if only] or the German *if only* [wenn doch]. These are actually conditional subordinate clauses. The threat mentioned above, *if you do that* [wenn du das thust] is also a subordinate clause. These clauses become congruent with their function and appear to us as main clauses. Similarly, in *quamvis dicat* [even if he says] the subjunctive is originally conditioned and subordinate to *vis*, similarly with *licet* [even if]; nevertheless, this subjunctive verb has become far more important since *quamvis* and *licet* were demoted to particles. In this way the subordinate element, by enhancing its value, can become the superordinate element for the main predicate, and the subordinate clause can become the main clause.

With consideration for the purpose of the speaker, conclusions are thus drawn in the mind of the listener from rather scanty indications and from the relations of value of the groups of thoughts made conscious individually. These make possible the comprehension of what is said, and they also infuse the stammering indications and signals of the speaker with a content which qualifies language for the noblest tasks of intellectual life. The mechanization of these component sequences and the atrophy of the basic meaning, the transformation of the etymological meaning into a functional one (a process which is so often absurdly lamented), this process of dying is the true consummation of the life of speech.

The Action

XI

ONE construes without reflection Caesar's famous words *veni, vidi, vici* [I came, I saw, I conquered] in a sense of a chronological series: *First I came, then I saw, and then conquered* [zuerst bin ich gekommen, dann habe ich gesehen, und dann gesiegt]. Evidently the syntactical form of these sentences and their type of relationship offer no special clue for this reading. Although formed in exactly the same way, *excessit, evasit, erupit* [went out, escaped, broke loose], is not understood as a chronological series; on the contrary, these three verbs appear as designations of the same fact. In the sentence *I remained at home and read* [ich blieb zu Hause und las], we interpret both actions as occurring simultaneously.

Apparently the order of several actions among one another is determined by the listener according to the actual content of the verbs which designate the actions; one asks how they can be connected, and then connects them accordingly. The plausibility of this method of association is concluded from the experience the listener has had with the given actions. Thus a chronological order of actions can only be construed by the listener when the actions are familiar in their content, their course, and their causal relationship. If the actions are unfamiliar, the speaker will then have to give further guidance.

However, if the actions are developed successively, then we generally require that the earlier action be named in the former position; otherwise we have the logically objectionable feeling of a hysteron proteron. The temporal succession of the listener's thoughts then basically corresponds to the temporal course of the actual actions. The temporal succession of the linguistic signals thereby becomes a signal and thus itself a means of presentation.

Now this law is, of course, not without exception; successive action words do not always summon the corresponding actual course of action to consciousness. We frequently indicate an earlier action parenthetically first as a supplementation because it serves as exposition of the action of the predicate; for example, *when he took off the overcoat, he wore a beautiful dark jacket* [er zog das Kleid aus, er trug einen schönen, dunklen Rock]. We proceed in this manner in all of those cases where, by means of a supplementary correction, temporal, causal, and concessive subordinate clauses have arisen, following the two patterns:

(1) *Caesar crossed the Rubicon,—he had decided* [Cäsar überschritt den Rubico,—der hatte sich entschlossen]—from this the relative subordinate clause: *who had decided* [der sich entschlossen hatte].

(2) *Caesar crossed the Rubicon,—who was that? he had decided—* [Cäsar überschritt den Rubico,—wer war das? er hatte sich entschlossen] —from this the Latin relative clause with *qui*.

These sentence connections can only become subordinate clauses, (1) because the listener arranges known actions according to their relationships, (2) because he differentiates between action which is actually valuable for the message, i.e., the predicate of the message, and that which is only a preparatory expositional action. The exposition is not the purpose of the message, but only a serving aid for the predicate, and thus subordinated to it.

The reason for the proteron hysteron, in order to use this expression for the successive form of the narrative, is a psychological one. If we are told or related something, the valuable thing is the entirety of the story, not the individual sentences or the particular action; the complete feeling of value appears only with the conclusion of the message. Obviously the assumption of the listener that something valuable is being communicated to him must be present from the very beginning of a story, and with this also the expectation or even the suspense for the continuation of a story already begun to be told. If we are not now given the later chronological development, but rather a former action, then disappointment of the suspended expectation appears, a feeling of discomfort which is only bearable if the hysteron proteron helps us to understand the entire course of the action, as is the case with supplementary exposition.

But this feeling of discomfort is not completely overcome by the awareness that the supplementary correction furthers us in our understanding, as long as the hysteron proteron in these forms even comes to consciousness. *One can thus observe the tendency in speech to dispose of the hysteron proteron, and indeed also of such exposition.* Thus one can observe that the clauses which have arisen from supplemental exposition are placed more and more at the beginning in the formation of sentences. For example, if the clause with *quom, cum* has arisen from the interrogative adverb, *when* [wann], then this question could originally have been placed only after the superordinated clause: *Caesar Rubiconem transiit. Quom? (when) viderat* [Caesar crossed the Rubicon. When? he saw]; likewise with *postquam, quando, ut, ubi, quia* [after, when, how, where, why]. And nevertheless, the usual order of these clauses is such that the subordinate clause is placed in front of the main clause, because it generally indicates an earlier action.

In an artistically delivered story, however, both the proteron hysteron and the hysteron proteron may be found, the latter only as a supplementary exposition (In its disgusting exaggeration, the hysteron proteron has been criticized severely by Immermann in *Münchhausen*.) The former appears as the correct and reasonably arranged method of narration.

Both forms lead to the same results of understanding. But the order of the thoughts, and, along with this, the inferences which lead to understanding, and even the stylistic impressions are different. With a hysteron proteron, the purpose of the message is more slowly and less mechanically revealed. In certain circumstances this form is therefore more piquant and even more suspenseful. It is more suspenseful, for example, when, in a story without exposition, the author is successful in so arousing the reader's interest in a character that it seems worthwhile to the reader to search for further elucidation. This narrative form frequently occurs in our modern fiction; I call attention to Storm's *Immensee*. In this novelette our interest is awakened for the character of an old man, before we are informed of his memories of youth. Thus, it is exactly that which formally would be understood as exposition which really has become the main subject of the story, the logical predicate. A similar situation occurs in the same author's novelette *Drüben am Markte*.

Even though Storm knows how to tell a story admirably, it cannot be denied that, at the part when it reverts to earlier times, that is, where the expectation of a continuation of the action begun is frustrated, a considerable feeling of discomfort arises. This frustration is only gradually overcome through the suspense of the new story.

On the other hand, however, the well-arranged form is somewhat naive and childish, often even pedantic; it is the well-known form of the fairy tale, which commences with *Once upon a time there was a man* [es war einmal ein Mann]. Horace's instruction in the *Ars Poetica*, not to begin with *ab ovo* [from the egg], proves that even the stylistic sensibility of the Roman poet was not pleased with the completely thought-out form of narration. Horace naturally meant in his requirement that the poet should commence as close as possible to the really important action, to lead with *medias res*, as Homer did, and to let all earlier elements be inferred or be given exposition through supplementary indications.

XII

*B*Y MEANS *of tense forms speech indubitably offers a valuable aid for the correct construction of temporal order*. Both the ancient languages and the Romance languages have an advantage in comparison to German, because they differentiate the aorist, the imperfect, the *perfectum historicum*, and the *passé défini*. But the time relationship is, of course, intelligible from the objective construction of the listener, even without this differentiation.

The forms of the subordinate clause are equally important for expedience and assurance in understanding temporal relationships, but they have arisen gradually from main clauses and have developed in the course of time within the individual languages to mechanical and congruent designations of time. Thus without them the understanding of temporal relationships would still be possible.

The tenses of the Indo-Germanic languages are first of all not even forms of expression for the arrangement of successive action, but rather expressions for the temporal relationships of the speaking subject to the actions. Therefore, when there are two past actions, of which the first is earlier than the second, for example, *veni, vidi*, the first will not be designated by the pluperfect, and the second by the aorist, but rather both by the aorist. This is because the speaking subject stands in the same temporal relationship to both. The pluperfect designates the relationship of a past, or preferably, of a completed action to the consciousness of a person no longer present, about whom the present and speaking person reports. Let us call the speaking person A, the action B, the person about whom is reported A p. (p. = perfect), and the action, which is related to the consciousness of A p., B p. The relationship is then A : B = A p. : B p. A p. and B p., as objects of the report about A, are the indirect speech in the sense mentioned before; B and A are the direct speech. With this, one can call the pluperfect the indirect reporting form of the perfect, and the imperfect may be called the indirect reporting form of the present. Past actions use the aorist as a direct reporting form.

Only in the subordinate clause in Latin, German, and Romance languages will the pluperfect and imperfect be used to arrange past actions; for example, *When Caesar had crossed over, he moved* [als Cäsar überschritten hatte, zog er]. The transformation in meaning is realized in this manner: since the completed action of B p., which at first designates only a relationship of consciousness to A p., is closely related in the aorist with the direct report and subordinated to it; it thereby gains a temporal relationship to A. One calls this the pre-completion, or the pluperfect. This development is thus first completed in subordinate clauses, but not in Greek, because in Greek the aorist remains in clauses with ἐπεί, ὅτε, etc., as it would also remain in main clauses. In Latin this form of expression also remains in the temporal clauses, with the exception of the clauses with cum. Therefore, the forms *ubi, ut, postquam, ubi primum, cum primum* [when, as, after, as soon as, as soon as], take the perfect indicative, i.e., the aorist. And also the German preterite in those clauses where the so-called exact means of expression should require the pluperfect, is to be regarded as the remains of this construction; for example, *When he came, he sat down* [als er kam, setzte er sich].

The repeating, iterate subordinate clauses, which in Latin require the pluperfect and the perfect, in Greek take the optative and the subjunctive with ἄν respectively. They are thus certainly understood as conditioned in the main clause by the consciousness of the subject. And it will also be the same way with most of the subjunctive subordinate clauses with *cum*, which require the pluperfect in opposition to the rules of temporal clauses. Similarly, in unreal conditional clauses, instead of the imperfect subjunctive, the pluperfect subjunctive gradually appeared. The Greek imperfect and the aorist contain the origin; the former places the action in relation to A p., the latter (the aorist) in relation to A.

Obviously then, there was originally, neither for the main clauses nor in the subordinate clauses, a tense suitable for the arrangement of temporal relationships. The usage of the pluperfect for this purpose must be counted as an advance in the distinctness of means of speech.

The future designates no more than a later stage in the developmental series of the action—later than something already mentioned. In *veni, vidi, vici* every succeeding action is later than that which preceded it, and yet certainly none of these would be expressed with the future tense. The future designates the future time as seen from the consciousness of the speaking person A, i.e., an action, intended or desired by this person, or induced and therefore expected. For example, *I will be home at ten o'clock* [Um 10 Uhr werde ich zu Hause sein], because I plan to be or want to be; *It will rain today* [es wird heute regnen], an inference since the rain appears as the consequence of certain conditions which are already present. It is not unusual that the form of desire, the subjunctive, is used as the appropriate form for all of the future. The futural meaning of the subjunctive in Homer's poems, the Latin future of the third and fourth conjugations, and, probably, the Greek future with σ, for example λύσω [I will loose], is nothing more than the subjunctive aorist with a shortened connecting vowel, and for this reason the subjunctive is naturally missing.

Also within the future actions, a chronological order is designated in Latin by the *futurum exactum*; in Greek if the earlier action is expressed in a subordinate clause, there is no corresponding expression, because the *conjunctivus aoristi* with ἄν cannot be used as such, nor the *participium aorist*, at least originally. But let us here discontinue this special investigation.

I know of only one case where the *plusquamperfectum* also serves the purpose of bringing about a chronological order in the main clause. It is the pluperfect we have already mentioned, which as an exposition is placed in front of as well as behind the predicate action; placed behind, for example, *He wore a garment which he had bought in A* [er trug ein Kleid, das hatte er in A gekauft]; placed in front, at the beginning of a story, for example:

> *Forte per angustam tenuis volpecula rimam*
> *Repserat in cumeram frumenti.*
> (Horace. *Epistles* 1. 7. 29)
> [Through a narrow crack in the grain basket
> Squeezed a little fox.]

It is frequently the same in German. Moreover, the pluperfect is used before a clause with *als*, Latin *cum* with the indicative, the *cum* of the concluding sentence or *cum inversum*: for example, *no sooner had he said that, than the door opened* [kaum hatte er das gesagt, als die Thüre aufging]. It is possible, in this case, to have the pluperfect in the preceding position, because the listener is aware that something valuable should be communicated to him. He places the action of the pluperfect before the predicate of value, and he induces simultaneously that this predicate of value must be a direct report about something which happened in the past. How similar this means of expression is to the subordinate clause has been indicated above. The grammatician's designation *cum inversum* or *cum in Nachsatze* [in the concluding sentence] clearly demonstrates that even coarse sensitivity can discern the logical concluding sentence in the action of the pluperfect.

Otherwise, the tense of the main clause served to determine the relationship of the action to the temporal stage of the person present. The special use of the augment was employed by the Indo-Germanic languages, and is present in Greek and Old Indian (Skv). If it is correct that the prefix syllables *a*, ε actually meant *at that time* [damals], and I myself do not doubt it, the listener could then deduce the past, because *at that time* [damals], as opposed to *now* [jetzt], would be sensed. But this could no longer be sensed as an indication of a definite earlier time, when one thought of the preceding clause as a sign of the preterite. Similarly, in German we speak of *at that time* [dunnemals] or say *it was at that time* [das war damals] with the meaning *earlier* [früher], and the Latin *olim* [at that time] is probably derived from the pronoun *ille* [that there].

If several preterite actions were now named one after the other, originally in any case, it would have been sufficient to use this preterite sign once, because in this temporal augment the force of the preterite indication would be retained long enough. Thus we also say: *at one time the Greeks went to Troy, besieged the city for ten years, and conquered it* [einst zogen die Griechen nach Troja, belagerten die Stadt zehn Jahre und nahmen sie ein], without having to repeat the temporal designation *at one time* [einst] with each individual action. In this way, all of the expositive means are always used only once and then related by the listener to all the following utterances in a continuous linguistic series. If one forgot the inherent meaning of the temporal augment, and if the preterite form were in any way different from the present form in the formation of the ending and the stem, then both forms, with and without an augment, of the same meaning would be used *next to each other*. This condition is present in Homer's poems and in Sanskrit, until either the form with an augment (Attic and Common Greek) or the form without an augment (Latin, German, etc.) prevails.

The most important means of speech for the indication of chronological order is thus the cultivation of the subordinate clause. In connection with this, the transformation of the meaning of the tense is also important, as long as the tense of a subordinate clause does not only indicate the chronological order of the speaker's temporal situation, but also indicates this for the action of the main clause. Speech thereby begins to gain the advantage of temporal connections. But this, however, only puts the smaller pieces of a larger story in relation to each other. The sentences themselves must again be construed by the listener in their temporal relationships, exactly in the same way as in the main clauses we have discussed above, for example *veni, vidi, vici.*

For arranging these larger members, speech has also created *arrangement words*, such as *thereupon* [darauf], *then* [dann], *now* [nun], *again* [ferner], *meanwhile* [indessen], *in the meantime* [unterdes], Latin *deinde, tum, autem, interea, interim, postea.* In Greek the ambiguous ἐδ prevails over all other forms of linkage, such as εἶτα [then]," ἔπειτα [thereupon]. It is very difficult, however, to link all the members in this manner, or at least it never happens, because the consequence would be a feeling of pedantry. In the end then, even with the use of the most orderly connections, the construction of the chronological order from the substance of the action is mostly left up to the reader or listener.

And is then the clause linkage so exact, or could it be so exact in all cases, that the temporal relationships could be completely determined? If I say: *when Caesar had crossed the Rubicon, he penetrated into Italy* [als Cäsar den Rubico überschritten hatte, drang er in Italien ein], is there contained in the linkage form even the smallest indication of how long the intermediate time is between the two actions? I relate *someone is reading* [jemand liest] and continue *meanwhile there was a knocking at the door* [indes klopfte es an die Thür], and there is no indication of how long he read. If one tried to do justice to all the questions which could be posed about the exact fixation of time one would encounter insuperable difficulties. The speaker gives only the chronological elements which are important for the comprehension of the entire predicate. The other elements of time are only approximately indicated, or are omitted entirely.

XIII

*T*HE *way of connecting and relating the subject to the verb, and the verb to the object, must also be construed by the reader. The words themselves do not indicate this.* How terribly different the relationships can be thought of in the various connections of words, for example, *to have: he has a house, a book, an illness, a headache, a sharp mind, black hair* [haben: er hat ein Haus, ein Buch, eine Krankheit, Kopfschmerzen, eine scharfen Verstand, schwarzes Haar], or *to make: he makes a jour-*

ney, mistakes, a table, leaps [machen: er macht eine Reise, Fehler, einen Tisch, Sprünge].

The correct construction of this relationship may only be possible when the listener already has some background knowledge of, for example, the financial situation, the condition of health, and the mental capabilities of a particular person. Thus, from actual, known relationships, not from the present linguistic information but rather from previous experience we supplement an expression which supplies but little to its complete content.

The type of movement of the acting subject is also completely different in every activity; for example *A eats, A lives, jumps, hits, writes* [A isst, A lebt, springt, schlägt, schreibt]. *And just as varied is the way in which the object is affected by the activity*; for example, *I see the man, I hit him, admonish him, nourish him* [ich sehe den Menschen, ich schlage ihn, vermahne ihn, nähre ihn]. But all of these relationships are indicated by a specific grammatical form, by the nominative as the subject case, and by the accusative or dative as the object case. In the passive voice the nominative is the indication of the object.

Indeed, language itself offers only an extraordinarily small number of indications about the relation of the action components to the action as a whole; yet it is precisely these few ways of connecting which form a significant part of the content in the action clauses. In this case it is the same as in the listener's conclusions discussed above: at the beginning these conclusions are drawn slowly, until habituation mechanizes them; and then the listener and the speaker *believe* that the supplementations gained by inference are expressed in the words of speech themselves, because the mechanized series of conclusions no longer cross the threshold of consciousness.

The linguistic indication of an action with a subject and an object is a series gradually passing in time, which is thus not brought to the listener's mind as an entirety, but in individual parts. In this case there can be two processes: (1) first the action is given, that is, called to the listener's consciousness, and then the particulars of the subject and the object, or (2) first the indication of the subject and of the object is given, then the indication of the activity.

(1) *Dare librum fratri decet*. Or, *dari a me librum fratri decet*. [It is fitting to give the book to the brother. It is fitting for me to give the book to the brother.] The first process by which the linguistic indication of an action is brought to the reader's mind is illustrated in the above examples. The act of giving, i.e., a type of movement which goes from one person to another and conveys an object to the latter, is what the listener is first conscious of in these examples. This movement or activity as such

was obviously never present. It is seen or observed only in the definite case, when a definite person gives another definite person a definite object. Only by the well-known process of unconscious abstraction does one comprehend the individual moments of movement simultaneously as a unit, and the subjects and objects as universal people. But without these subjects and objects the activity lacks all limitation, all form. From the very beginning they must be included as the determining points of the activity when thinking about the action. Thus, given an utterance *he gives the book* [er gibt das Buch], one can ask *to whom then* [wem denn], because one necessarily includes this point of reference as a limitation.

So, if we hear *dare*, and if we understand the activity, we think straight away of a subject person, an interested person, and a neutral object. However, we think of all of these points as indefinite, and, therefore, as points about which we would like to ask some questions. The connection of these points is conveyed to us by the activity *to give* [geben]. If we are further given the dative case, its function will be to indicate the person concerned, whom we had to think of when supplied *to give* [geben]; similarly with the accusative and the nominative cases. Thus, the abstract picture of movement, with its indefinite and abstract constituent points, is raised to a definite and concrete picture, i.e., the indefinite points are corrected and transformed to definite points. The process is, therefore, similar to supplementary correction which we discussed above.

Because of the frequency of this process in our own mother tongue, only seldom do we still sense this psychic transformation. We do sense it, however, in foreign languages, in which we are less fluent. Nevertheless, in testing whether this process also takes place in the most fluent understanding of speech, we find that our expectations are disappointed if the points necessary for the construction are not indicated. We are missing something, and we know exactly which point of relation to specify. For example, if the sentence: *we give to you* [wir geben dir] appears incomplete to us, we then ask: *what?* [was denn].

The second process by which the reader is informed of an action with a subject and an object is illustrated in the following example: (2) *Frater librum tibi dat.* [The brother gives you the book.] Here, the subject, the object, and the interested person precede the word of action. The form *frater* is sensed as the subject, according to the sound form, i.e., the listener thinks: the brother is acting or doing something. An indefinite object *something* [etwas] is made definite by the subsequent *librum*. The dative case likewise arouses the expectation of an act, which will take place in the interest of the named person. In this case it is the action which is indefinite at first; the way in which the subject and object are to be connected must initially also be completely indefinite. This relationship first becomes definite by the quality of the action; as soon as the word of activity is given, these abstract, indefinite relationships receive their definiteness. Thus here too, the picture thought of as indefinite and completely abstract is amended by the subsequent supplementary correction.

In this case, our consciousness of speech also gives us proof that this process really does exist, even though it usually takes place unconsciously. If a verb were placed after the accusative and dative, which could not be connected with the case, there would enter a strong feeling of frustrated expectation, which we would indicate as an offensive grammatical mistake. For example, if in Latin *hoc remedium aegroto* [this remedy for the sick] were followed by *utor* [I use and ablative] instead of *adhibeo* [I administer and Acc.], we would be disappointed and have the discomforting feeling of a grammatical mistake.

XIV

I THINK it can be seen from the analysis given above how important this progressive construction of the action is for the whole of the life of speech. The expectation of elucidation of an indefinite, unclear relationship is stimulated in the listener. With this a bond is formed, whereby the individual parts are soon incorporated as members of a sentence whole. If the expectation is fulfilled, then one has the feeling that the message has been completed.

The accomplished speaker is in a position to *nourish an entire series of expectations at the same time.* For example, let us examine the following sentence: *When Caesar, who had subdued Gaul, had crossed the Rubicon, he advanced in a short time to the heart of Italy* [als Cäsar, der Gallien unterworfen hatte, den Rubico überschritten hatte, drang er in kurzer Zeit bis zum Herzen Italiens vor]. With the words *when Caesar* [als Cäsar] an expectation is immediately aroused, and as this remains unfulfilled the word *who . . . Gaul* [der Gallien] arouse yet another expectation and then with *had subdued* [unterworfen hatte] the first expectation is still unfulfilled. Indeed the first aroused suspense of the expectation continues and does not even end with the words *had crossed* [überschritten hatte]; here the expectation is maintained by the form of the subordinate clause. The fulfillment of this expectation is brought only by the main clause.

But perhaps this main clause doesn't even contain the really important part of the message. It might possibly be given only after a hundred or a thousand clauses, for example, as it is in a novel, and the expectation of such an important message continues, until the important part is actually communicated. In this way then the aroused expectation forms the inner bond of the sentence, of the paragraph, and of the linguistic work of art.

Those languages which are not inflected apparently must leave much more to the listener's construction than the inflected languages. However, these also leave much unclear and unsure which can only be clarified by the entire content of the message. In German one says not only *I throw the stone* [ich werfe den Stein], but also *I throw at the man with the stone* [ich werfe den Menschen mit dem Steine]; in both cases the linguistic expressions are quite similar, but the relationships to be thought of are completely different. Clarity in each individual case is given only by reflection about the character of the object and the intention or the consequences of the activity. In Latin *castra munire* can mean *to raise a fortified camp* [ein befestigtes Lager aufschlagen] as well as *to fortify an extant camp* [ein vorhandenes Lager befestigen]. When Horace says;

> *Velox amoenum saepe Lucretilem*
> *Mutat Lycaeo.*
> *(Odes* I. 17. 1)

[He quickly leaves the Lycaean mountains
For the pleasantly situated Sabine.]

he then means the opposite relationship, as with the words:

> *nunc mitibus*
> *Mutare quaere tristia.*

[Now to seek to change
Bitter words to sweet.]

In this case, the listener can only be certain if he makes a causal connection between the action of *munire* and *mutare* and the other preceding and following actions.*

If one is listening to a story or another linguistic communication, one will often make the observation that *one knows words beforehand, even before they are spoken,* or one can at least give synonyms for them with assurance. Indeed, when the speaker gets stuck in a conversation the listener often helps him out. Often the listener can tell the speaker the word for which he is searching in vain. For example, imagine the following

---

* *Editor's note:* Here Wegener explains briefly that the ambiguous meaning of some words and passages can only be resolved in context.

being related: *when I to Berlin* [als ich nach Berlin], we could assuredly insert a verb of motion like *come* [kommen], *drive* [fahren], *go* [gehen], *travel* [reisen]. The listener has thus supplied the activity of motion from the *terminus ad quem*. The ease of such a supplementation is increased to the extent that (1) the situation of the action to be communicated is known to the listener, and (2) the connection of certain words is isolated and mechanized. Thus the Romans of the classical period would have supplemented only an official name and, first of all, *decemviri* [the ten men]. The word *quod felix* [that bring good fortune] arouse the well-known supplementation by themselves. In this connection, an instructive observation is how much we abbreviate and imply; for example, Latin *S. p. qu. R.* [Senate and the Roman People], *u. s. w.* (3) The ease is also increased to the extent that, with the character and the situation of the subject given, the choice of a possible action is narrowly limited. The Greek ποταμὸς ἐκδίδωσι [the river surged forth] can only have one object, the water. If one calls *stop* [halt] to a carriage driver, the object cannot be in doubt; *mounting* [das Aufsitzen] can have only one goal for a horseman.

I do not want to go into further detail here but simply to point out the fact that in such cases in which a determining point of the action or the entire action are supplemented by a built-in necessity, *certain abbreviations of linguistic expression* have emerged. I have indicated above the absolute usage of the transitive verbs; it is to be added that intransitive verbs have developed in the same manner from transitive verbs. It is known, moreover, that in the Latin *ablativus absolutus passivi* the logical subject will not be linguistically indicated, but will be supplemented from the context, for example, *Caesar Gallis victis in Italiam rediit* [Caesar conquered Gaul, returned to Italy]. The whole area, which one often encompasses with the name ellipsis, requires an accurate classification of the individual material. However, the principles are clear, and it appears to me that they have been exhaustively illustrated.

In the case of the verb the point of relation, acting subject, and affected object must be thought of at the same time. This is also the case with the substantive indications of an action which require supplementation: for example, *dying* [das Sterben], *death* [der Tod], *life* [das Leben], *the walk* [der Gang], *the trip* [die Reise], *the blow* [der Schlag], *the throw* [der Wurf], πρᾶξις [doing] *exercitatio*, etc. This is especially the case with the *substantivis actionis* and *actoris*. The supplementations of the subject and object brought to these are in the genitive; only the connection, thus the word's ability to be construed, can show how the function of the genitive noun is to be regarded. The immediate feeling places these genitives parallel to the verbal subject and object, and afterwards calls them subjective and objective genitives. It is thus only one step further, when these words actually pass over into their verbal character as infinitives and participles, and assume a verbal construction as infinitives and participles. In them, instead of in the verb, is also found the well-known transfer of the relative meaning to the absolute.

XV

IF WE see a man digging, working as a potter, or making a table, we probably perceive actually no more than that he sinks the shovel, kneads the clay, or that he is planing and sawing. But we express our knowledge gained from perception as *he is digging, he is making a table* [er gräbt, er macht einen Tisch], and so on. In sensual perception we perhaps distinguish clearly every thrust with the shovel, every push of the plane, and every turn of the lathe; but if we must explain the activity, we do not indicate a multiplicity of movements, but rather single actions as the collective entirety of those individual movements.

It is completely different, however, when we do not understand the activity. Then we say *he is continuously turning a disk, stabbing into the earth* [er dreht immerzu eine Scheibe, sticht in den Boden], and so on. But this understanding can only lie in the consciousness of the purpose with which the acting person is pursuing his activity. *We first recognize and understand actions through the purpose of the activity, so that the activity becomes the purpose of the action. The purpose is thereby the bond by which we condense a series of movements to an entirety.*

Likewise planing, digging, and turning are actions, since certain means and movements must be employed in order to attain the respective goals. Indeed, the movement itself can be this goal, but one assumes reasonable purposes for human activity, i.e., those which can be regarded as worthwhile for the egotistical or moral human being. Only under certain special conditions can the movement in itself have such a purpose. Therefore, one would not consider a purposeless movement as an action in quite the same way as, for example, digging, beating, jumping, swimming, running, walking. With these movements one will always look for the purpose which lies beyond them; in other words, one regards them as merely instrumental.

This conception apparently has its basis in the mechanization of the activity. One no longer usually feels that walking is itself a goal for which certain means must be set in motion. One could call such activities or actions *mechanized actions* which occur automatically and which no longer leave a trace of a spontaneous desired activity, conscious of a purpose.

It is of the greatest importance for linguistics that we sort out such activities. First, *they form the building blocks from which the complicated actions are linguistically composed*. Second, they are the cause for the differentiation of *two types of subjects* (a) *spontaneous*, intentional, and acting consciously with a purpose, and (b) *automatic*.

Let us first of all concern ourselves with the last fact. It would be hardly conceivable that an impersonal object could assume the speech forms of a personal being, and that the activities of a personal subject could be predicated of an impersonal one, if the personal subject were always to be thought of as spontaneous and rational in the clauses of activity. On the other hand, it is quite easy to transfer the forms of automatic movements which we perceive in our own actions to the animated object. *So moves the indicator* [so geht der Zeiger] of the clock from hour to hour, without our thinking about the fact that it must have had the intention of moving itself; likewise *so runs, springs the globe, the ball* [läuft, springt die Kugel, der Ball] across the plain, and so on. I know quite well that this is not the only basis for the use of the metaphor, and I will later have an opportunity to comment more fully on the figure of speech. But I do regard the mechanization of action as a powerful lever in conveying the area of the objective and impersonal into the area of the free personality, so that the forms of the latter become the general pattern forms of the former area.

By means of this mechanization, it is possible that the personal forms of the subject are also related to the verbs of sensational condition and pain, exactly as it is with the verbs of external action; *to sense pain, sorrow, hear, sleep, lie, stand* [Schmerz empfinden, dolere, hören, schlafen, liegen, stehen] are not external activities or actions.

Moreover, we sense no contradiction when the passive verbs have the affected objects in the nominative case. This fact has also probably been facilitated in the Indo-Germanic languages as many of their object designations already had assumed the personal form of the nominative, a phenomenon designated as the personification of objective groups. The neuters of the *o-stems* can, however, take the accusative, but not the nominative, for example, *templum*, ἄντρον [temple], *magnum*, ἀγαθόν [good]. If they assume the nominative, their personality thus becomes masculine *magnus*, ἀγαθός [good]. In the Indo-Germanic languages, the neuter appears to have been used originally only as an object, because it is lacking the self-determining power of motion. For this reason, in the so-called nominative of the neuter, either every ending is missing and the simple stem will be related, or the masculine form of the accusative is chosen. The movement of an object thus appears to be thought of always as caused by a personal subject, and only the later differentiation between automatic movement and automatic subject makes it possible for those material objects to become automatic or mechanical subjects. I do not want to argue with the fact that analogous forms of the stem have also played a part in this type of grammatical personification, but had this formal similarity of the stems encountered a complete difference in meaning and function, the assimilation would have been difficult to effect. It also cannot be forgotten that people's opinions about what should be considered personal or impersonal are quite diverse, and vary according to their cultural level.

Of the great and continuous series of human movements and activity, the individual actions are merely the means of obtaining more purposeful objectives. The activities of *placing* [Stellen], *lying* [Legen], *sitting* [Sitzen] are first determined by the most inferior purpose of each activity's object. If I want to understand the expression he lays the *book down* [er legt das Buch hin], I must think of the purpose and from it visualize or think of the movements which find their limitation when the purpose is realized. Limitation by the immediate goal, for example, *I lay the book upon the table* [ich lege das Buch auf den Tisch], gives the purpose a more definite form, and at the same time gives the activity as a means a more limited form. *I write a letter* [Ich schreibe einen Brief], in this case the most immediate goal is the letter itself; it clearly determines the form which the activity of writing will assume. As we have observed above, the object thus itself also determines the form of the activity.

In the Indo-Germanic languages, the forms for the object are alike. Sometimes the object can equally well contain the thought of the immediate goal of the movement. The differentiation of the various functions which this form serves in certain connections, does, of course, have to be constructed. Moreover, this construction cannot be completely avoided even when we use prepositions for the immediate objective and the eventual purpose. This is because the *effected* object already mentioned above is nothing other than the purpose of the activity, for example, *he builds a house, he writes a book* [er baut ein Haus, er schreibt ein Buch], τειχίζει τεῖχος, *castra munit* [raises a fortified camp]. We must, however, differentiate this from the *affected* object.

It is interesting to notice wherein the actual difference of these objects lies: *if the effected object is the purpose of the activity, then the affected object is always the spatial goal of the movement.* For example, *I hit the man* [ich schlage den Menschen]; the movement of beating has as its spatial goal the man, *I see the house, I eat the meat* [ich sehe das Haus, ich esse das Fleisch]. Thus every activity has in its movement the affected object as a spatial goal. It is, therefore, natural that the spatial object* and the affected object have the same linguistic forms. Because the effected object indicates the purpose, although the purpose may be thought of in the form of a spatial goal, it is only natural that there is in this case also an agreement in the linguistic form.

We nevertheless sense a difference between the affected object and the spatial goal. *I hit the man* [ich schlage den Menschen] was thus originally *I hit at the man* [ich schlage nach den Menschen]. In the first example we really do feel that the activity has actually attained its spatial goal. However, in the second case we only sense that the activity is trying to attain the goal, without being informed of whether it succeeds. The following chapter should elucidate this problem.

XVI

W E HAVE seen that in order for the listener to understand an action he must always think of its purpose. *In the eyes of the listener this thought about the purpose gives the activity the direction toward its completion*, i.e., towards the limitation of the activity. The condition in which the activity finds its conclusion, thus the condition of completion, is the one aspired to; from this comes the connection of the verbs of intention with the perfect infinitives in ancient Latin and in Middle High German, with *wollen* [want] and *sollen* [should]. And, therefore, the indication of the beginning of an action necessarily arouses the listener's hope and expectation that the goal will be attained.

I kill [ich töte], *interficio* in the present tense means chiefly *I employ the means to bring about the death of a person* [ich wende die Mittel an, den Tod einer Person herbeizuführen], likewise *I lay the book down, I write the word* [ich lege das Buch hin, ich schreibe das Wort]. Thus the *presentia* and, correspondingly, the *imperfecta* are actually *de conatu*: *I seek to kill, to write, to hit* [ich suche zu töten, zu screiben, zu schlagen]. In spite of this, the form of the present tense signifies to us that the means have realized their purpose. In Latin and Greek, therefore, one has differentiated the *praesentia* and the *imperfecta de conatu* as special grammatical usage forms. *The spatial goals of such praesentia with this*

---

* Just as the names of cities, to the question, whither? are in the accusative in Latin, likewise the isolated forms *domum, rus,* the preposition with the accusative to the question, whither?, the poetical use of the simple accusative to this question posed by Homer and other Latin poets proves that this case was originally the means of expressing the immediate goal.

transfer of the meaning must be mechanized to attained goals, i.e., *to affected objects; the purposes of the action must become realized purposes,* i.e., *results of the action or effected objects.* This is the solution to the inconsistency between the goal and the affected object which appeared above.

In German the meaning of the future was developed from the meaning of the incompleted movement, which is aspiring to a future goal; for example, *I am going to the next inspection, I am going to church tomorrow, I am still going to do that* [ich gehe zur nächsten Musterung, ich gehe morgen in die Kirche, ich thue das doch]. Apparently, in this case as in the one which preceded it, the movement and the purpose are condensed to one momentary unit which can be thought of either with the time of the means of the movement completed in the present, or with the time of the purpose as completed in the future.

The phenomenon is exactly the same when *praesentia* with inceptive forms, such as διδάσκω [to teach], εὑρίσκω [to find], no longer indicates the beginning of the activity, but the whole course. What is more, some present compounds whose original meaning must have been inceptive assume futural meaning, whereby the condensed action is projected into the future; but the beginning is no longer sensed as belonging to the present. To these belongs the German compound future. *I will do* [ich werde thun] is a form of expression which originally must have indicated *I am now setting forth to do* [ich entwickele mich jetzt zum thun]. Also belonging to these is the Latin future with -*bo* such as, *amabo, monebo, ibo,* from the stem of the Greek φύω [to bring forth], Latin *fui.*

Etymologically, the German present passive is similarly formed: *I am beaten* [ich werde geschlagen], in which, initially, only the beginning of the activity is indicated; but the subsequent course is clearly sensed today with consideration of the goal.

We may assume that *through this process the Indo-Germanic languages developed their perfect tense.* In this form of the past tense no element indicates absolute completion of activity. Reduplication of the same word in free unmechanized speech affords a similar blending effect (as does the rhetorical *iteratio* and *duplicatio*), since free use of this duplication may mean repetition of action and increment in intensity as well as emphasis of continuing reality. Duplication is also found in the present and aorist tenses. How the present tense may assume the exact meaning of the perfect past is shown sometimes in the usage of a whole group of Greek verbs, such as ἀκούω [I hear], κλύω [I hear], πυνθάνομαι [I experience], αἰσθάνομαι [I perceive], γιγνώσκω [I know], μανθάνω [I learn], λέγω [I say], etc., Latin *audio, video* [I hear, I see], German *Ich höre, sehe, erfahre, bemerke* [I hear, see, experience, notice].

The double meaning of the continuing activity and the completed action as a state of being are likewise shown in the *nomina actionis* and *actoris*. Two examples of this would be *exercitatio*, meaning an activity of exercising as well as a state of having exercised, and *murderer*, *thief*, meaning the person executing the murder as well as a person in this state or of this character.

How much the present ongoing and the completed meaning of an action generally overlap is further illustrated in the French present passive *je suis aimé, I am loved* and in the same type of formation in Old German. It is furthermore illustrated in the meaning of a group of Greek perfect verbs, such as ὄδωδα [I had a smell] from ὄζω [to have a smell], δέδια [I feared] and δέδοικα [I feared] from φοβοῦμαι [I fear], οἶδα [I know], *I know* [ich weiss], πέφρικα [I bristled], and the German *Praeteritopraesentia*.

States of being form the conclusion of a series of movements; in certain situations then *the preceding movement will be construed by the listener in reverse from the designation of the state of rest* and be sensed along with the designation of the state of rest. One says about a wrestler who has fallen to the floor *there he lies, he is thrown down* [da liegt er, er ist hingeworfen]. Familiar forms of expression: πάσχω ὑπό τινος [to be treated by someone], ἀποθνήσκω meaning *I am killed* [ich werde getötet], ἀκούω meaning *it is said by me* [es wird von mir gesagt]. In Latin and German it is from the connection of the substantive verb and the adjective of the state of being that the passive perfect and the pluperfect are formed, such as *interfectus est, mortuus erat* [he has been killed, he had died]. On the other hand, states of being are designated by the action directed at a goal, such as Latin *cognovi* [I have learned]; and, very often, this is so in the Greek perfect tense.

XVII

BUT we must examine further the influence of *the expectation of a goal* or purpose of an action upon the linguistic presentation. This expectation is aroused by the suggestion of an action, and its influence is very significant.

Thus one relates *the war was declared, the first battle was bloody* [der Krieg wurde erklärt, die erste Schlacht war blutig], or *in the first battle were killed* [in der ersten Schlacht fielen], and so forth. It is not said whether belligerence actually followed the declaration of war; this sequel is assumed as self-evident because the goal of a declaration of war is simply the waging of war. Unless mention is made to the contrary, from the purpose involved one infers that hostilities have been realized. One could almost say with grammatical terminology that the present has been advanced to the perfect.

I received a letter that a friend had died [Ich erheilt einen Brief, dass der Freund gestorben sei]. That the letter was read is assumed as self-evident from the purpose of the letter. Without this *vaulting type of narration* it would be nearly impossible to bring a long story to a conclusion.

This fact gives us, furthermore, a new point of view for the *development and the change in the meaning of words*. When given a word which designates the beginning of an activity, if the further development leading to a goal is thereby considered, then the later stages of development can also be sensed as the content of the word. The Roman thinks actually not only of contact, upon hearing *intacta virgo*, or *untouched Virgin* [unberührter Jungfrau], but also of the further consequences of this; likewise with the German expression: *er hat das Mädchen nicht berührt* [he hasn't touched the girl]. Given *integer*, whose derivation is surely *in* and *tango*, certain consequences will always be thought of: of breaking, therefore *unconsumed* [unversehrt], or of besmirching and defiling, therefore *uncontaminated, pure* [unbesudelt, rein] in character. In the German *angreifen den Feind* [to attack the enemy], those consequences will always be thought of which follow the attack on the enemy, the fight itself. Similarly, *to handle the matter correctly* [die Sache richtig anfassen] may give instructions for an activity which are requisite for its execution.

The understanding of a story or any other linguistic communication thus emerges from (1) conclusions about subsequent factors in the development, (2) conclusions a posteriori from what actually lies ahead. For examples of this rule one should refer to the beginning of Goethe's *Hermann und Dorothea*. How very many conclusions *a posteriori* must be drawn, in order to acquaint oneself with the person who is speaking, the situation of which he speaks, and the facts which precede the beginning moment of this story. One should also refer to Uhland's *Klein Roland, das Nothemd*, and innumerable other stories of this type.

It is self-evident that such conclusions *a posteriori*, if they are repeated and mechanized, can be included in the meaning of the word, as was the case in the examples given below: κεῖμαι [I am driven] as perfect passive to τίθημι [I put], ἀποθνήσκω [I am dying] as passive to ἀποκτείνω [I kill], ἐκπίπτω [I fall] and φεύγω [I flee] as passive to ἐκβάλλω [cast out, exile].

It is hardly necessary to give a special presentation to prove that the listener's anticipation and *a posteriori* conclusions are not drawn from the words themselves, but can be created by the experience gained from the appropriate action. When the experience is lacking, then understanding of the linguistically indicated action will itself be failing. *The meat is being cooked, the meat is well done, the dog is being beaten* [das Fleisch wird gekocht, das Fleisch ist gar, der Hund wird geschlagen]; this communication can only be understood when one knows the purpose of the cooking, and then recalls from experience which means best serve this purpose. With the word *well-done* [gar], we must be aware of the state of the meat when it is prepared for eating.

He who knows nothing of the manner in which a railroad train gets underway, will also fail to understand this message: *One shriek of the locomotive and the brother had disappeared* [ein Pfiff der Locomotive, und der Bruder war verschwunden]. *For the understanding of a linguistic designation of an activity then, one needs the knowledge of the developmental factors and of the activity's goal.*

Those conclusions directed at the subsequent situations in an action are produced by expectation. *This expectation originates from the frequent experience that an activity usually continues in a certain fashion.* This expectation plays a great role in the whole inner relationship of factors, as we have partly shown above. We must observe still another effect of expectation.

In the example given above *war was declared* [der Krieg wurde erklärt], we can continue *but it never came to war* [aber es kam nicht zum Kriege], or *it came nevertheless* [es kam jedoch], or *nevertheless it came* [doch es kam], Latin *sed* [but], *tamen* [nevertheless]. That is, we say that the listener's expectation of the actual outbreak of war does not necessarily follow in this case. The speaker should therefore have consideration for the listener's expectation of a connection between his sentences. Otherwise an asyndetone, the joining of sentences without expected connections, would make it difficult for the listener to understand.

The connection can also be concessive. In Latin *quamquam* [although], *etsi* [even if], *licet* [granted that], *quamvis* [however much] and *quam vis* [ever so much] clearly refer to the mental state of the listener, originally *as you very much would like* [wie sehr du willst]; the addressed person is but the listener. In this case, Greek could have the adversative word ἀλλά whose basic meaning is clearly *in another way* [in anderer Weise], from that which the listener would naturally hear or expect. The actual meaning of such a connection is thus: *War was declared* [Der Krieg wurde erklärt]; *it came differently than you* or *one suspected* [es kam anders, als du, or man, vermutest]; *it didn't come to war* [es kam nicht zum Kriege]. The concept *in another way* [in anderer Weise (ἀλλά)] cannot be connected with the words: *War did not come to pass* [es kam nicht zum Kriege], because it is not the sentence which is altered, but rather the expectation of the listener. Both sentences, *it happened differently* [es kam anders] and *the war did not happen* [der Krieg trat nicht ein], are in the end fused into one by the linguistic consciousness, as soon as the function of ἀλλά [but] is merely sensed, namely, the function of contradiction.

If the sentence read *War was declared, and thus it came to war* [der Krieg wurde erklärt, und es kam also zum Kriege], the expectation entertained would thereby be confirmed. The continuation is thus nothing more than the beginning, but rather just like it, and this is the meaning of *thus* [also]. One therefore uses the adverbs *so, thus, therewith* [so, also, somit], Latin *ita, itaque*, and Greek ὥστε to express this relationship corresponding with the expectation. The German *so* [so] in a subsequent sentence also originates from this usage. Indeed, the asyndetone would in this case also be sensed as conclusive through the use of a constructive, conclusive form.

The other concessive means of expression are also based on this expectation. German *doch* from *dô uch* [there, also] means *also in this case* [auch in diesem Falle]. Thus in the example above, *however, it didn't come to war* [und doch kam es nicht zum Kriege], means *also not in this case* [auch in diesem Falle nicht] when one should have expected it; similarly *dennoch* [nevertheless]. The formations with *auch* [also]—*auch wenn* [even if], *wenn auch* [although], καὶ εἰ, εἰ καί, *etsi, etiamsi*, and those with περ, καί περ mean also *although the war was declared, even then it didn't come to war* [auch wenn der Krieg erklärt war, so kam es nicht zum Kriege]. That is, they emphasize that both facts are valid, but that expectation cannot connect them with each other. It is the same in the German *obgleich* [although], meaning *if thought of in the same way* [wenn in gleicher Weise gedacht]. With *quamquam* and *quamvis* is meant that however valid one case may be, it does not invalidate the other. These concessive sentences are thus formations of speech which the speaker develops with regard for the expectation of the listener.

If we now no longer think of the comparatively basic meaning of those expressions, but rather of the subsequent or conflicting function, then we will be mainly confronted with the repeatedly observed fact that the expressions have become congruent with their function. But this function itself is already a transformation or special formation of the expectation. This is because the relationships which have aroused in us the expectation of a certain further development, now appear to us as the reasons themselves for this further development. *The psychic state of expectation is thereby changed into the logical conception of a causal relationship*; and the expectations we have gained by experience are, in their totality, the forms and the patterns by which we connect everything that happens in the world.

How incomplete and imperfect the experience is upon which are built these expectations and thereby the consciousness of causality at this time needs no special attention. The deficiencies of experience are indeed the main source of all mistakes. These deficiencies are a most dangerous source in that even the most deficient experience arouses the expectation for the development of an action, and forms the consciousness of causality. From this come the many foolish and childish connective forms shown in superstition and in the so-called mythical thinking of peoples. But we do not want to pursue the deficiencies in this method of connection any further. Nevertheless, we have established the fact, so extremely important for the life of speech, that from this experience there results an expectation of a definite further development of the action, and that from this develops *the pattern, by which we believe we must connect the sequence of the action.*

With this transformation of expectation the listener loses the feeling of suspense inherent in the expectation; with the contradiction he loses the feeling of disappointed expectation. Instead of this, the listener senses only the unemotional awareness of logical agreement and logical contradiction.

Given the character of those experiences, there often appear enough *breaches of the pattern*, because the expectation is often based upon such incomplete and deficient experience that it must be false. How interminably frequently in a story occur those sentences with *nevertheless* [aber, doch], how often the plot develops differently than one expects! Thus that expectation pattern is only conjectural, and it does not have the character of strict adherence to solid law.

XVIII

ON THE whole, the listener seldom becomes aware that his conclusions about the further development of an action are uncertain and only conjectural. If, in a story, the fact which we have expected follows the fact which has aroused our expectation, then the speaker's conclusions correspond immediately with ours. And, if one hears in quick succession the phrases A *promised to come, but didn't* [A versprach zu kommen, kam aber nicht], then the listener doesn't have time to become conscious of the suspense of expectation, nor to surrender to the uncertainty of whether A will come. But as soon as he is given time to sense this expectation he will also sense the uncertainty of his conjecture, and the question will arise *will he probably come* [wird er wohl kommen]?

If I read from Cicero *he feared that he would lose his political influence* [er fürchtete, dass er seinen politischen Einfluss verlieren würde], then, if the speaker leaves him time for the suspenseful expectation, the listener waits expectantly for the further development. But if the speaker continues right away *and he actually lost his influence* [und wirklich verlor er seinen Einfluss], then the listener has only the sensation that Cicero had correctly foreseen the trouble, and that he was also stricken with it. The expression *and actually* [und wirklich] has then in itself only one meaning: *what appeared to Cicero as possible had become so in fact* [was dem Cicero als möglich erschien, ist thatsächlich geworden]. In such a case in Latin, it would be stated either with a simple *et amisit* [and he lost], and thus it is left up to the listener to decide whether his fears were just or not; or one could add a confirmative *vero, profecto* [in truth]. This addition originally could have served only to answer the expectant question of uncertainty of the listener with a *yes, in truth* [ja, wahrhaftig], or, more correctly formulated, to confirm the conjecture of the listener.

The same phenomenon is found in the verbs of hoping, promising, taking an oath, threatening, and conjecturing, in which the realization in the future is assumed, but is expected with some uncertainty. We may assume that the Roman's linguistic consciousness with those *et vero, et profecto* was in the end the same as the German's with *und wirklich* [and actually], i.e., that it was sensed as a message of actuality. Thus in this case is shown, as in the Greek ἀλλά, the German *also* [thus], *the transformation of a subjective state of sensation to the conception of an objective real relationship*. The cause of this lies in the speed of narration which makes it impossible to have a feeling of suspenseful expectation or to ask a question.

When the listener loses the feeling of suspenseful expectation the expression loses an important factor in its stylistic effectiveness, precisely that suspenseful feeling. If the reason for the loss is the speed of the communication of facts so that the suspense cannot develop, then the artistic form of the presentation must change in order to give the listener time to cultivate the expectation to its fullest force, because the suspense in the expectation is exactly what is of greatest importance for an artistic story.

If it were important to the author to arouse interest for those dangerous times of Cicero and for Cicero himself, he would not merely say *Cicero was afraid of losing his influence, and he actually did lose it* [Cicero fürchtete seinen Einfluss zu verlieren, und er verlor ihn wirklich]. Rather, he would present in detail what thoughts, feelings, and desires were alive in Cicero. The fear would thereby be spread out, the listener would retain the feeling of expectation longer and, thereby, become more suspenseful. It is precisely in plot that the stylistic difference between analytical and synthetical form of presentation becomes very significant. For example, in Goethe's *Hermann und Dorothea*, the simple fact that Herman is afraid that Dorothea could reject him causes the poetic presentation: (Klio)

But the youth remained, and with no sign of joy he listened to the messenger's words, which were heavenly and comforting, sighed deeply and spoke: "We came with a swift carriage, and perhaps we will return home slowly and ashamed; because since I have waited I have been seized here with anguish, suspicion, and doubt and everything that wounds only a loving heart. Do you believe that if we simply come, the girl will follow us because we are wealthy, whereas she moves around destitute and exiled.

Undeserved poverty itself gives prize. The girl appears to be contented and active, and thus the world is hers. Do you believe that a woman of such beauty and manners was nurtured without ever exciting *the good youth?* Do you believe that up until now she has sealed her heart from love? Don't go that far so quickly! To our shame we should softly steer the horses around toward home. I fear that some youth is in possession of this heart, and that the gallant hand has reached out and already promised fidelity to the fortunate one. Alas! here I stand before her with my proposal humiliated."

[Aber der Jüngling stand, und ohne Zeichen der Freude
Hört' er die Worte des Boten, die himmlisch waren und tröstlich,
Seufzete tief und sprach: "Wir kamen mit eilendem Fuhrwerk,
Und wir ziehen vielleicht beschämt und langsam nach Hause;
Denn hier hat mich, seitdem ich warte, die Sorge befallen,
Argwohn und Zweifel und Alles, was nur ein liebendes Herz kränkt.
Glaubt Ihr, wenn wir nur kommen, so werde das Mädchen uns folgen,
Weil wir reich sind, aber sie arm und vertrieben einherzieht?
Armut selbst macht stolz, die unverdiente. Genügsam
Scheint das Mädchen und thätig, und so gehört ihr die Welt an.
Glaubt Ihr, es sei ein Weib von solcher Schönheit und Sitte
Aufgewachsen, um nie den guten Jüngling zu reizen?
Glaubt Ihr, sie habe bis jetzt ihr Herz verschlossen der Liebe?
Fahret nicht rasch bis hinan! Wir möchten zu unsrer Beschämung
Sachte die Pferde herum nach Hause lenken. Ich fürchte,
Irgend ein Jüngling besitzt dies Herz, und die wackere Hand hat
Eingeschlagen und schon dem Glücklichen Treue versprochen.
Ach! da steh' ich vor ihr mit meinem Antrag beschämet."]

On the other hand, in the expression *Cicero feared* [Cicero fürchtete], we know nothing of the individual sensations which are determined according to the character of the situation and of the person. Indeed, we do not even analyze the expression *to fear* [fürchten] in its general connotations: *to expect* [erwarten] and *evil* [Übel]. This series of thoughts proceeds so mechanically and quickly, *he expected an evil* [er erwartete ein Übel], that we are no longer conscious of the individual factors, even less of the thought factors in to *expect* [erwarten] and *evil* [Übel], and so on in continued analysis. We are accustomed to reproducing these series of thoughts so quickly that we sense them as a compact unit, as a group of thoughts.

Fear has thereby become for us a special kind of conception or conjecture. If we observe the Greek and Latin way of constructing these verbs we will perceive that this condensing of the thought process was not always present. In both languages a final clause with μή, *ne* is *followed by negative* μή ού, *ne non, ut* and the conjunctive. The particles μή and *ne* are mere negations, and, therefore, they are powerless to form a subordinate clause. The sentence: *timeo ne veniat* was thus divided originally into two main clauses: (1) *I fear* [ich fürchte] (2) *he should* or *may not come* [er soll oder möge nicht kommen]. As long as this connection is sensed in its etymological meaning, then, along with the thought of fear it must also be considered that the prospect of future trouble arouses the desire or will to repulse the trouble. Thus, along with the trouble itself there must be sensed this characteristic of repulsion. All of these individual thoughts have become bound and condensed into a group by mechanization. The clause of intention has become a mere supplementation of the transitive verb, thus an object clause. On the other hand, in the etymological sense, the form of the expression is the same as that of the artistic form of presentation when the prohibitive desires of a scared person are presented. In such a presentation, the sympathetic expectation of the listener would be much more suspenseful than in the mechanized expression.

A similar phenomenon is offered by the Latin verbs of prevention, which are accompanied by *quominus* or *ne*. An expression like *impedio eum, quominus* or *ne veniat* or *prohibeo* with the same construction etymologically means: *I hamper him, he should not come* [ich hindere ihn, er soll nicht kommen]. Neither *impedio* nor *prohibeo*, of course, in these earlier times was a completely sufficient expression for the German *hindern* [hamper], but rather they designated the expressions of an activity from which the prevention had to be inferred; maybe *I entangle someone's foot, he should not* [ich verwickle Jemandes Fuss, er soll nicht] = *impedio*, or *I hold someone back in his forward motion* [ich halte Jemanden in seiner Bewegung nach vorn fest] = *prohibeo*. In this case we are only concerned with showing that the content of the thought aroused in the listener by the mechanized expression is much weaker now than in the time when the etymological meaning was sensed.

The same holds true for the other Latin verbs accompanied by *ne* and also, to a degree, *quo minus.* Etymologically, there is a considerable difference between both means of expression; for example, *non deterret sapientem mors, quominus in omne tempus rei publicae consulat* [Death does not deter the wise man from making (so that he might not make) provisions for a period of time in all matters of the republic] (Cicero, *Tusculanarum Quaestionum* 1. 38. 91). The sentence with *quominus* is either an indirect interrogative sentence, like the Greek sentences with ὅπως, and indicates how someone should not do something; or the sentence is formed with the relative usage of the pronoun *qui,* like the German *damit* [with it], and supplies the information that the action of *deterrere* [to deter], is the means by which someone is prevented from doing something, thus *prevented by the intimidation of sorrow* [durch das Abschrecken am Sorgen verhindert]. The sentences with *ne,* however, the linguistic utterance of the hindering or preventing subject in direct speech. For example, *It was forbidden by the Pythagorians for it to be pruned, lest they eat the broad bean* [Pythagoricis interdictum putatur, ne faba vescerentur] Cicero, *De Divinatione.* 1. 30. 62) was originally *they should not eat* [sie sollten nicht essen]. The ruling verb is superfluous in these sentences as long as the sentences are direct utterances of the speaking person. However, it becomes necessary if the sentence with *ne* contains a report about an expression of another person's desire. And with this, each sentence is the exposition for the other, corresponding to the form of finished presentation. The verbs frequently used in these constructions have naturally forfeited their etymological meaning. For example, *recuso* is surely taken from the language of the courts, and the traditional technical judicial meaning *to reject a complaint* [eine Klage ablehnen] or *to protest against a complaint* [gegen eine Klage Einspruch einlegen] is probably the basic one. *Interdico* meant originally *I speak between them* [ich spreche dazwischen], so that the speaker is separated from his purpose. This is the final result of the historical linguistic development: *the action determined by its definite purpose is thought of quite generally no longer in the definite form, as it was in its etymological designation.*

This process is so regular that we can give several more examples: *to decline an offer* [ich weise ein Anerbieten zurück], nobody thinks any more about the declining gesture of the hand; *to reject something* [ich lehne etwas ab], the meaning of the leaning is forgotten; *I concede this* [ich räume dies ein], *concedo, permitto,* no one thinks any more about

232 The Life of Speech

spatial clearance; *I describe the house orally* [ich beschreibe mündlich das Haus], *describo*, who still senses the distinction between writing and oral description? *I disregard this point* [ich lasse den Punkt bei Seite], *omitto, praetermitto*, and so on.

As long as the actual meaning was clearly sensed when hearing the expressions, then the individually determined designation of the action must have given the reference for the general type; for example, from *to disregard* [bei Seite lassen] the general category for *to consider unworthy* [für unwert halten], from *describe* [beschreiben] to *portray* [darstellen]. On the other hand, if the etymological meaning had disappeared then only the general category of the expression would be understood. The expression coincided with and was congruent with its function, and the more general it became, the weaker.

I think we understand how a *timeo, ne* and related expressions originally aroused a much longer and more slowly proceeding succession of thought in the listener than they did after the appearance of congruity. This is because (1) the content of the so-called ruling verb was mechanized to congruity, and (2) the independent main clause with *ne* became a subordinated supplementary member for the ruling verb, a mere object. Along with this were shortened (1) the time to present the sentences, and (2) the content of the syntactical form in which the sentence was clothed. Furthermore the expression of desire was no longer sensed. Thereby, *throughout the expression, the possibility of the development of suspense in the listener's expectation had to be reduced*, for example, if the fear were realized.

XIX

B UT let us now leave this question and return to the investigation of how the listener understands the communication of an action.

We have seen how in the connection of subject, object, and activity a continued correction takes place. We have observed the significance of the idea of a purpose for the bringing together of the motions to *one* action, and also the great importance of expectation for the connection and relation of actions to an uninterrupted succession of activities. The only remaining question is how and with which means of speech does the listener construe the individual action?

In all of the Indo-Germanic languages there is a multitude of *de-*

nominative verbs, that is, those verbs which are formed from a noun or adjective by a derivative affix; thus in German are found *ackern* [to plow], *kutschen* [to drive a coach], *fussen* [to be based on], *stiefeln* [to boot], *satteln* [to bridle], *pflügen* [to plow], schriftstellern [to write], *tischlern* [to do joiner's work], *mauern* [to lay bricks], *röten* [to paint in red], *ergänzen* [to fill up], *kürzen* [to shorten], *schwärzen* [to blacken], *künden* [to announce], *ebenen* [to level], *öffnen* [to open], *trocknen* [to dry], *bessern* [to make better], *verschlechtern* [to make worse], *entzweien* [to divide in two], *einen* [to unify], *einigen* [to unite], *donnern* [to thunder], *bevölkern* [to populate], *blättern* [to turn over the leaves of a book], *begeistern* [to inspire], *rändern* [to edge], *zertrümmern* [to smash], *duzen* [to thou a person], *ihrzen* [to address a person as ihr], *schattieren* [to adumbrate], *grundieren* [to ground], *stolzieren* [to flaunt], and many others. Some French denominatives are: *barricader* [to barricade], *pallisader* [to fence in], *voyager* [to travel], *fourager* [to forage], *signaler* [to signal], *embarasser* [to embarrass], *cuirasser* [to arm with a cutlass], *actionner* [to rouse up], *perfectionner* [to bring to perfection], *occasionner* [to occasion], and so on. There are also Italian derivatives of this type as well as Latin derivatives like the following: *comare* [to gossip], *cenare* [to sup], *curare* [to care], *cumulare* [to accumulate], *numerare* [to count], *regnare* [to rule], *vagari* [to wander], *laetari* [to make joyous], *maturare* [to mature], *calcare* [to lower], *pacare* [to make peaceful]; *aegrere* [to be sick], *albere* [to be white], *salvere* [to be cold], *lucere* [to be bright], *lactere* [to become milk], *erudire* [to make an end], *finire* [to bound], *grandire* [to make great], *ineptire* [to act foolishly], *insanire* [to be mad], *ferocire* [to be ferocious]. There are also Greek derivatives such as: τιμάω [I honor], ἀντιάω [I meet], ἀριστάω [I eat a meal (not dinner or supper)], ἑστιάομαι [*sic*] [I am a guest], νοέω [I see], ὀκνέω [I delay], εὐδαιμονέω [I prosper], σωφρονέω [I am sound of mind], φορέω [I bear], χρυσόω [I guild (make golden)], δηλόω [I show], γυμνόω [I strip (naked)], ἐλευθερόω [I set free], βασιλεύω [I rule], φονεύω [I murder], πομπεύω [I escort], δικάζω [I judge], θαυμάζω [I wonder], τειχίζω [I build], πλουτίζω [I enrich], μηδίζω [I act like a Mede in manners, language or dress], ἑλληνίζω [I imitate the Greeks], βαρύνω [I burden], ἡδύνω [I sweeten], and others.

If I say *he saddles the horse* [er sattelt das Pferd], *he plows the field* [er pflügt den Acker], *he dries the wood* [er trocknet das Holz], *he leafs through the book* [er blättert im Buche], *he adumbrates the drawing* [er schattiert die Zeichnung], *he levels the path* [er ebnet den Weg], the expression will be understood. But what is actually communicated by the verb to the understanding of the listener?

The verbal derivative affix of *satteln* [to saddle] gives us the notion of activity, but which activity? No definite one, but rather activity in the most general sense. By means of the substantive stem we are given saddle [Sattel], an object of this activity. The whole formation thereby etymologically designates *to undertake an activity with the saddle* [eine Thätigkeit mit dem Sattel vornehmen], or perhaps more suitably *to undertake the activity with the saddle* [die Thätigkeit mit dem Sattel vornehmen] because the determining and limiting factor *Saddle* [Sattel] is in the first position and already in our consciousness before the general designation of the activity is distinctly heard. Both components are related to each other as the logical predicate *saddle* [Sattel] is to the logical subject *the undertaking* [das Thätigkeitssuffix]. According to the already frequently observed law of the old Indo-Germanic word arrangement the logical predicate stands in front of the logical subject.

Since nothing was said to the listener in that formation about which activity was to be thought of with the saddle, he must gain understanding of this (1) from the very general conception of activity and (2) from an object which could be thought of in connection with this activity. If the object *the horse* [das Pferd] is added, the listener thereby is given a new point of reference by which he can determine and limit the activity to be perceived on the saddle.

If we say *he plows the field* [er pflügt den Acker], we are first of all given again the most general of all activities to be perceived of with the plow and, as a further point of reference and limitation, the object of the field. In this case too, we find the same fact observed above in the relationship of subject, object, and verb. *The content of an activity has to be construed by the listener in that he connects certain points of reference of the activity.* The way of connecting them has to be known by him. They are not given to him.

To give a simile, it is the same as with a geometrical problem: we are not given a complete triangle, but rather three points on a plane and the demand to construct a triangle. Therefore, we ourselves must then find the connecting lines according to our knowledge of a triangle. Or if we are given three points on a plane and the term *circle*, we must then construct the connecting circular line ourselves. Now, in the same way that the mathematical figure of the lines seems to be the most important part for perception (although this is not given in the above examples), it is equally true that the activity of connecting is the important factor for the action. It also is not given, but rather must be discovered, just as the solution to that geometrical problem.

If I say *he unifies the quarrelers* [er einigt die Streitenden], *he levels the path* [er ebnet den Weg], *he supplements the book* [er ergänzt das Buch], *he opens the door* [er öffnet die Thür], then the distinguishing characteristics for recognition of the action by the listener are (1) the activity, thought of in general terms, (2) the designation of the state of being, such as *level* [eben], *unified* [einig], *open* [offen], *complete* [ganz], and (3) the object toward which this activity should be directed. Let us first try to construct the relationship of these factors. The activity should be directed at the object in such a way that this object is brought into the given state. For example, the door should be handled in such a way as to make it ajar. Therefore, the action is not communicated to us, but rather must de deduced by us.

If we say *he writes* [er schriftstellert], *he joins* [er tischlert], *he saddles* [er sattlert], and so on, then besides the general activity, a category of persons is named: *writer* [Schriftsteller], *joiner* [Tischler], *saddler* [Sattler], a category which has been mentally classified according to the occupation. The listener thereby receives two personal designations of the subject, and the category designation of the predicate. The personal designations are both loosely positioned in the relationship, as if one said *he is a joiner* [er ist ein Tischler]. The listener must construe the personal designations correctly. He would not construe *writer* [Schriftsteller], *joiner* [Tischler], *saddler* [Sattler], in this case as in the case of the inanimate objects *plow* [Pflug], *field* [Acker], *saddle* [Sattler], but rather as people who are also personally engaged. He therefore infers the connection: *he acts as a writer* [er handelt als Schriftsteller], and so forth. I do not need to point out that such verb formations, which designate a special characteristic or a special category of people, can always be newly formed in a free fashion. In this way the verb *zastrowen* [to act like Zastrow] became common because of the notoriety of the Zastrowian crime. The same thing happened with the crime of Dr. Preuss, *preussen* [to act like Preuss].

From this observation we have discovered *three ways by which a certain action can be understood*: (1) by providing *the object* moved or affected by the action, such as *to saddle* [satteln], (2) by providing the purpose of an action, *to level* [ebenen], *to unify* [vereinigen], (3) by providing *the people whom we are accustomed to seeing engaged in a certain type of activity*, such as *to write* [schriftstellern], *to join* [tischlern].

We have seen above that the affected objects are actually the spatial goals of the activity, and, therefore, the first type of action designation could be named according to these spatial goals. Nevertheless, as a consequence of the mechanization of the activity and the separation of the form of expression we now differentiate sharply between the affected object and the spatial goal. That is, we would rather designate the action by means of the affected object. But the limitation of the action by means of spatial goals is also a very frequent way of designating actions. In Germany, the vernacular expression *to make for the city* [nach Stadt machen], *to make for Berlin* [nach Berlin machen], is probably very well-known. *To make* [machen] is the verbal expression of the activity in the general sense. The determining factor is only found in the spatial goal *to the city* [nach Stadt], *to Berlin* [nach Berlin]. It is probably the same in the Latin *proficisci*, a derivative of *facio* and the determining factor *pro* = forward. The German *entzweien* [to divide in two] is a derivative from the old *in zwei* [in two]. The expression thus originally designated the aim, but it is now conceived of as the determination according to the purpose, because we sense *entzwei* [in two] as a designation of state. The French formations which are probably in this group are *amasser* [to heap up, to bring together en masse], *amatir* [to mat, leave lusterless], *amaigrir* [to make lean], *amariner* [to man a vessel], etc.

In the same way that the spatial goal and the affected object actually coincide the purpose and the affected object also coincide. And since we are not only concerned about individual verbs in our investigation of the understanding of action we must also include the well-known connections such as the Latin *Romulum regem fecit* and the Greek ποιεῖν βασιλέα [to make king], a connection in which *Romulum* is the affected object, *regem* is the effected object, or the purpose, and the designation of the purpose is congruent with the German expression *zum Könige machen* [to make King]. In this case, the word for the activity is quite general, and the special type of activity must be deduced. But it is just as necessary to draw a conclusion with the more precise activity designations such as καθιστάναι [to land a ship], ἀποδεικνύναι [to have been in want of] *efficere* [to bring about], *creare consulem* [to make consul], *reddere caecum* [to make blind], *declarare* [to make known], *designare consulem* [to designate as consul]. This is because the appropriate connection with the activity to be understood is much more precise than given by the verb.

In this case we are thus faced with the phenomenon similar to that of the noun. The two major types of psychological substance are now analyzed into two-substances, the personal and the impersonal, such as *youth* [Jüngling], *Negro* [Neger], and so on. Thus *the most general type of activity can be analyzed into many subordinated genera and species.* Instead of *to saddle* [satteln] originally in the sense of *to begin to do with the saddle* [sich mit dem Sattel zu thun machen], one can also say *to put the saddle on the horse* [den Sattel dem Pferde auflegen]. *To lay* [legen] and *to put on* [auflegen] are subordinated genera designations of the action. Instead of *to adumbrate* [schattieren] one can say *to draw the shadow* [den Schatten zeichnen]; instead of *to address a person as "ihr", "du"* [ihrzen, duzen: ihr sagen, du], *to say "ihr", "du"* [sagen]; instead of *to make for Berlin* [nach Berlin machen], *to travel, go, drive to Berlin* [nach Berlin reisen, gehen, fahren].

It is of course obvious that supplementations are just as necessary with this type of designation as with the most general type of designation of activity. For example, *to put the saddle on the horse* [auf das

Pferd den Sattel legen] should designate a completely different type of activity than *to put the book upon the table* [das Buch auf den Tisch legen], or *to put the rug upon the floor* [die Decke auf den Fussboden legen]. We first have to supplement this special type of activity from the character of the point of reference and further from the purpose: for example, how we have to grasp the saddle, the book, the cover; how high and with how much force we must lift these things; how to spread out the cover; how we have to fasten the saddle so that the rider can use it, so that the cover fulfills its purpose. *To travel to Berlin* [nach Berlin fahren] designates for someone who lives near the railroad line something completely different than for someone who must travel with a coach or use his own vehicle. *To travel to Hamburg* [nach Hamburg fahren] is for the American or Englishman something completely different than for a resident of Leipzig.

This special species must therefore be supplemented and deduced by what is provided in the subordinated types of action designations. If this has been precisely designated then the individual type must be deduced, i.e., the exact way in which the appropriate subject performs this activity. We will come back to this point.

But we have still almost completely forgotten a class of limiting points of the activity, *the local limiting points*. At most we have only named their spatial goals. *The trip goes from Hamburg to London* [die Fahrt geht von Hamburg nach London]; in this sentence the *terminus a quo* is just as important for the designation of the action as that of the *ad quem*. *I fetched a bucket of water from the spring* [ich holte Wasser aus dem Brunnen]; in this case the *terminus a quo* is of the greatest significance for the limitation of the activity. *He went across the street* (er ging über die Strasse], *through the corn* [durch das Korn], *under the bridge* [*unter* der Brücke durch], *over the mountain* [über den Berg]; *he lived in Berlin* [er lebte in Berlin], *ate in garden* [ass im Garten] are all local imitations of the action, through which their peculiar character is first designated.

Thus added to the points of reference already named in understanding the activity are the local points of reference. Including a number of other points, we could incorporate these points into the class of *adverbial determining factors*. These also determine the activity's type of conception. Thus, for example, *by the sword* [durch das Schwert], and *by the noose* [durch den Strang] with *to kill* [töten], are very significant for the type of action. It is not necessary at this time to investigate these limiting points more closely, because we have seen how understanding is deduced from points of reference in general.

But it should be pointed out that a great number of these adverbs are local determining factors or have developed from the local meaning into modals. For example, the Latin *qua* is actually local, but sometimes modal, and always so in *quasi*. To understand this process, one should compare it with the German expressions *auf dem Wege des Frevels* [on the way of sacrilege], *auf dem Wege der Gewalt* [on the path of power], *auf den Bahnen der Sünde* [on the paths of sin]. Moreover, one might compare the usage of the originally local prepositions such as *per litteras* [through books], *per vim* [through power]; Greek διά [through] ἐκ [from].

XX

WE RESPOND emotionally to the objects of the outer world with wishes and desires, feelings of rejection, joy, pain, anger, or other strong affect, and the emotional stance may figure as supplement in the description of action or mental state. These German expressions are from the vernacular: *ich wollte nach Hamburg* [I wanted (to go) to Hamburg], *ich wollte fort von Hause und in die Fremde* [I wanted (to go) away from home and take to the road], *das Packet soll nach Berlin* [the package is (to go) to Berlin], *ich möchte fort, nach X, raus, ins Freie* [I want (to go) away, to X out in the open].

We are dealing here with connections of verbs of desire having local or spatial points of reference, connections which are conceived of by the listener in the sense of *I would like to get, drive, convey thither* [ich möchte dahin gelangen, fahren, transportieren], and *I would like to go away from* [ich möchte fortgehen von]. However, only the desire and the goal or departure point are linguistically designated. According to the way in which the desire's point of reference is realized, the listener then supplements the desired, wished-for, or required activity.

Exactly the same supplementation is supplied by the listener when an object is given with these verbs. In the sentence *I would like the book* [ich möchte das Buch], *to have* [haben] or *to buy* [kaufen] is supplemented. In the sentence *I want a bowl of soup* [ich will einen Teller Suppe], *to have* [haben] or *to eat* [essen] is supplemented; similarly with *I wish, would like ink, meat* [ich wünsche, möchte Tinte, Fleisch], [er soll einen Teller Suppe].

We have seen in the first investigations that human emotional processes are expressed quite directly by a special type of tone modulation, tempo, and intensity in the presentation. It is self-evident that the form

of the *Actio* of these emotions, as we have called it, cannot always replace the verbs for these emotions. For *this emotional outbreak is always
immediate and direct*, and it always has the speaking subject as its object
of the action. Thus a replacement by the emotional tone is only possible
in those cases when the speaker himself is also simultaneously the subject of those emotions. The form can be transferred to the reporting
speech, as we observed earlier, only according to the laws of formation
of indirect speech, thus with a change in tone and an exposition to the
report.

We previously discussed those imperative sentences solely consisting of
an object, such as *my boots* [meine Stiefeln], *roll* [Butterbrot], *a piece of
bread* [ein Stückchen Brot]. These sentences were, above all, statements
about the painfully lacking object. But they were sensed by the listener
as demands; for example, *to bring the boots* [die Stiefeln zu bringen] or
else *to clean* [zu putzen], *to give* [zu geben], or *to cobble (them)* [zu
flicken]; *to prepare and give the roll* [das Butterbrot zurecht zu machen
und zu geben]; or *to take the hat out of the closet* [den Hut aus dem
Schranke zu nehmen]. These demands are basically to insure the crying
subject's being given the desired object in a manner suitable to him.
Naturally, according to the perceptive or conscious situation or, as we
now say, according to the perceptive or conscious point of reference,
another action may thereby be intended and undertaken. For example,
book [Buch] means to read from it out loud. *The pictures* [die Bilder]
means to show them. *Another glance* [noch einen Blick] means to look
at an object or a person once again. *A swallow* [einen Schluck] means
to take a swallow.

One can differentiate here. On the one hand, there are affected and
effected objects which should be given in this means of expression. On
the other hand, there are objects of the action or inner objects which
should be given by the action itself, for example, *a puff of the pipe*
[einen Zug aus der Pfeife]. When looking at a pencil, *one more time*
[noch einmal] means to write or draw with it; similarly *another push*
[noch einen Druck], *another trip* [noch eine Fahrt].

Moreover, there is a contextual difference in whether the affected or
effected object is demanded of the speaking or addressed person, although there is no linguistic difference involved. *Another roll* [noch
ein Butterbrot] can thus be a demand upon the listener, and then *to
take* [nehmen] will be inferred and supplemented in a way corresponding to the object.

It is the same for demands with a local goal. *To Berlin!* [nach Berlin!] called out at the ticket counter is understood as *give me a ticket to
Berlin* [geben Sie mir ein Billet nach Berlin]. In the same way, of course,
the person being waited upon could be told *to the salesman!* [zum Kauf-

mann!]. The latter construes this as a demand to go to the salesman or to take something there. The shout, *here with it!* [her damit!] is probably meant in the sense of *come here with it* [komm damit her], but may be understood as *give that here* [gib das her]. Naturally there is no difference among the other local determining factors, such as in the point of departure of a movement: *down from the chair* [runter vom Stuhle], *away* [fort], *out* [raus], *out of the house* [aus dem Hause], *from the horse* [vom Pferde], *away with the books* [weg mit den Büchern], *away with the wine* [fort den Wein]; or with an object with the *terminus a quo* and *ad quem*: *your hands from your pockets* [die Hände aus den Taschen], *hand from the butter* [Hand von der Butter], *the sword in the sheath* [das Schwert in die Scheide], *the book in the closet* [das Buch in den Schrank].

In these examples, also, the demand can have a twofold relationship. Either it contains a command for the addressed person, or it can also be a demand of the speaker to himself, or to himself and to the addressed person together. Self-address should be judged by those principles which we have developed for monologic spech. However, the address of the speaker to himself and another present person is the basic form of *adhortativus*; for example, *away from here* [fort von hier], meaning *let* [lass] or *let's go away from here* [lasst uns fortgehen von hier]. That this demand also includes the speaker must, of course, be inferred by the listener.

Here are several more examples for the other local designations: *through the gate, over the table, in the closet* [durchs Thor, über den Tisch, im Schranke] (should be searched); *with the broom* [mit dem Besen] (should be swept), and so forth.

We also recognize the demonstrative as an imperative; for example, *here!* [hier!], *madam!* [gnädige Frau!], *there!* [da!], or often in the dialect *there!* [ta!] Upon hearing this, one simply supplements *take* [nimm], *you take* [nehmen Sie], *you eat* [essen Sie].

Also the *vocative* is an imperative and is understood as a verb, i.e., as an expression of action: *you!* [du!], *you there!* [du da!], *you!* [Sie!], *hey there!* [Heda!], *Hallo!* [Holla!], *Carl!* [Karl!]. According to the situation one supplements this imperative as *listen* [höre], *take* [nimm], *come* [komm], *wake up* [wach auf], or as a warning *don't do that* [thue das nicht] or as a stimulation to be attentive or obedient.

Also the question is by nature, as we have seen, imperative. When Götz shouts: *What news from my dear henchman?* [Was für Nachrichten von meinen lieben Getreuen?], *do you bring* [bringst du] is supplemented in agreement with the character of the object and the situation of the subject. One walks into a room and asks: *What, fire in the oven?* [Was, Fuer im Ofen?] or *heated?* [geheizt?], *new chairs?* [neue

Stühle?], *already?* [schon?], *the lamp?* [die Lampe?], *at work?* [bei der Arbeit?]. In each case the listener supplements another action. When Götz shouts: *My people, where are they?* [Meine Leute, wo sind sie?], the question *my people* [meine Leute] is sufficient for this situation, and the addition *where are they?* [wo sind sie?] is supplementary correction. Local questions are *to Berlin?* [nach Berlin?], *from Hamburg?* [von Hamburg?], *through the forbidden gate?* [durch das verbotene Thor?], *on the new street?* [auf der neuen Strasse?].

The emotions of joy and pain lead to the same means of expression and to the same type of inference and supplementary understanding from the listener. *Victory, Victory!* [Sieg, Sieg!] is sensed as *I, we have won* [ich, wir haben gesiegt]. *The Father!* [der Vater!] means *is here, has come, is coming, will come* [ist da, ist gekommen, kommt, wird kommen], *a letter!* [ein Brief!], *marriage!* [Hochzeit!], *a cake!* [ein Kuchen!]. *Today, to the Müller's!* [heute zu Müllers!], means *we have been invited to the Müllers, are going to go to Müllers,* oh, or! [weh, weh!], *the lion!* [der Löwe!]. *In prison!* [ins Gefängniss!], means *we are to go;* Götz shouts: *The apples of my eye in prison!* [in Ketten meine Augäpfel!]. Here follow several more of Götz's complaints: *Woe, alas! his wounds, a low fever!* [Weh, weh! seine Wunden, ein schleichend Fieber!], *Alas woe! Poison from my woman!* [Weh, weh! Gift von meinem Weibe!], *My Frank, led away by the abominable one!* [Mein Franz verführt durch die Abscheuliche!].

One can shout with emotional disparagement: *Pooh, these wretches!* [pah, diese Elenden!], *ugh, this retired life!* [pfui, dieses Stilleben!], or *fie on this retired life!* [über dieses Stilleben!], *swindle!* [Schwindel!], *nonsense!* [Unsinn!], *humbug!* [Humbug!]. These predicates of an action, of people, or of conditions, can be and actually are sensed as complete sentences, and are understood as verbs of judgment; for example *they work at swindle, nonsense* [sie treiben Schwindel, Unsinn].

As examples for *other emotional outcries,* the following phrases should be sufficient. The bailiff says to Götz: *I will accompany you* [ich werde Euch begleiten]. Götz answers: *Very honored!* [Viel Ehre!]. *Thanks!* [Dank!] *Many thanks!* [vielen Dank!], French *merci!* Italian *grazie! He or I!* [er oder ich!] From Egmont: *Then it happened, bim, bam, back and forth!* [Da gings, rick, rack, herüber, hinüber!]. *One more step and you're done for!* [noch einen Schritt, und ihr seid verloren!]. *In vain, the neighbor strides to France!* [Umsonst, der Nachbar schreitet nach Frankreich!]. In indignation he shouts, *I don't want to go to France!* [ich will nicht nach Frankreich!]. *One crack and the house disappeared* [ein Knall, und das Haus war verschwunden], *a war and nothing remained* [ein Krieg, und nichts bleibt übrig], *a bridge, and I am saved!* [eine Brücke, und ich bin gerettet!]. *That to me!* [Mir das!], *to chide me!* [mich zu schelten!], *unhappy me!* [me miserum!], *woe this life!* [vae victis!] All of these are passionate outcries, from which the listener infers various phenomena.

XXI

FROM these forms of direct and spontaneous emotional utterance, it is above all clear that *for the understanding of associated action there is absolutely no necessity for certain special words which we call verbs.* When the speaker is presently active or suffering in front of our very eyes, the actions will be inferred which, according to experience, cause or remove this emotional state.

The points of reference of the action associated with this immediate manner of communication may now be properly divided into only two large classes: (1) *the subject,* and in the end that is *the self-conscious man alone* and (2) *the objects,* which are either personal or impersonal. Belonging to these two classes are all local points of reference to the action, not only the local goal as an affected object and the purpose as an affected object, but also the point of departure, the points through which the action extends, and the point of rest of the action. They are all touched by the action, and *they are all objects of thought of the self-conscious speaking subject.*

While the listener is certainly aware of only himself, this subjective mode of thinking and feeling is nevertheless present in every other person. And although the listener can only see the speaker as an object which is facing him as a perceptual picture and with whose mentality he has sympathy, he understands this object and its mental states only as far as he can equate these mental states with his own. He then interprets according to this analogy, in that he thus transposes himself into the mind of the speaker. Since this human process of mentally equating oneself with another person is one of the most common of all, it must also be one of those which are most strongly mechanized, and, which, therefore, proceeds unconsciously most of the time.

In this way the speaker again becomes a subject for the listener. The true and actual subject can thus only be *I,* that is, the first person. For the first person, the next subject will be the second person, which is for the first person *once again* an object, thus a *secondary subject. Tertiary subjects* are those of the third person, as far as they are present as causes of action in the consciousness of the first and second person. A fourth degree would be found in those subjects present in the consciousness of a tertiary third person. A fifth degree would be found in those which a fourth degree third person self-consciously senses and conceives of as causes, and so on in an endless gradation. In the same way, the objects [of all these subjects] are arranged in degrees.

If this relationship were brought to vocal utterance its lucidity and simplicity would be thereby extraordinarily compromised; but mechanization is also helpful in this case. The speaker loses his awareness that, in addition to their function as subjects, the second and third persons function simultaneously as objects. One can just imagine the endless chain which would arise if this awareness were not lost. For example, if one wanted to say: *Cicero said that his enemies wanted to destroy him* [Cicero meinte, dass seine Feinde ihn vernichten wollten], then one would have to say: *I (the speaker) have Cicero in me as an object of memory; I imagine of this Cicero that he had his enemies as conscious images in his mind and that he imagined of them that they, who had him as an object of consciousness, who also were subjects for Cicero himself, that they wanted to destroy him* [Ich (der Sprechende) habe in mir den Cicero als Erinnerungsobjekt, diesen Cicero stelle ich vor, dass er seine Feinde als Bewusstseinsbild in der Seele hatte, und dass er seine Feinde vorstellte, dass sie, die ihn zum Bewusstseinsobjekt hatten, der wieder Subject für den Cicero selbst war, vernichten wollten].

The simplification of linguistic expression consists of the speaker's transferring his consciousness of the subject, which he has experienced concerning himself, to other subjects. He thereby steps out of the picture completely, although a trace of the relationship is still preserved in the differentiation of the persons, of which the first person is the primary, the second and third persons are secondary and tertiary subjects. But this trace is mechanized and so shortened that one is no longer conscious of it.

The *transference* itself, however, is nothing more than the *insertion of the first person's forms of speech into those of the second and third*, i.e., *the forms of direct and immediate speech are transformed into a report*. Thus, as we have seen, changes in the emotional tone appear, and expositive explanations about the situation become necessary.

One should now ask which are the forms of the direct and immediate emotional expression. This question has been fully discussed in the preceding section and in the first discussion. This form of expression is the word-sentence.

The next question would be what are the means of exposition of the report. These means are those which make it possible for the listener to understand a logical predicate of which the context is given neither in his perception nor in his immediate memory.

This answer is, of course, a very general one; it really cannot be defined specifically, although it can probably be illustrated. In a report, first the action is completed, and in such a way that the consequences are no longer perceptively present as a condition; the action is that of the aorist. Second, the person who acted is no longer present as an acting person, and, therefore, is not the person immediately sensing or affected by the action. For example, if the first person reports one of his own previous actions, the emotional states of that time and their linguistic expressions are not present. Therefore, they must be indicated by words which can summon objectively the emotional state to the listener's consciousness, rather than enacting it as present; for example, words for *to be angry* [zürnen], *to speak* [sprechen], *to complain* [klagen], *to be pleased* [sich freuen]. And if the emotional state is not present, then the indication of the acting, speaking, angry, complaining subject will also be missing and this absence may require linguistic indications. Third, those persons who were in the presence of the previously acting subject, if there were any, are no longer present and must be indicated. Fourth, likewise, the persons who cannot be counted as second persons, to which the action is related, must be indicated. Fifth, the objects in the broadest sense of the word, that is, the local points to which the action is also related, must also be indicated.

Yet, from all of this we may see no distinct difference from direct speech. What was indicated in direct speech? Only the logical predicates. In reporting speech, however, the logical subjects will also be indicated. For example *Victory, Victory!* [Sieg, Sieg!] was direct speech, and the listener knew who was speaking, who had the sensation of joy, and who was victorious. A sentence can say reportingly: *A yells: Victory, Victory!* [A ruft: Sieg, Sieg!] In this case, *A yells* [A ruft] would be the exposition. But if we want to report that A was once victorious, then we must say: *A was victorious* [A siegte]. What is the exposition here in the reporting speech? First, the subject, secondly, the elements by which the victory is placed in the past. In this case then, the syllable *-te* (past tense suffix) or in Greek ἐνίκησε [it was resolved], the derivative components, whereby the stem νικη- becomes the third person of the aorist.

If I call *my boots* [meine Stiefeln], in indirect speech, that becomes *A yelled: my boots* [A rief: meine Stiefeln] or *A demands (my) his boots* [A fordert (meine) seine Stiefeln]. The exposition in this case is *A yelled* [A rief], *A demanded* [A forderte]; the change from the direct *my* [mein] to *his* [sein] occurs at the same stage as the change of emotional tone. I do not need to explain the same processes which occur in the other parts of the exposition: *The plague upon you!* [Pest über dich!] would be in a report *A wished the plague upon B* [A wünschte die Pest über B]. *Here with it!* [her damit!] in a report would be *A ordered B to bring the object X* [A befahl B den Gegenstand X zu bringen]. As we have already seen, certain expositive components become necessary for the foundation of the situation of perception and remembrance, and, therefore, also by such situations: *here with the book* [her das Buch].

Of course we must not forget that the report is also possible in the present tense. It is possible when notification is given of a person not present, thus the third person of an habitual action. It may also appear when an action occurs at another place, while the speaker gives the information; for example, *A lies* [A lügt] meaning, is accustomed to lying, or *A is now going hunting* [A geht jetzt auf die Jagd].

Therefore, the sentences of action with the precise forms of the verb actually become necessary only at the level of the report, and the forms of the report must be understood simply as indirect speech. In the reporting sentences we now come across the object, the local points of reference, and the indications of condition as supplementary designations of the verb; these were not the original circumstances. Originally, as we have seen, these points of reference were in direct emotional speech as sentences, word sentences. They were at first put together independently of the expositive elements by the report, but they were then amalgamated with the expositive elements and became parts of the sentence, according to the laws of the development of indirect speech.

Only with this conception of the origin of the sentences can what has been previously discussed be fully understood. The sentences with *timet, ne* and the related Latin sentences with *ne* were clearly the combination of an expositive verb and direct speech *he fears: A shouldn't come* [er fürchtet: a soll nicht kommen], *he refuses: A shouldn't receive* [er weigert sich: A soll nicht erhalten]. While direct speech itself already shows the developed form of reporting speech with a special verbal form, direct emotional speech says only: *A, not the book* [A, nicht das Buch]. *Utar aliqua re* [that against something], χρῆσθαι τινι [to use something] are most probably to be likewise explained by this construction. The direct statement says *with the axe* [mit dem Beile]; reporting speech adds the exposition *uti* and χρῆσθαι [use], and the instrumental remains with it.

Verbs of intention originally took the infinitive in the Indo-Germanic languages, as demonstrated in German, Greek, and Old Latin. The isolations of this construction may be seen with *volo* [I want], *nolo* [I do not want], *malo* [I prefer], *cupio* [I desire], the verbs of termination. These had the opportunity to be expressed in direct speech, although they were often used in a report. If we now consider that the infinitive in direct emotional speech is often an expression of desire or an imperative, and that it was once actually a noun, then it also becomes probable that it has been retained from direct speech. For example, *not to go* [nicht gehen], *to go* [gehen] direct; *he wished not to go* [er wünschte nicht—gehen] indirect. Only in this way can the negation in Greek verbs be explained; for example, that of preventing with the infinitive, ἐκώλυσεν αὐτὸν μὴ ἰέναι: *not to go* [nicht gehen] *he prevented him* [er hinderte ihn].

If we now see that action will always be revealed from given points of reference, if we see further that direct speech is lacking this action designation or can very well dispense with it; we will then have to make *the development of the verb dependent upon the development of the report, and we have to regard the given points of reference, thus the objects, as the only possible factors from which this could develop.* Also etymologically, we find in the verb only a mechanized compound of nominal components; for example λέγο-μεν [we say] λόγο-s [the saying, nominative] λέγε-τε [you say] λόγε- [the saying, vocative].

Aside from the stem which we have designated as the logical subject, the elements of composition are expositional elements. There was no cause for an exposition with the first person singular of the present and the future, because in every case the first person singular itself had to be the speaking and sensing person; accordingly, in most of the verbal formations, the expositive element -μι was lacking. Correspondingly, the primary subject was lacking the inflectional elements ἐγώ, *ego* and the secondary subject was lacking *tu*, σύ as in the vocative.

The stem, which was the basis of the verb, then administered functions similar to those of the infinitive. Corresponding to this, we find these nominal forms after the verb of saying in indirect speech: for example εἶπεν ἐλθεῖν [he said], *er sagte* [he said] = exposition, direct ἐλθεῖν = *to come* [kommen] = *I am coming* [ich komme]. Also this infinitive is retained from direct emotional speech.

XXII

IT IS well-known that in his *Laokoon* Lessing considered the meaning of the action as an agent of poetry and discussed how this action takes place with regard to its use in poetry. We owe a great deal to the laurels of this great man as well as to the prestige which this brilliant investigation enjoys. We shall enter into this investigation as far as the purpose we are pursuing allows.

Lessing says (*Laokoon*, XVI. 98. Hempel, ed.):

It is true that the imitations of painting use completely different means and signs than poetry; the former are figures and colors in space, the latter are articulated sounds in time. If the symbols must have an indisputably comfortable relationship with what has been described, then symbols arranged next to each other can also express only objects which are next to each other or whose parts exist next to each other. Symbols which follow one after the other, however, can likewise express only objects which follow one after the other or whose parts follow one after the other.

[Wenn es wahr ist, dass die Malerei zu ihren Nachahmungen ganz andere Mittel und Zeichen gebraucht als die Poesie, jene nämlich Figuren und Farben in dem Raume, diese aber articulierte Töne in der Zeit; wenn unstreitig die Zeichen ein bequemes Verhältniss zu dem Bezeichneten haben müssen: so können neben einander geordnete Zeichen auch nur Gegenstände, die neben einander oder deren Teile neben einander existieren, auf einander folgende Zeichen aber auch nur Gegenstände ausdrücken, die auf einander, oder deren Teile auf einander folgen.]

Lessing is talking here about the means of poetry; but what is true for this means is true for all of speech. The means of poetry are thus: articulated tones in time, imitation and an unquestionably convenient relationship with what is designated. From these three premises it is concluded that the object of imitation must agree with the means of imitation in its temporal succession in its chronological course.

The conclusion can only really be valued if the premises are correct; but we do not want to pose the question in such general terms as *is speech an imitation of the presented object*? Rather, we would ask at this time if *the linguistic presentation of the action is imitation of the action itself*? Up to now our investigation has taught us that the presentation of the action leaves the construction of the action up to the listener and provides him with only the points of reference, from which he must, as it were, simultaneously solve the mathematical problem of connecting them with the corresponding lines.

We spoke about the saddle of the horse; how is it possible that one can imitate an action executed by the inaudible muscle movements of a man who touches a sensitive animal with an inanimate object? I can understand that one says that speech imitates the surge of the ocean, the whistling of a storm, the swishing of a bow; but how a means of tone should be capable of imitating an inaudible action, is beyond my comprehension. Certainly those sounds emanating from many actions are not articulated; but the means of speech are articulated tones! If speech is thus to be relegated to imitation, and if the purpose of speech is only to imitate objects to which the means have a convenient relationship, then speech and poetry can only reproduce an articulated sound. Where else then are articulated sounds to be found except in man's speech?

Furthermore, we have already seen that in those cases where speech imitates apparently articulated or even inarticulated sounds, the imitation deviates widely from the original; and yet these reproductions of strange sounds, which in the end have become unrecognizable, become effective means of speech.

But so much for imitation! Lessing is perhaps dependent in his expression upon only the unfortunate theory of the ancients, especially of Aristotle. What he probably meant by imitation is what we call description, as his further presentation seems to show. Of course, his proof is immediately annulled, as soon as the theory of imitation is overruled. *But is the presentation of an action really a description of it?*

To describe an action means to analyze all of its individual factors and to enumerate these factors one after another. Imagine if it were to be described how Diomedes walks into battle; we would expect of the poet in doing this to inform us which muscles the hero sets in motion, how often this muscle movement takes place, by how many feet he stretches his legs, how he moves his arms along with this, how many minutes he needs for this, and so on. That would be description of the action, but never poetry. Obviously there would have to be factors described, which Lessing forbids the poet to describe, because the motions of the arms and the legs would occur simultaneously. The hero's walking requires a ground or a field, and this would also have to be named in the designation of the activity. The movements would be influenced by legguards and armor, and these objects could not remain unmentioned in this situation.

Or let us choose an example from Lessing, *Ilias* V, Canto 722. I am using the part from the Jordan translation.

722   Hebe then immediately shoved onto the wagon's iron axle
      Wheels, rounded in ore, counting eight spokes. The rims
      Are imperishably formed of gold; as a tire over that
725   A pounded cover of ore, astonishing to look at;
      Silver hubs cover both ends of the axle;
      Weaved strips of gold and silver form the driver's seat,
      Which is held fast by a double railing as a breastwork.
      In front of him stuck the silver shaft. At the end it
730   Bound the golden yoke and firmly hooked the beautiful
      Golden hames on to it. Now the nimble racers were brought by
      Hera under the yoke, yearning for fight and the cry of battle.

722   [Hebe schob da sogleich auf des Wagens eiserne Achse
      Räder, gerundet aus Erz, acht Speichen zählend. Die Felgen

Sind unvergänglich geformt aus Gold; der darüber in Reifen
725 Angetriebne Beschlag von Erz, erstaunlich zu sehen;
Silberne Naben umlaufen die beiden Enden der Achse;
Streifengeflecht von Gold und Silber bildet den Fahrstuhl,
Welchen geschweift ein Doppelgestäng als Brüstung einfasst.
Vor ihm streckte sich aus die silberne Deichsel. Ans Ende
730 Band sie das goldene Joch und hakte an diesem die schönen
Goldenen Kummete fest. Nun führte die hurtigen Renner
Hera unter das Joch, nach Streit verlangend un Schlachtruf.]

Lessing remarks about this (*Laokoon*, XVI. 100. Hempel, ed.):

If Homer had wanted to let us see Juno's chariot completely, then Hebe
would have to put it together piece by piece in front of us. Instead, we see
the wheels, the axles, the straps and halters, the seat, and the shafts, not so
much as they appear altogether, but rather as they are brought together by
Hebe's hands. For the wheels alone the poet employs a whole line and points
out to us the eight brass spokes, the golden rims, the brass bands, the silver
hub, everything by itself. One might say that since there is more than one
wheel, then there should be given as much extra time to describe each one of
them as their special appearance required.

Will Homer uns den Wagen der Juno sehen lassen, so muss ihn Hebe vor
unseren Augen Stück vor Stück zusammensetzen. Wir sehen die Räder, die
Achsen, den Sitz, die Deichsel und Riemen und Stränge, nicht sowohl wie es
beisammen ist, als wie es unter den Händen der Hebe zusammenkömmt.
Auf die Räder allein verwendet der Dichter mehr als einen Zug und weiset
uns die ehernen acht Speichen, die goldenen Felgen, die Schienen von Erz,
die silberne Nabe, Alles insbesondere. Man sollte sagen: da der Räder mehr
als eines war, so musste in der Beschreibung ebenso viel Zeit mehr auf sie
gehen, als ihre besondere Anlegung deren in der Natur selbst mehr erfordert.

Basically then, Lessing admits in the case of the wheels that the poet
presents them simultaneously, in order to describe them more dramatically. The reason for this is just as bland and incorrect as the whole
imitation theory from which it is created. What is more, the action of
building is neither imitated nor described; the actual words of Hebe's
activity are (722) *Hebe schob* [Hebe shoved], (729) *ans Ende band sie
das goldene Joch* [she bound the golden yoke on the end], (730) *und
hakte an diesem* [and hooked onto this]. The action of shoving in this
case consists mainly in taking; the wheels must be taken from some
place, be lifted up, carried somewhere, placed in the appropriate position
so that they can be shoved, and then be fastened. There is not a trace of
all this in the presentation. And if it were said, how and in which position, with which muscle exertion and movement did Hebe perform the
individual activities? How are the feet and legs placed? If Homer had
described all of this he wouldn't have been Homer.

Moreover, it is clear that such a description, given by a poet or prose writer, would be no more vivid than Haller's description of the flowers of the Alps, which Lessing rightfully dismisses as poetically unsuccessful.

Thus, not merely the reason Lessing gives to explain why poetry can only describe actions, but even the assumption that poetry is capable of vividly describing actions is false.

The solution of the problem which Lessing attempted was probably impossible, given the deficient psychological knowledge and education of those days. Therefore the statements are less those of the great critic than those of the times in which he lived. But there are also the statements of contemporary times, which so often thoughtlessly repeat Lessing's theory or attack it with dull weapons, even though there are now many more means available to answer the questions than there were at Lessing's disposal.

XXIII

*I*S IT *then impossible to describe actions?* In the literal sense of the word, certainly. We are not capable of vividly understanding an exact description of an activity which presents the individual processes, and equally incapable of giving one.

The activities of walking and lying down, when analyzed into their individual components and impulses, would either be incomprehensible to the listener, or at least would lose all of their vividness. Nevertheless, up to a certain degree, an analysis of an activity remains vivid; for example, *he took the wheel, raised it, turned it toward the axle, and placed it upon it* [er nahm das Rad, erhob es, wandte es nach der Achse hin und steckte es darauf]. Walking is itself very hard to analyze; but with Homer's βῆ δ' ἴμεν it could be correspondingly said *he strode out and walked, raised his foot and strode* [er schritt aus und ging, erhob den Fuss und Schritt]. If we wanted to analyze *to stride* [schreiten] further: *he raised the right foot, stretched it forward, placed it on the ground again* [er erhob den rechten Fuss, streckte ihn nach worwärts, setzte ihn wieder zu Boden]. Thus we would no longer be describing vividly, we would only be explaining dryly and in a troublesome way. The listener would lose the suspense and his interest; the latter because something unnecessary had been given, the former because, in his expectation, he was already far ahead of the speaker's words.

We immediately sense that there can only be causation for such an analytic means of presentation when we assume that the listener doesn't know what *to stride* [schreiten] means. This is barely conceivable, and if it ever did occur, then we would prefer to show a person how it is done. Thus, we have shown that *in the analytic description of an action, certain limits cannot be exceeded*: (1) limits which are determined by the familiar acquaintance of the listener with the activity, (2) limits which differentiate the completely unconscious, purely mechanized aspects of the activity form the consciously purposeful movement.

Thus among the various types of activities in our consciousness there are the most simple activities present, which themselves can no longer be described, but rather can only be employed as building blocks of description. In general one can at least say that the mechanism of bodily movement can no longer be individually described, but rather that certain larger groups of muscle activity, such as movement of the leg, the eye, the head, the arm, and the hand may be regarded as the basic building blocks of description. These larger groups were formed in us and mechanized to automatic movements unconsciously; therefore, they can no longer be easily analyzed into their basic elements. It is just the same with the elements from which are combined the larger groups and activities of our minds. For this reason physiology and psychology, with their analytical descriptions, are only understood by the expert, not by the layman, not even by the educated layman.

Of course physiology and psychology are in actuality understood by many people; thus also these two most elementary basic activities of man are comprehensible through analytical description. Indeed they are! The question is only by what means. The answer can be given right now: by any means which enable one to understand activities which are unfamiliar to him as a listener. However, these means are not subsumed in continued analysis.

Let us first of all establish: *all mechanized movements, which we assume are also automatic for the listener, will no longer be analyzed in their component parts*, except for the purpose of making conscious what we do unconsciously and automatically.

These simple activities are the motions previously designated as the building blocks of the presentation of an action. To us they seem to be the simplest of all activities, but they aren't really. Rather, they are further composed of even simpler automatic movements. Thus we may use the convenient expression, molecules of action as compared with atoms.

Now what makes this atomistic process so difficult to understand? In a description from the mechanics of the human body, for example, in the description of the pronunciation of *a* or *r*, we must be told: *one places the tongue on the alveoli, opens the glottis* [man lege die Zunge an die

Alveolen, öffne die Stimmritze]. We know the actions of laying and opening quite well, but not the points of reference. We are not completely familiar with the alveolus and glottis, and, because of this, the special activity which is required in this special case is unknown. We have here exactly the opposite relationship from that expression of action which we found above. There the points of reference were known, and the action was supplemented without difficulty, even when it was not communicated. In this case the designation of the action is given, the points of reference are unknown, and we don't understand. This is because activity does not exist without relation to the points of reference; a verb without its objects is only an abstraction which says nothing.

The instruction about the sound physiology is therefore not understood because the points of reference are unknown. Surely one can describe these: the alveolus is the back part of the upper gum. The listener can't do anything with this instruction either, because he has never consciously observed how the tip of the tongue is laid on this part of the mouth, nor what effect this has upon the ear when this is aspirated. On the other hand, if he had really laid his tongue there according to the instructions and then aspirated, the action would then become comprehensible to him, but comprehensible only because he experienced the action consciously.

Thus, only those actions or activities experienced consciously can be understood by the listener. If one thought, for example, of trying to make clear with words how the fingers are to be rested upon the shaft of a pen to a person who has never held a pen nor seen anyone write, it would become obvious that this movement, just like every movement, is a succession passing in time, and that it is certainly recognizable in no other way than by the eye and the sense of touch. *Therefore, a notification of an action can only be understood by that person who has visually or sensually perceived the activity in another or consciously experienced it in himself.*

XXIV

BUT this view seems to lead to contradictions with the facts. *Who has ever seen the action of Faust, Iphigenie, or The Iliad with his own eyes?* Nevertheless we think we understand the action and are probably right, at least to a certain degree.

Let us look at the beginning of one of Homer's tales about Achilles' anger (Song I. 8):

Which of the immortals incited them (Atreus' son and Achilles) to
   hostile enmity?
Leto's son and Zeus. Because he, angry at the king,
Sent ruinous plague through the army; peoples sank:
That is because for him Chryses was insulted, his priest,
Atreus' son. Because he came to the hearty ship of Achaia,
Freely to buy the daughter, and brought eternal solution,
Wearing the laurel ornament of the striking Phoebus Apollo,
Over the golden staff; and he implored all Achaiens,
But most of all the Atreides, the two army princes of the people . . .

[Wer der Unsterblichen reizte sie (Atreus Sohn und Achilleus) auf
   zu feindlichem Hader?
Leto's Sohn und des Zeus. Denn der, dem Könige zürnend,
Sandte verderbliche Pest durch das Heer; es sanken die Völker;
Drum weil ihm den Chryses beleidiget, seinen Priester,
Atreus Sohn. Denn er kam zu den rüstigen Schiffen Achaia's,
Frei zu kaufen die Tochter, und bracht' unendliche Lösung,
Tragend den Lorbeerschmuck des treffenden Phoebus Appolon,
Über dem goldenen Stab'; und er flehete allen Achaiern,
Aber zumeist den Atreiden, den zween Heerfürsten der Völker . . .
                                                            (Voss)]

   Obviously the entire action is unknown to us, but among the individual actions there is not one with which we would not somehow have
become acquainted from experience: *to incite men to anger, to be angry*
[Menschen zum Zorne reizen, zürnen] is an activity we can easily understand. *To send the plague* [Pest senden] will not be familiar to most
readers of the *Iliad* from personal experience, nor will *to freely buy a*
man [frei kaufen einen Menschen] be familiar to many people, nor *to*
wear a laurel ornament [Lorbeerschmuck tragen]. Nevertheless, we believe that we understand these actions. Evidently we think of *to send the*
plague [Pest senden] with the analogy of *to send a contagious disease*
[ansteckende Krankheit senden]; *to freely buy a man* [frei kaufen einen
Menschen], with the analogy of cattle auctions or any other auction; *to*
wear laurel ornament [Lorbeerschmuck tragen], with the analogy of
wearing an *oak wreath* [Eichenkranz] or *wearing other leaved orna-*
ments [sonstigem Baumschmuck tragen].
   We do not, however, want to imply that through these conceptions
the comprehension of the listener is always complete. For the understanding of a foreign or temporally distant story there are also a great

number of historical, ethnical, and antiquarian facts which must be known. We are only concerned with how we believe that we understand such actions. *Understanding by analogy with a known process is understanding with a model, a simile.*

Such models can appear as completely sufficient or as only partially sufficient. In the former case, we have the feeling of complete recognition; in the latter case, we have the feeling of only approximate recognition, the feeling of only being able to conceive of something similar to what is meant.

Recognition of the action regarded as complete, which has been arrived at with a model, is not always, however, really complete and sufficient. This can be ascertained by looking at pictorial descriptions of ancient events in paintings or drawings of the sixteenth or seventeenth centuries. Of course, the listener or reader usually doesn't notice the deviations of his conception from the original action.

It would also be wrong to believe that those models are the same by which people of the same cultural level imitate a presentation of an action for its understanding, thus the importance of the subject, the objects, and the particulars of space.

The people discussed in a story, if unfamiliar to us, are first of all *visualized by us according to a model.* The characters of a situation actually are mentally visualized. If we are told something about an unknown living person, and we later see this person, then we would say *I imagined the person in that manner* [so habe ich mir die Person gedacht] or *I didn't imagine him thus* [nicht gedacht], *I imagined him large, small, blond* [ich habe sie mir gross gedacht, klein, blond]. The anticipated picture we form of a person does not merely originate when his external appearance is described, but also when certain of his inner, ethical, and spiritual character traits are known to us. This is because these traits are not completely dissociated from their relationship with bodily appearances. Given these inner traits, everyone imagines those external traits of the person as he has become acquainted with them in certain other individuals. The proof of this psychic process is seen in the way in which we, and especially the naive man, judges a stranger. The appearance of such a person probably reminds us of some traits of another person; this known person then provides the model according to which we judge the inner qualities of the new person.

One may listen to how naive people, especially women, judge the hero of a novel. One regards him as lithe and blond; the next, with a beard; the third, without a beard; one, with blue eyes; another, with dark eyes, and so on. If they want to characterize him more specifically, then they say that he is like a well-known person with similar characteristics. If a Frenchman is describing the head of Achilles, one will certainly recognize the suggestion of the Gallic features in his presentation, if an ancient pattern has not already supplied the model. In any case, when historical models are lacking, the artist's national type will be prominent.

The formation of such models occurs by the well-known psychological means of abstraction. The handsome men and beautiful women, the scoundrels and villains, the lovers, the Spaniards, the Greeks, the Italians are arranged together as groups in our minds. Similar features connect and strengthen each other, dissimilar ones inhibit each other. With the forming of these general pictures one should not discount *the relationship of the intensity of the individual pictures to each other,* from which such groups are compounded. *The degree of intensity* is first dependent upon *the degree of interest* we have for the individual picture concerned. For the formation of a model of a good mother or good father the picture of one's own parents will always be of salient significance.

Moreover, we must distinguish *in what order the individual pictures enter our minds.* It is indeed well-known that we recognize a familiar thing even when we only see a few parts of it, because we then fill in the other parts. This supplementation is only possible if we have a firm and complete image of the object. If individual parts of this image are associated by us with individual parts of another image, then the whole picture emerges. From this it follows that the connection of related images seldom occurs so that all similar parts are connected with each other and that all dissimilar parts inhibit each other. We see, for example, only particular parts of a new person and supplement them from the general picture we already have. This supplementation is nothing more than putting parts of the picture we have had previously in place of the new picture.

But this process does not first make its appearance when the general picture has been derived from a vast multitude of individual pictures. Every picture from which we apperceive an earlier one supplies parts and features for the picture which is to be newly apperceived. Therefore, the question of which pictures first appear in our mind is a vitally important one for the formation of models. Those most decisive for the models of people are thus those which have first been completely worked out as pronounced pictures in the child's mind. In addition, these people as a rule have the advantage of the greatest sympathetic or antipathetic interest in the mind of the child.

These models of ours are exactly the same in format as the ideals of character of the artist who draws and sculptures. Also the often-discussed trait of naive observers, especially women, of wanting to discover similarities everywhere, finds its origin in this type of psychic mechanics. In this manner are originated all of those models we mentioned above for hero, scoundrel, villain, curmudgeon, fiancé, stepmother, witch. One must only question whether these categories don't correspond in large degree to certain personal perceptual pictures which one feels can really lay no claim to generality.

We might remark here that we first become acquainted with many of these categories *through graphic presentation* or from written stories with illustrations. Naturally, from the illustrations the first visual experiences will adhere most firmly once again and provide the model for later characters. Thus for me the heads in Beck's stories of ancient times form the models for Odysseus and Achilles, and the illustrations of *Hansel and Gretel* in Grimm's fairy tales form the model for witches. The pictures of people obtained from such engravings may interact basically with those of living perceptual pictures for the formation of such models.

XXV

EXACTLY the same thing can be observed *with the objects and the spatial settings of the action.* If we read about *bread* [Brot], *wagon* [Wagen], *chalice* [Becher], *Wine* [Wein] in Homeric tales without any special knowledge of ancient times, then we conceive of these objects according to the model of contemporary bread, wagons, and so on. We therefore immediately supplement with contemporary manipulations the actions related to these objects. For this we need no special discussion, since it is generally known.

But what is the situation with the spatial scenes of the action? One should examine, for example, how one conceives of a chapel, ranger's lodge, a palace, a castle, a peasant's hut, the ocean's shore, or a valley in the mountains. At least I have noticed that when I consider a situation or spatial distribution of places or buildings in a story I am reading, I realize that I am simply transferring the pattern of the ranger's hut or the chapel from the models first formed by me to the ones in the narrated action with which I am presently concerned. Indeed, this happened to me just about a year ago with the ranger's hut in Spielhagen's novel *In Reih' und Glied*, and likewise with the chapel in the same story.

But along with this we notice deviations, deviations which are determined according to one or several *established patterns for movement.* I read in one of Heyse's novelettes that a Swiss man coming from Bologna

was traveling on a dusty turnpike and passed by a country house. As I
later examined how I had mentally arranged such actions, I found that
the country house lay to the left of the traveler and the highway. Odysseus goes to Circe, and for me her palace has been to the left of Odysseus
since my youth. Odysseus goes to the divine swineherd; for me, he goes
directly up to the house. From there he passes, on his way home, an
altar lying to the left; he arrives at his palace lying to the right. He has
to walk along the wall surrounding his courtyard; then he turns right
into the door, walks up to the house. The hearth in the house again is
to the right; but the dog is to the left of the courtyard. Hermes encoun-
ters Odysseus, on his journey to Circe, from the right; Athena meets
the returning Odysseus on the right. Calypso goes looking for Odysseus
from the right. Calypso goes looking for Odysseus at the seashore and
finds him sitting to the left. The homestead which Ingo passes in Frei-
tag's *Ahnen vom Grenzkamm* is to the left for me; the turn he makes
in order to get to Mr. Answald's farm goes to the left; the stream with
which Ingo is engaged flows to the right of his path.

I don't dare combine these personal perceptual forms into a general
rule; but, as it appears to me, everything which lies to the left is that
which is incidentally observed along the way, whereas everything which
is to the right or in front of the traveler is that for which he is intentionally looking. However, there are found on the way many incidental
points coming one after another, so that for me a change often takes
place, the first lying to the left, the second to the right. A change also
takes place when several sideward movements occur within a series or
continuation of movements, in certain circumstances.

It is also very problematical whether this way of looking at things can
be made into a rigid rule, even for a single individual. It is not the purpose of this discussion to search for such a rule. We have only imparted
these considerations to prove that there are present in our minds established spatial patterns, according to which we understand spatial
communications, and that we likewise have mental patterns for our
movements in space, according to which we understand and supplement communications of movement. It is of great importance that we
learn how we arrange the spatial relationships of an action according
to our own patterns of movement.

It is obvious that these patterns of movement are formed from the
automatic human forms of movement, and that, further, probing the
history of these means of formation is even more difficult that with those
of the patterns already discussed. It appears certain to me that the way
the right and left arms are habitually used is of importance. I don't want
to forget to point out one expression which occurred to me many times
during these studies: *to leave something to the left* [eine Sache links

liegen lassen]. Linguistic expression might also be conditioned in many ways by this pattern; for example, *he is the right one* [er ist der rechte] and *to the right* [rechts] have an identical stem. The goal is straight ahead, what is right is straight, and what is not right is a sidewards movement (compare French *droit* [right] and *tort* [wrong], *Recht* [right], *rectus*).

The same patterns are formed for *other fixations of the action*, which we have termed *adverbial*. These are *the points of reference of the intensity—quantitative and qualitative*. If we say *to cough strongly* [stark husten], *to run strongly* [stark laufen], we thereby indicate the coughing and running have exceeded a certain norm, precisely the correct norm, the *normative*. This normative is quite varied for all the different actions. A great intensity of tone may be indicated for coughing, but little for thunder, the roaring of the sea, of a lion, and so forth. We regard a man's running speed as considerable, but it appears insignificant when compared to the speed of a dog, a horse, or a locomotive. So these normative pictures of degree are determined by the character of the subject and the kind of activity.

A big child is small compared to an adult male, who is small compared to a tree, which is small compared to a tower. Thus we have normal pictures of quantity, which are likewise determined according to the character of the subject and of the action. The different subjects must therefore have an average size in our minds; likewise with *much* [viel], *little* [wenig], *often* [oft], *seldom* [selten].

Besides the quality, to use a convenient expression, are found the same normative patterns, which are determined according to the character of the subject and the action: a man is *handsome* [schön] because of completely different features from that of a lion; a knife is *bad* [schlecht] which doesn't cut; weather is *bad* [schlecht] which doesn't abet our purposes; *hot* [heiss] is a different temperature on a summer day than the warmth of a room in winter, and so on.

Thus all human groups of thoughts produce such normative and average pictures; we now only lack those for *action and activity*. Maybe one of us has never seen how someone partakes of his midday meal while sitting in an armchair and eating from a small table, as was the custom of Homeric heroes. Nevertheless he would know how to visualize this action. We have the pattern for *eating* [essen], and in this pattern is included the taking of the food, putting it in the mouth, mastication, and so forth. Of course, we eat cooked and roasted foods with instruments, unlike the ancients; therefore we must fancy away forks and spoons. The pattern of eating which now appears is that used with bread, fruit, and other foods. Eating from a table at the side is understood according to the pattern by which one takes away something from such a table.

Thus, as I have called them above, *the molecules of activity are the components of action which are always unchangeable, and are always formed according to the same pattern. On the other hand, the larger complexes of these molecules are varied in their composition, but in such a way that the sequence and the transfers from one molecule to another are again constructed according to definite patterns.*

The following sequence is inconceivable: to put the food first into the mouth, and then to take it from the table. We have learned from experience that *the sequence is generally determined by the purposes of the action and by the laws of causality. Along with this, the form of the larger action complexes also remains determined.* Only individual particles can be modified under certain circumstances in this sequence if their succession is not necessarily determined causally by the purpose. Therefore, if we say *the Homeric Greeks ate without forks* [die Homerischen Griechen assen ohne Gabeln], then the listener surely knows which part of the entire action complex is being touched *without forks* [ohne Gabeln], i.e., the food. Thus, the succession is determined by the particular *without forks* [ohne Gabeln]. With this the whole connection of the group remains intact.

From such patterns and laws of causality we know how to reconstruct even larger action complexes, for example: *he ate* [er ass], *left the Hall* [verliess den Saal], *went to the seashore* [ging zum Meeresufer], *boarded the ship* [bestieg das Schiff]. We know all of the patterns which illustrate for us the transitional movement from one element of the series to another.

But does everyone have such a pattern for every activity? Most assuredly not for many technical actions, and, therefore, the description of most technical activities is incomprehensible to most laymen. I need only recall Schiller's description of the action in bellfounding. Everyone who has had to explain the poem to students realizes the difficulties involved in understanding it. *Thus, only when the individual actions in the story are copied by the listener according to certain patterns, and when the connection of these actions is likewise constructed according to patterns and laws of causality which give the purpose, can one count on the listener's comprehension.*

If, on the other hand, the molecules of activity are combined to a merely accidental aggregate of actions without the binding putty of causality, then the perception and comprehension of the whole is rendered very difficult. For example, we can, of course, understand the sequence of actions enacted in a strange cult or festival ritual in its individual molecules; but these fall asunder incoherently, or as Lessing puts it, they all roll down the mountain up which the narrator has painstakingly rolled them. The listener cannot combine from them any vivid picture. The same happens to them as happens to the parts of a description of a pretty girl, a stately man, or a flower. This because there is lacking the putty of causality, and along with this, as we have seen, the binding magnet of expectation.

XXVI

WE HAVE seen how the points of reference are simultaneously the elements from whose connection develops the electrical current of the action in the listener's consciousness. In the same manner the purpose of the action arouses the electrical current of expectation, which, becoming prominent as a law of causality, also switches over missing elements, and includes more remote ones. We have seen further how the assimilation of these elements and currents takes place according to certain inner mental patterns. However, we must acknowledge that, within the sequence of molecular elements, there remain certain possible permutations, which we have designated as accidental and independent from the causality. We have further noticed that in the consistency of the molecules there was a certain variability. Thus, there was a possibility of changeability in the pattern, such as the Greeks of Homer not using fork or spoon, nor sitting in front of the table but rather next to it. All of these deviations from the pattern are deviations from "the universal picture," and the universal picture is what is general. Thus, these deviations are the particulars of the action, We must, therefore, pose and answer the question: how are we to understand individualization?

All nouns are designations of genus, such as *the man* [der Mensch], *the table* [der Tisch], *the country* [das Land], *the bench* [die Bank], *the mountain* [der Berg]; only proper names are, at least for certain circles in the language community, designations of individuality, such as *Cicero, August, Friedrich, Berlin, Bavaria*. In addition to these, we have those few words for beings and things which are like a name and are found only in certain instances. Such words include *God* [Gott] (although this word is also a designation of genus for polytheists), *devil* [Teufel], *hell* [Hölle], *heaven* [Himmel], *earth* [Erde], *underworld* [Unterwelt], *world* [Welt].

The individual character of these words proves that *a word's charac-ter of individuality is determined solely by whether we conceive of several or one individual thing in connection with it.* If several individ-ual things are connoted by one word then it must become a general pic-ture, a type of abstraction, and thus be related to something general.

A noun can neither be individualized nor become a designation of a concrete single person or thing by means of attributive connection with an adjective. For example, *the beautiful table* [der schöne Tisch], *the beautiful chair* [der schöne Stuhl], *the big man* [der grosse Mann], is always only a subdivision, a species of that genus *table* [Tisch], *chair* [Stuhl], etc., which summons all of the individual beings as a multi-plicity to our consciousness, to which the characteristics are passed on.

The verb also summons something completely general to our con-sciousness: *to rule* [herrschen] is predicable of many subjects and many objects; likewise, *to walk* [gehen], *to run* [laufen], *to listen* [hören] and all verbs. *The big man rules over the little men* [der grosse Mann be-herrscht die kleinen Menschen] can also be a general sentence.

The adverbial expressions like *very* [sehr], *little* [wenig], *violently* [heftig], *so* [so], *differently* [anders], certainly designate a general quan-titative or qualitative modification of being or acting. They once again are only the species of a genus: *very strong men, to desire violently* [sehr starke Menschen, heftig begehren], and so on.

Therefore, there would be only one possibility of designating some-thing individual—the proper names. However, we can discuss a certain bridge, a certain school, a certain closet without giving its name. Fairy tales hardly ever give names; but, of course, we think of the kings, ogres, fishers, and peasants as distinct individuals. Therefore, without regard to proper names, *with the general means offered us in our words of speech*, it must also be possible to delineate and understand individual things, people, and activities.

With the exception of the two people named in the title, the characters in Goethe's *Hermann und Dorothea* were given no name by the author. Nevertheless, there has hardly ever been such a masterful individualiza-tion as with the figures in this work. The innkeeper of the Golden Lion confronts us right at the beginning of the story with a speech, and then the author tells us: *Thus spake comfortingly to the woman the host of the Golden Lion, who was sitting under the door of the house in the market place* [So sprach, unter dem Thore des Hauses sitzend am Markte, Wohlbehaglich zur Frau der Wirt zum goldenen Löwen].

A speech with a specific content and in a specific form can only be spoken by a single individual. *The host of the Golden Lion* [der Wirt zum goldenen Löwen] will hardly have become a special general cate-gory for just any man, although one can surely imagine that someone could say *the hosts of the Golden Lion cheat the people* [die Wirte zum goldenen Löwen prellen die Leute]. Thus this someone claims that among innkeepers those of the Golden Lion have a special character, and that from the aggregate of innkeepers these are excluded as a separate species. But it is inconceivable that the Lion innkeeper, sitting in the gateway of the house in the marketplace and speaking to the lady, could possibly be excluded as a special category in anyone's mind. This also because the preterite is reporting a past fact.

It is thus already apparent that *all designations of genus meant to be thought of individually must obtain a set of attributes, which are thought to be present in no one's mind as attributes of a general category*. It is apparent, however, that these categories may not be the same for everyone.

In the example we have given *such attributes* were (1) *place: under the door of the house on the market place* [unter dem Thore des Hauses am Markte]; (2) *time:* the preterite *spake* [sprach]; (3) *conditions* which only obtain with the same people transiently: *sitting* [sitzend]; (4) *relationships* which are not present with every person: the woman as wife and her company with the man; (5) *action*, as can only take place once: the innkeeper's speech.

With the exception of the last one, these attributes would not singly be in a position to individualize: *under the gate the man thinks about the gate custom* [der Mensch denkt unter dem Thore an den Thorzoll] —that could be anyone. The connection with a preterite could also be understood in this sense: *earlier the man under the gate thought about* . . . [früher dachte der Mensch unter dem Thore an . . .].

A fixed limit for the individualization of an object or a person cannot be given, since everyone has a different number and a different delimitation of the categories. Nevertheless, *this approximate limitation is sufficient: comprehension of individualization is attained when an individual is demarcated by local and temporal attributes, by attributes of character and relationships with other beings, and by attributes of degree and quantity in such a way that they could no longer probably be the constituent attributes of a general category.*

If it is said that *In a big city a man lives* [In einer grossen Stadt lebt ein Mann], the listener doesn't know at first if one is speaking of a specific individual or of man in general, because one single attribute is not yet sufficient for an individualization. It might thereafter be said: *one lives cheaper* [lebt man billiger] *or more expensively than in a small city* [teurer als in einer kleinen Stadt]. But the continuation could just as well read: *a man, who has done much good* [ein Mann, der viel Gutes gethan hat]. *Only then would the listener gradually become aware that one is speaking of an individual, and that this occurs because of the continued restriction of limitation of the concept of the genus which he first heard.*

If we disregard the word order in our example and proceed with *a man* [ein Mann], then this expression is limited in its location by *in a big city* [in einer grossen Stadt]. It is further limited temporally and in its activity by *lives* [lebt], and further by the completed action *who has done much good* [der viel Gutes gethan hat]. The restriction consists of the group of thoughts, at first too generally regarded by the listener, gradually considered in more limited terms and thereby corrected; *the continued limitation is thus also continued correction.*

Correspondingly, it has been shown that the action is understood by means of continued correction. Naturally this principle is also valid in the following case: the more quickly and fluently such a spoken succession elapses, the less perceptible are limitation and correction to the listener.

One, therefore, knows that we sense no disappointment if we are forced to think of the genus first conceived of as something individual in what follows. But in addition to the fact of mechanization there is a new factor protecting us from disappointment, a factor known to us from what has already been discussed. We observed that we conceive of everything according to definite patterns. Indeed, these patterns as they possessed individual pictures were frequently stripped of individual features by means of abstraction. Nevertheless, the form of a specific individual picture was simultaneously the basic sketch from which only individual features, lines, and strokes were deleted; others were later inscribed therein, according to later pictures. The pattern for a witch was a specific witch, that of a man was a specific man with multifarious, blurred, and variable features. The general picture, of course, thereby always retains the character of a vivid individual picture, but only with the property that, in this form, there are clothed a multiplicity of individual beings. We have affixed the general attributes not to the formless groups, but rather to the solidly-fashioned ideal pictures.

Therefore, in our understanding of the general expression *man* [der Mensch], this idealized pattern of a genuine human figure emerges in our mind. Yet, if we should later think of this general man as a father, a hero, a noble youth, or a beautiful virgin, then there must necessarily occur a modification and reformation of this picture.

The more general a pattern, the fewer features this common picture contains. There is then no difficulty if this picture gradually obtains an expression of power or goodness, a mighty beard, a rosy face, dark locks, or blond braids, or if the figure is extended or diminished. The fewer features we conceive of with the picture, the more indistinct the picture is for us. If we see a human figure in the distance, then perhaps those attributes only first perceived are sufficient to recognize that the figure is human. As it comes closer we perceive new attributes; it is a woman. The figure comes even closer; it is a young woman. Later we recognize the color of her hair and her features in full detail. This sharply and clearly defined picture of the woman remains the same as that one first indistinctly perceived, but not appointed with a multitude of united features.

And it was not disappointment that we sensed during this event; on the contrary, our expectation was aroused. As the figure appeared in the distance, one asked: who might that be? With every step closer, the recognition became more complete, and as the figure stood clearly in front of our eyes, the expectation was gratified. *Continued modification of the picture is thus continued recognition and continued gratification of expectation.*

Everyone knows from his own experience that the first expositive particulars in a story are received with less interest by the listener or reader than the later action. How often has one heard, for example, that a reader has become involved in the extensively-sketched expositions of Walter Scott's novels. These expositions are designed to make the listener familiar with the individuality of the characters. Thus the interest and the suspense grow with more intimate knowledge of the characters and the situations in which they are involved.

Now, one can further observe that *by no means all characters,* of whom we have at one time heard in a story, *are developed as established and vivid individual pictures in our minds.* A great many characters in the story have no more individuality in our minds than the general feature *man* [Mann] or *woman* [Frau]. There is a twofold reason for this phenomenon. First, to the understanding of an individuality there always belong several features; the larger the number of these features, the more complete the individual picture is for the listener. Secondly, not all characters claim our interest to the same degree. However, when the interest is small or nonexistent, then the group of aroused thoughts surfaces with very little strength from the mass of other groups. We are only dimly aware of it and of the pattern from which the individual picture should be produced.

Thus is shown (1) *a gradation in the clarity and vividness of the individual pictures produced by the listener,* and (2) *that this gradation in the degree of clarity is determined by the interest of the listener in the character.* Therefore, the greatest clarity and vividness of these pictures will be obtained if the storyteller is successful in producing the highest degree of the listener's interest. Success is conditioned (1) by the nature and the character of the attributes given, and (2) by the way in which these attributes are provided by the storyteller.

The most energetic interests, as we have seen, are *the egoistic interests*, in the broadest sense of the word, i.e., the strivings connected with feelings of joy and discomfort and concerned with the sustenance and gratification of our ego. Our thoughts are, thus, fixed firmly on our enemies and benefactors. One gladly hears his enemy censured and his friend praised. He gladly hears the words which advance his personal spiritual endeavors. Since there is no lack of interest in this case the speaker easily attains vividness. These interests are called special interests and, thereby, are peculiar to only small groups in a language community. The advancement of baser egoistical interests may be regarded as immoral, however every person has these interests for himself alone.

If we ask about the *universal interests*, those common to all men, which the storyteller and, above all, the poet has to consider, they are those interests which arouse the same feelings in us as do the egoistical ones. However, they do so without our sensing a desire for the advancement of our own ego, a discomfort in inhibition, or a fear about the endangering of our own person. These are the *sympathetic feelings* of man, feelings of the same quality as the egoistical ones, but differentiated by the relationship: the egoistical feelings are related to the feeling subject itself, the sympathetic feelings are related to other people. Formally, this process is the same as the one discussed above, where the primary subject is replaced by the secondary and tertiary ones; simultaneously accompanied by a state of being indirectly interested, as the insertion of the tertiary for the primary subject was in indirect speech.

These sympathetic feelings of fear for another person, of hope, of joy, and of pain in the mind of someone else, come about by means of corresponding states of being into which the fellow human being is transposed. They occur in such a way, however, that we too would have those feelings if we found ourselves in the same state of being. Man's states of being are, however, conclusions of events undertaken by him. The situations which arouse our fears and our hope are precisely those which arouse our wish that the suffering person will be transported to a situation arousing our joyous feelings. In short, these feelings are aroused in us through actions, which, as a consequence, bring about states of suffering and joy in a stranger.

If the storyteller is then successful in arousing the listener's feelings in regard to an unfamiliar character, then the listener's interest is greatly increased, and, because of this interest, the individual picture or pictures will be easily raised from the mass of the other thoughts. *Thus when the attributes of individuality are closely related to our sympathetic feelings, our interest is increased. This is only possible with actions which lead to certain states of suffering, and the poet may thus depict only such actions. Lessing's demand was, up to this point, completely correct; only his reasons were mistaken.*

Nevertheless, free, *completely free, is the construction of these individual pictures, a free act of the listener.* It would be foolish to believe that the poet could, with his methods, force the listener to produce a picture completely and precisely. The patterns of the listener are different from those of the poet, and only according to our own patterns do we produce and construct these pictures. Therefore, Lessing is right again when he challenges the qualification for the description of personal pictures. The act of the poet, his whole great performance, lies in his forcing the listener consciously to conceive of independent, completely personal, individual pictures with full strength, with full vividness, in short, with full interest.

From this occurrence a whole group of postulates for the poet's art could be derived, but I only want to mention a few of the basic demands. If interest is founded upon the stimulation of feelings for the good or bad condition of a heroic person in a story (for example, for the bad condition of the scoundrel or antagonist), then the poet must oblige these aspirations and gratify them, because these aspirations produce expectations of hearing more about the further course of the state of suffering. If these further particulars are omitted, then the expectation is frustrated. Furthermore, since it no longer gratifies the strivings, interest is lost for the rest of the story. We can designate the demand contained in this as the demand for the *unity of the action.* From this demand the other *demand for the strict guidance of the action* is derived. From the complex surrounding situation of the characters and the action, one must impart only that which is necessary for comprehension of the action and for arousal of interest, because with every particular given we attach expectations. For example, if we were told about the building of a house, not because it was important for the further course of the action, but merely because of its architectural interest, then our expectations associated with the house would remain frustrated. We would feel restrained in our striving to experience more about the expected progress of the associated action.

Since, at this opportunity, I do not plan to pursue the questions raised about the sphere of poetry, I would like merely to draw attention to the following concrete instances: if the listener is forced to entertain interest for poetical characters, he then freely constructs for himself everything necessary for the perception of an individual picture. For this he needs no particulars or information from the poet. As an example of this, I am using Uhland's *Rache.*

The servant has stabbed the noble lord,
The servant would gladly be a knight himself.

He has stabbed him in the dark grove
And has sunk the body in the deep Rhine;

Has put on the shining armor,
Upon the lord's horse he has swung openly.

And as he wants to spring over the bridge,
The horse stops and rears up,

And as he gave it the golden spurs,
It flings him wildly down into the river.

With arm, with foot he steers and battles:
The heavy armor forces him under.

[Der Knecht hat erstochen den edeln Herrn,
Der Knecht wär selber ein Ritter gern.

Er hat ihn erstochen im dunkeln Hain
Und den Leib versenket im tiefen Rhein;

Hat angeleget die Rüstung blank,
Auf des Herren Ross sich geschwungen frank.

Und als er sprengen will über die Brück',
Da stutzet das Ross und bäumt such zurück,

Und als er die güldnen Sporen ihm gab,
Da schleuderts ihn wild in den Strom hinab.

Mit Arm, mit Fuss er rudert und ringt:
Der schwere Panzer ihn niederzwingt.]

This poem is an example of individualization purely from the interest for the action. The characters of the servant boy and of the knight are otherwise in no way differentiated by limitation from other servant boys and knights.

As a further example of the strict guidance of the action which forsakes the imparting of parts of the situation unimportant for the action, I present the beginning of Goethe's *Braut von Corinth*:

To Corinth hither from Athens
Came a youth, still unknown there.
He hoped he was suited to be a citizen;
Both fathers were related as guests,
Earlier had already called
Little daughter and son,
Bride and groom.

[Nach Corinthus von Athen gezogen
Kam ein Jüngling, dort noch unbekannt.
Einem Bürger hofft' er sich gewogen;
Beide Väter waren gastverwandt,
Hatten frühe schon
Töchterchen und Sohn
Braut und Bräutigam voraus gennant.]

Every reference to time is missing here, but later we are told in the action itself all that is necessary. All information about the background of the youth, his education, nationality, and also about his route is also lacking. About the situation is said only what is valuable for the action, according to the immediate necessity that everything said must have value, either in itself or in regard to a higher predicate. There is no performance of any action itself, and yet we understand what is communicated about action according to our own action models.

XXVII

WHEN the listener lacks a model it is useless to want to outline to him a description with a picture, because he lacks the capability freely to conceive of one. Therefore, he is not in a position to perceive either a spatial body or an action.

There is a means, however, to awaken his comprehension, a means we have already mentioned: *when the appropriate patterns are lacking, then one resorts to related patterns* and causes the listener to infer the object and the motion by analogy. This means is the *simile*.

It is wrong to believe that the simile is peculiar to poetry alone; it is one of the most common of all means of speech. Imagine if one wanted to depict more precisely the path a ship makes at sea, or a pedestrian on land. One would then perhaps say *the ship travels one mile to the east, makes a sharp curve to the south, travels 40 yards in this direction*, and so forth. Or one would call the route, the space which the ship travels over, circular, oval, or square.

The designation *oval* is clearly a simile with an egg. Everyone will know to what extent a motion in one plane can be compared with an egg, and thus will correctly perceive the motion according to one aspect of the pattern of the egg. The egg is used as a simile, because one assumes that the listener has a mental pattern picture of an egg. The length of the motion is measured by *foot* [Fuss], *fathom* [Klafter, Lachter], *pace* [Schritt], *ells* [Ellen], or *miles* [Meilen]. The foot was originally a human foot, a perceptive picture, the extension of which can at any moment form an idea, either because it is firmly imprinted in our mind, or because we can visualize the picture using our own foot. On the other hand, the normal foot-length is a pattern which we have only in our consciousness. This pattern will for most people be similar to a ruler, and with it the length of trip is measurable. Likewise the *ell* [Elle] was originally the forearm, the *fathom* [Klafter] was the length of outstretched arms, and the *mile* [Meile] was 1000 Roman paces.

Frequently the length of a spatial movement is determined by the time it takes to reach that distance: *an hour away* [eine Stunde], *five minutes away* [fünf Minuten]. The metaphorical use of these and similar expressions is quite familiar: *a rifle-stot (away)* [ein Büchsenschuss], *a pipe (full) of tobacco* [ein Piep-Toback], *a hound's bark* [ein Hunneblaff]. The designations of the compass directions are basically metaphors, originally comprising comparisons with the course of the sun: *Orient (rising sun)* [Oriens], *Occident (falling, or setting sun)* [Occidens]. Metaphors denoting the times of day were also originally comparisons with the course of the sun: *evening (levelling of the sun)* [Abend], *morning (early rays of light)* [Morgen], *noon* (originally *ninth hour from sunrise* as computed by Romans) [Mittag], *midnight (middle of darkness)* [Mitternacht]. And when we designate a direction with *right* [rechts], or *left* [links], we are comparing the direction of the movement with regard to the position of the stronger and the weaker hand.

And what do we do when we want to describe a building? We speak about the arrangement of the windows; they are so many feet apart from each other, a metaphor; so many meters high, a metaphor. We define the vaults with the metaphor of a mathematical circle, as we do a barrel vault with a simile of a barrel. For an onion tower the metaphor is taken from the plant world.

But the elementary sensual and nerve sensations cannot be described; they can only be indicated by comparison. The color green is for us *grassgreen* [grasgrün]; we speak of *brickred* [ziegelrot], *pitchraven black* [pechrabenschwarz], *steelblue* [stahlblau], *rosered* [rosenrot], *vinegarsour* [essigsauer], *fruitacid* [obstsäure], *honeysweet* [honigsüss], *bitter as gall* [gallenbitter], and so on. And if we analyze the above-mentioned simple elementary nerve and muscle processes of the psychic phenomena into their atoms, we see that we take the designations from the area of activity lying just on this side of the border separating the unconscious: *the muscles move, they twitch, they are stretched, contracted, the thoughts obstruct each other, something occurs in the mind* [die Muskeln bewegen sich, sie zucken, sie werden gestreckt, zusammengezogen, die Vorstellungen hemmen sich, es geht etwas in der Seele vor].

But I want to stop here. It is indeed obvious how very significant this designation by means of borrowed patterns is for the principles involved in the development of word meaning, semasiology. It was also explained in the first discussion how a figurative designation gradually becomes congruent with its actual function. It is further known how decisively important the metaphor has been for the artistic form of presentation in prose and poetry. It must also have become evident from the studies undertaken that questions of rhetoric and poetry must be answered from the same points of view and rules as questions of grammar.

In conclusion, I will give a *short compilation of the most important general findings* of the studies undertaken.

We have seen, first of all, that speech develops from ethical needs, from the need to influence the mind of another person in a way which appears valuable to the speaker, whether it be with an imperative, a question, an indication, or an invitation to realize elements of consciousness.

Comprehension of this influencing of the mind takes place by means of inferences drawn by the listener from the situation, from certain linguistic indications of the speaker, and from emotional phenomena. He deduces the speaker's states of suffering, and from this deduction he feels motivated by the ethical force of sympathetic feelings to help the suffering person. He obeys the inferred commands; he answers the posed question by looking at the perceptive picture indicated. Thus, at the speaker's behest he reproduces a picture of consciousness, a pattern. According to the extent that the speaker can arouse the sympathetic feelings of the listener, to this extent is cultivated the listener's interest and, consequently, the clarity and vividness of the pictures summoned to consciousness.

The listener's inferences are mechanized by frequency and practice, are compressed to the most spontaneous processes, and take place unconsciously. The command to realize a perceptual picture is combined with the command to reproduce a picture of remembrance, as is the predicate of a substantive group with the noun. New predicates based on this group are again combined with it in the same way as attributive relationships, and so forth.

All elements of speech are originally sentences. These sentences are graded according to the illustrative value they contain for what is actually valuable in the communication. They become subordinate clauses, words, or components of words, like suffixes and prefixes. According to this theory, the simple word is constructed and arranged like the sentence, like the paragraph, and like a compact linguistic work of art.

There are two large classes of speech elements to be differentiated, the exposition and the predicate. There are also two forms of arrangement: (1) with the predicate in the first position and then the exposition, the naive form of supplementary correction, and (2) first the exposition and then the predicate. The first arrangement prevails in the older formations, inflections, compositions, attributive connections, appositions, and subordinate clause formations. The second arrangement prevails in modern speech formations and signals an ethical advance.

The expectation of the message's predicate, of the actually important predicate and the subordinated predicates, forms the inner bond whereby the listener joins together the elements of speech. It forms the foundation for the logical causal coherence, the apperceptive means for the understanding of following predicates.

Expectation and the idea of the purpose of the groups of movement are important factors for understand the action. From them, and from the pattern pictures obtained from the abstraction of experience and of everything formed by the content of our experience, we infer the action. From our experience of the real content of the imparted activities we infer the general or individual character of the groups and series from which the message is formed. And from experience we make conclusions about the relationship of subject, of objects, and of activities to each other; only from the content of the objects do we infer the content of the activity.

Our exact speech comprehension is based upon inferences. At first these inferences come from very simple elements, such as the emotional tone, the mimical means. But eventually they spring from complicated ones, such as the word, the sentence, the paragraph, and, finally, the finished work of art. With deductions we are in a position to recognize from the emotional tone, the emotional state of the personal present, and we are able to understand the context of the words used as a means for a sentence. From the distortion of the emotional tone we conclude that one is reporting about the state of a third person. We have indirect speech, and with it a huge supply of linguistic utterances, including reflex sounds like onomatopoetic sounds, through which we are reminded of situations; these are the predicates. The primary objects become secondary subjects; with this, speech attains the simplicity and transparency of a report.

All of these groups and chains of conclusions are shortened by mechanization, and the linguistic means become congruent with their function. They are not congruent immediately; nevertheless, speech contains both congruent and incongruent means for the same functions, i.e., means by which the shortened or extended groups of inferences in the listener's mind are set into motion. The stylistic differences of speech are determined by the diversity of these groups of inferences.

The same phenomena found in the area of syntax are found again in poetry and oratory. Therefore, the treatment of these areas cannot be separated from that of the area of syntax. On the contrary, the phenomena are much clearer in an analytic presentation than in mechanized syntax. The analyzed form, however, is the object of poetry, rhetoric, and stylistics. The word is a compressed sentence, and thus the rules of form belong to the area of syntax.

Speech is based upon human intercourse, upon egoistical and sympathetic feelings. Its life is deeply engrained in the conditions of society and of the individual. Speech is human intercourse, and only those linguistic processes which we as listeners have understood can serve us in our speaking. Therefore, the problem of the understanding of speech must be in the foreground of a philological investigation.

In rough outlines these are approximately the major findings of the investigations undertaken. If I have been successful in showing the unity of grammar, rhetoric, stylistics, and poetry and in proving that precisely from such an approach in treating the compressed and analytical forms of speech with the same points of view important results can be obtained; if I have further succeeded in demonstrating that in all of these questions, the keys to the solutions are held in the hands of ethics and psychology, then I would believe that I have achieved something. For my part, I should also like to promote the view in grammarians' circles that the actual task of a scientific grammar consists of discovering the basic relationships and laws from which the individual linguistic phenomena are produced. The individual phenomenon in the sphere of a single language may lay no more claim to a higher value for the science than does the single fact in mineralogy that in one region or another is found quartz or galena. Research of course needs reliable statistical material; however, such statistical material is dead and useless without the invigorating points of view and ideas which are revealed by the general approach.

Appendix and Supplement

[additional commentary on
points made in the text]

Page 126. That this law should also be of decisive significance for the history and development of speech is quite obvious. The fact is quite generally known that for the Indo-Germanic languages the highly-accented syllables have retained their true integrity more than the unstressed syllables. One should compare French *homme* with Latin *hominem* [man], *fûtes* with *fuistis* [you were], also the expansion of German unstressed *e* obtained in place of other vowels. Furthermore, the dialectical disposal of this also remains in older, fuller vowels.

As far as I can determine, the causes for loss or mutilation of unstressed syllables in the speech of an accomplished language community are several. The most common cause may be a greater uncertainty in muscle feelings for those parts of the word which are more weakly stressed. This is because the weaker the acoustical sensation, the less will be the accuracy in the imitation of the phonic image, i.e., the weaker will be the power of the sound pattern present in the mind. This may be proven. All of the movements of a drunken person become uncertain, the movements of walking, of writing, and, likewise, of speaking. It is in this state that the psychic direction of the motor nerves has become uncertain, of course in different gradations. Those movements most highly mechanized will be executed with greater certainty than those less mechanized. Thus, in this case, someone can perhaps walk tolerably well; whereas reading, playing the piano, and other technical skills have become impossible. In the state when stammering begins, the strongly-stressed syllables will be spoken with relatively more certainty that the more weakly-stressed syllables. This is decisive proof that the mechanization of pronounciation is further advanced in those syllables than in the ones more weakly-stressed. Since mechanization is a consequence of frequent practice of a movement, it is then comprehensible that the production of the weakly-stressed syllables is less mechanized than the sound movement of the strongly-stressed syllables, because the latter were spoken earlier than the former.

The second reason is that even when the pronounciation of the unstressed syllable is imperfect, in most cases we still understand the word. Indeed, probably very often the listener hears only the stressed syllable, when he actually has the feeling that he has heard the whole word. That this is very often the case can be observed by anyone from his own experience. Confirmation of this fact comes from the similar psychic sphere of optical perceptions. It is well-known here that we do not even notice small deviations in appearance from a former condition, but rather we recognize the person or thing as identical with the picture we have of it in our memory. Furthermore, we never execute the recognition of a known visual object according to all of its perceptible characteristics, but rather only according to several especially significant ones. It can also be assumed with certainty that deviations in the elements of a word or sentence which are less important for comprehension will not be noticed in the acoustical perception of speech groups. Clear-cut proof for this is the fact that we seldom or never notice the mutilation of the unstressed forms of the article or the copula *is* [ist]. There are many other words, which have suffered similar losses because of sentence accent, such as *n Tag* [mornin'], instead of *guten Tag* [good morning]. We do have, however, an established, normal picture in our minds for these words, and we do more justice to them in cultivated speech when we have to watch ourselves.

One might perhaps believe that the few years in which we spoke the stressed syllables longer than the unstressed would not be noticeable as far as mechanization is concerned. This would be a mistake. If one observed all the other cases of mechanization one would realize the importance of precisely the first years of a child's life for mechanization. Uncertainty in the usage of syntactical forms by a speaker impeded by alcohol for example takes place more easily than uncertainty in the choice of words. The vocabulary first used by the child is altogether the most mechanized part of the vocabulary and in usage predominates over all synonymous words in ease of reproduction. Therefore elegant words are more difficult to manage than common ones. We express ourselves with greater ease about groups of thoughts with which we have become familiar in our early childhood than about those acquired later. Yet, after a while frequent usage brings a certain weariness or at least reduces the enjoyment of some words, just as candy and other childhood pleasures are apt quickly to lose their appeal.

As a supplement to the fact that we comprehend and recognize the words of a speaker, we notice that in small circles whose members are close to each other, for example within *one* family, within *one* village, one very often observes that the words in the conversation of these members are far more imperfectly articulated and spoken with much less intensity of expiration than in the conversation of the same people with strangers. Each knows rather well the special peculiarities of each other's articulation, and each has peculiarities of his own. One therefore comprehends from the mere voice; one understands the speaker when he holds his hand in front of his mouth, when he yawns, when he has a pipe between his teeth or lips, when he is eating. One can therefore rightly say that the farther apart that men who are in linguistic intercourse with one another stand, the greater the value placed on exact articulation will be. What also contributes to the easy understanding of intimately connected members of a small community is, naturally, the identity of interests and, thereby often, the transparency of the situation for the purposes of speech and for the predicates of communication.

Page 126. The exchanging of sounds, such as *d* and *l*, *n* and *l*, *k* and *t*, especially of the alveolar and uvular *r*, is another process which has been active in the history of language. A gradual transition is not conceivable in these cases. Rather, only an exchanging in which the language community takes no offense at the similar acoustical sensation or with which it could certainly not exercise any regulating influence is possible. For the association of sounds see my review of H. Paul's *Prinzipien*, "Zeitschrift fuer deutsche Gymnasial-wesens," Jahrgang 36, p. 301, Berlin 1882.

Page 127. Compare this with my comments about human vocabulary according to one's needs, in the article about dialect research: "Zachers Zeitschrift fuer deutsche Philologie," XI, p. 468, Halle 1880.

Page 131. I have intentionally called this mood the supplicatory mood and not the optative. The reason for this is the following: with the wish, for example, *oh if he would only come* [ach wenn er doch käme], *utinam veniat, veniret,* εἰ γὰρ ἔλθοι and ἦλθε, and other forms of expression such as the request, the endeavor of the speaker to receive the named object is naturally present, but the requesting person makes the attainment of his aspiration dependent upon the will and inclination of the person to whom he is speaking. He is thus trying to win favor and goodwill of this person, and, therefore, believes that by his request he can exercise influence upon the realization of the aspiration.

With the wish, on the other hand, the appearance of the aspired fact must be thought of as dependent upon powers and conditions over which we believe we have no influence at all. An actual wish can therefore only be expressed (1) when the determining powers are spatially and temporally removed from us, for example, we wish that our absent brother would do something although we are aware that we are unable to exert an influence upon his will; or (2) when we believe the fulfillment of the aspiration to be dependent upon powers, in the face of which our intention appears completely ineffective. These are the laws of nature or, in certain philosophies of life, this is fate; for example, if in the winter time we wish *if I could only find flowers outside* [wenn ich draussen doch Blumen fände].

In any case the actual wish always presupposes an insight into the conditions of the incidence of an action, and in general a child lacks such insight. If the child wishes that his absent brother do something, he simply says *he should do that* [er soll das thun] and directs these words at the people whose help he is accustomed to call upon when he doesn't know how to help himself, usually, his mother and father. If one is walking with the child in the country, and the child becomes hungry or thirsty, he simply demands, without consideration, to eat and drink; and, at least up to a certain stage of development, all remonstrances of the parents, that one must first come to a house, are in vain.

Thus the child's insight into the limitations of his own will and of the will of those people with whom he must deal can only be gained very gradually. Ultimately there always remains the last resort: God can do everything, and man can influence His will. This childlike stage is not merely peculiar to children; it is also characteristic of naive men in lower cultures. It is only too well known how long it takes to recognize the ineluctable validity of the laws of nature and how long man has fought against those laws with prayer and magic. Thus children and men in childlike stages of development learn only with time to express the wish, i.e., conscious desire, and at the same time, realize that such desire is dependent upon incontrovertible and intangible conditions.

With this it is obvious that wish and condition are twins and that one form of the conception cannot appear without the other, because one may say that the sensitivity of aspiring man, i.e., the sensitivity of aroused selfishness, develops understanding for the condition and, thereby, for the concept of possibility and impossibility. The forms of condition are therefore the forms of the wish, or should one say it the other way around? The German *wenn er (doch) käme* [if he would (only) come], *Greek* αἰ, εἰ(-θε, γάρ) [Oh that, would that], and Latin isolated *o, si* are all forms of condition. The expression of a wish only becomes complete and distinct by adding the tone of desire.

By means of the tone of sensibility, similarly with the tone of the threat, the concluding sentence will be supplemented somewhat in the sense of: *that would be more beautiful, then I would be very happy* [das wäre schön, da würde ich mich freuen]. We actually no longer supplement this concluding sentence, but by habituation to this supplementation we already sense the content of the concluding sentence in the protasis, i.e., the conditional sentence has become the corresponding and congruent form of the wish.

How difficult it is, at least in Greek, to decide whether the condition is designated by the form of the wish, or whether the form of the wish is designated by the condition, is shown in the negation μή [not] in the conditional sentence. This has definitely originated, not from the purely objective designation of the condition, but rather from the condition in the form of aspiration. The Greek optative also designates the wish, the (realizable) condition, and the possibility; thus in this case, too, the forms of desire and the form of the knowledge of the possibility and of the condition are inextricably amalgamated. As has already been indicated, we must believe that the first realizations of condition and possibility developed from the obstructions and necessary limitations of human ability encountered by man's desire. Thus the desired action is initially conditional. Its realization, however, does not lie in the will of the person desiring.

If we know that a thing is not realizable, then we call the wish unrealizable, the condition unreal. But this is still not an actual wish, because this human emotional condition is now lacking the hope and expectation of possible realization of a wish. This wish has in fact become only a regret, a pure expression of sorrow that a thing either has not been realized or cannot be realized. It is, therefore, understandable that in Greek the wish form is not used for this condition. If, in these cases, we find in Greek the indicative, especially of the imperfect or aorist, and if Latin and German also use a form of the preterite, then this form is also psychologically understandable. For example, *if he had (only) come* [wenn er (doch) gekommen wäre], is a shortened conditional sentence, the tone of regret gives rise to the concluding sentence: *then it would be beautiful* [dann war es schön]. The sentence *if (only) man did not die* [wenn (doch) des Mensch nicht stürbe], could be understood as *then it would be* or *would have been wonderful* [dann wäre oder war es schön]; in Greek and German dialect *if men died not* [wenn die Menchen nicht starben]; French indicative conditional: *si les morts reve-naient . . . les pères et les fils ne se connaitraient pas* [if the dead returned . . . fathers and sons would not recognize each other]. Evidently the impossi-bility or unreality of an action is a maxim of experience, and the expression of the maxims of experience is suitably the preterite, as is the gnomic aorist in Greek.

In German and Latin however this condition is mostly designated with the subjunctive, although the German dialects often use the indicative, and, like-wise, in Latin it is present to express unreality. In this case we will have to regard the subjunctive as having infiltrated from the wish sentence, and we will have to assume that the unrealizable wish sentence has taken on the sub-junctive form of the related realizable wish sentence.

Moreover, in Latin and German the mood of wish is the subjunctive, not the optative, or stated more correctly, Latin and German have blended the optative and subjunctive as closely related forms of desire. Apparently the actual wish has thus not been that distinctly separated from the form of de-sire, by means of which we attempt to influence the will of another person. In certain cases, even for a more highly developed consciousness, both forms of desire are situated very close to each other: *peream, moriar, si, I want to die if* [ich will sterben, wenn]. As a prayer directed at a divinity, i.e., as a curse, the expression is one of the will. If the relationship with the divinity recedes, then the curse becomes a wish.

We have seen further that the wish gradually develops out of the inhibited feelings of the will. There is then nothing more obvious than that the expres-sion of the will is linguistically retained, but, according to the modified con-tent, it takes on a modified meaning to which the expression gradually be-comes congruent. And in this manner the German and Latin wish forms: *utinam-* and *o, dass (doch)* are to be understood. They are actually expres-sions of will, exactly corresponding to the romance imperative with French *que-*, Italian *che-*, because *uti-nam* is a final conjunction. The cultivated con-sciousness has thus in this way retained the forms of a childlike stage when it didn't know a wish but was impressed with the new content.

The corresponding Latin wish form is *ut dii illum perdant* [may the gods destroy that]. The Latin wish sentences with *dum, dum modo, modo* [yet, if only, only] were originally final sentences of will. It might also be pointed out that the many various desire forms of the wish and will are frequently not sharply differentiated in their verbal and nominal expressions; compare Greek βούλομαι [to wish] Latin *volo, voluntas*. It is further to be remem-bered that the wish form can easily be revealed as the imperative, as was done in the second discussion.

Page 132. At this time I would like to point out the importance which the knowledge of human sentence melody, of tempo, and of energy of speaking has for a scientific understanding of music. It need not be demonstrated that the form of linguistic sentence melody is very often utilized by music; I refer, for example, to the "Request" in Schumann's *Music for Children*, in which a distinct imitation of the question sentence melody of the speaker can be recognized. If we understand such a piece of music, which is, however, difficult without a program designation, then the consciousness of the situation in which such a series of sounds is linguistically customary, gives us the key to understanding. Thus in this case the model by which we can understand the series of sounds according to their content is the sentence melody.

We are accustomed to comprehending also the tempo and the energy of the intonation of a piece of music with the medium of the linguistic forms of passion and sensitivity, unless the linguistic text or an illustrating word of the music in the program instructs us that something else is to be thought of as the representative of the passionate movement or motive of the sounds. Thus in Schubert's "King of the Elves," we think of the form of movement of the instrumental accompaniment as the clatter of the horse, and we think of the horse as the motif of the sounds; in Beethoven's "Pastoral" the sounds will be construed as thunder and the shawn sounds of the shepherds.

If tempo and rhythm are firmly associated with certain of the forms of movement, such as the dance rhythms, then the dance situation will be summoned to the listener's consciousness and will give the means of interpretation. Or if certain harmonizations and series of sounds are constant for certain situations, such as the types of church sounds for the situations of religious edification, then these too must be summoned to the consciousness as material for such interpretation.

Except for these cases where the association with certain external situations gives the music a real and vivid content, instrumental music arouses only certain formal qualities of sensation with a range from pain to sorrow. Therefore, the listener can interpret tempo, series of sounds, and energy only as forms in such an arousal of feeling. Among these forms appear such sensations as melancholy, delight, and so forth. Thus, the listener must interpret those outward musical forms according to the example of human audibly expressed sensation in reflex sounds or as embedded in articulated sounds of speech.

Page 133. The perfect subjunctive *ne dixeris* [that you might not have said] is the relic of an older way of applying the subjunctive of the Latin perfect; this subjunctive is ageless. We know that in Latin the perfect aorist and the perfect tense of an earlier stage of speech have been blended; this is clearly proven by the aorist meaning of the Latin indicative historical perfect. If we regard subjunctive as of the aorist mood, then the usage corresponds exactly with the Greek prohibitive μὴ ποιήσῃς [not done] and this prohibitive is also limited to the second person. For the explanation of the Latin subjunctive perfect prohibitive, one could perhaps think of the application of the infinitive perfect in sentences of will; but the subjunctive potential of the present tense *dixerit quis* argues more persuasively for the acceptance of the ageless meaning of the perfect subjunctive. This application of the subjunctive is, as far as one can judge, connected to the old optative, which in Latin has fused with the old subjunctive in form and meaning. Both cases of the perfect subjunctive are isolations, as the grammarian Paul appropriately calls such phenomena. It is high time that one began to collect these isolations in the syntactical sphere of the old languages. If this were done, the opinion about the syntactical means of connecting would be significantly reformed, and the rules would, in many cases, have to receive a completely new framework.

Page 138. The story is from the *Sigurdarkwida III* and reads according to Simrock's translation:

> 47 Now come hither, those who want gold
> And those who seek lesser treasure from me;
> I give to each one, golden red necklaces,
> Bows and veils and glittering garments.

> 48 Softly they were silent and pondered over advice,
> Until they finally all gave us an answer:
> "However needy we may be, we still want to live,
> Remain ladies of the court and do what is right."*

> 49 Reflectively the brightly-jeweled one,
> Young in years now spoke the word:
> "Not a one should ungladly and unprepared
> Have to die for my sake.†

> 50 "But one day yet on your bodies will burn
> Scanty baubles, when you come to die
> And to visit me, not magnificent treasure."

> [47 Nun geht herzu, die Gold wollen
> Und minderes Gut von Mir erlangen:
> Ich gebe Jeder goldrothen Halsschmuck,
> Schleif und Schleier und schimmernd Gewand.

> 48 Stille schwiegen sie und sannen auf Rat,
> Bis endlich zur Antwort sie alle gaben:
> "Wie dürftig wir seien, wir wollen doch leben,
> Saalweiber bleiben und thun was gebührlich ist."

> 49 Sinnend sprach die lichtgeschmückte
> Jung von Jahren jetzo das Wort:
> "Nicht eine soll ungern und unbereit
> Sterben müssen um meinetwillen.

---

* Thus the unreasonable demand of dying with her for the presents is not even expressed because it appears so natural.

† Only this slight indication makes possible an inference about the conventions of that period.

50   Doch brennet auf euern Gebeinen dereinst
     Karge Zier, kommt ihr zu sterben
     Und mich heimzusuchen, nicht herrliches Gut."]

Page 144. As soon as the relative construction appeared as a congruent expression for the determination of a person or thing according to a definite action or quality, the relative clause could become prominent. A similar phenomenon presents itself in the inversion of the clauses of a sentence according to the laws of the proteron-hysteron.

Page 147. The English relative clause without a relative pronoun is the same as that German sentence of explanation with *weil, dass* [because, that], and has developed from the simple parenthesis.

Page 148. I am not generalizing this explanation for cases with a final *ut, quominus, quin,* although these conjunctions are also formed from the interrogative stem. In the text of the second discussion, the sentences with *quominus* and *ne* are examined. Certainly those sentences formed with *ne* are actually direct discourse, and the so-called governing verb with a high illustrative value is the exposition of the report; it is likewise the case with *quin,* for example, *non dubito, quin veniat* is actually *What, why shouldn't he come? I don't doubt it* [wie, warum sollte er nicht kommen? ich zweifle nicht]. Thus in this case too we are dealing with the transposition from a direct question.

In judging the final *ut* one will have to refer to the verbs *studii et voluntatis,* as they are appropriately called in secondary school grammars. In this case the construction of the verbs of worry, such as *curo, provideo,* with *ut,* remind one very definitely of the corresponding Greek verbs with ὅπως [how]; for example ἐπιμελεῖσθαι ὅπως [I should act]. And in this case, i.e. with the verbs of worried consideration, the construction as an indirect question is etymologically very transparent: *I anxiously consider how I should act* [ich überlege sorgend, wie ich thun soll]. This indirect question is developed from the direct question *how should I act, A worried* [wie soll ich thun, sorgte A]. Also in this case the so-called governing verb is the exposition of the report. This construction of *ut* is immediately understandable in verbs such as *consulo* [I advise], *prospicio* [I take care], *video* [I see], *contendo* [I contend], *laboro* [I make an effort], *nitor* [I strive], *operam do* [I make an effort], *id ago* [I do this], *id specto* [I see this], *nihil antiquius habeo* [I prefer].

It now appears probable that, formed on the analogy of all these verbs, all the related verbs in which an intention was sensed assumed this construction. This assumption appears ever more probable when we consider the constructions of the verbs *volo* [I want], *nolo* [I do not want], *malo* [I prefer], *cupio* [I desire], *iubeo* [I command], *veto* [I do not allow], which were isolated by the prose writers of the classic period. These are exactly like the Greek verbs of intention containing the infinitive and the accusative with the infinitive with unequal subjects. In the same company is the likewise isolated construction of *studeo* and the verbs of comprehending. Other verbs of requesting, demanding, allowing, advising, commanding, and challenging also contain the infinitive in the Old Latin. And as in so many other instances, in this construction the Augustan poetic language conforms to the Old Latin, because the poetic stylistic feeling in the time of Augustus is formed according to the language of the old epic and drama. And from the language of the Augustan poets, especially from Virgil, the stylistic feeling of later prose is formed. Tacitus, for example, derives his stylistic feeling from the early poets and he too uses the infinitive construction. Therefore, it appears probable that the means of construction with the final *ut*, which was only etymologically suitable for one group of verbs (those of worrying), gained a much wider range and not only combined with the other verbs of intention, but also appeared where now the German *damit* [thereby] is used.

Page 153. Naturally the frequent German expression *es kam Karl* [it came Carl, (Carl came)] can be included as a supplementary correction. Thus the impersonal indefinite *es* [it] comes first before the definite subject.

German and French use the personal pronouns *ich, du* [I, thou] and the Romance representatives of *ego, tu* in unstressed meaning. But in the other Romance languages it by no means has the emphasis. One generally assumes in Latin that only the personal pronoun is used with special emphasis. The assumption is wrong in this generality: it cannot be disputed that with *quidem . . . sed, indeed . . . however* [zwar . . . aber]; the personal pronoun will be added without emphasis, whereby *equidem* [to be sure] represents the combination *ego quidem* [I, certainly], for which in the second and third person *tu quidem* [you certainly] and *ille quidem* [he certainly] are chosen. It has furthermore become very dubious in my mind whether such an assumption for the Augustan poets is justified. To decide this question one would need a complete catalogue of plots, which I do not own, not even for any single poet. I give here some examples from which one can see that the exception is very suspicious: *non ego te . . . quatiam* [(I shall not rouse you) not I shall rouse you]; *non ego perfidum dixi sacramentum* [no deserters oath I've said]; *Carthagini iam non ego nuntios mittam superbos* [never by me shall message proud be sped to Carthage]; *nec dulces amores sperne puer neque tu choreas* [Spurn neither sweet loves, boy, nor dances]; *Arcanum neque tu scrutaberis* [You shall not investigate the secret].

It is these cases with the negation *non, neque* [not, and not] which often stands in combination with the personal pronoun, *non te* [not you (acc.)], *non me* [not me]; likewise, *hunc frenis, hunc tu compesce catena* [you, constrain this one with curbs, this one with fetters]; *tu pulmentaria quaere* [you, seek the relishes]; *tu cede* [you, proceed], sententious here throughout, could only doubtfully be thought of as with an emphasized meaning. This question deserves closer study and the purpose of this information was to stimulate such an investigation.

It is interesting that the old Indo-Germanic sequence of sentence elements is found again in the language of deaf mutes. Schmalz states "That which appears most important to the deaf mute is always put in front of the rest, and he thereby leaves out whatever appears superfluous to him. For example, in order to say *father gave me an apple*, he makes the sign for an apple, then the sign for father, then the sign for me, omitting the sign for give."

Corresponding with our results are: (1) the position of the logical predicate; (2) the action itself remains unexpressed and is supplemented from our own points of reference; (3) the points of reference are not in conformity with each other, but each time they are an independent movement in themselves, and as such they only have reference to the mimical subject. Therefore the sign for *I* [ich] is not distinctly different from the sign for *to me* [mir].

Page 154. I now provide without exposition several reliable examples of the comparative: Latin *aliud ego, aliud tu* [one thing I, another you], *different for me than you* [anderes ich als du], *aeque pauperibus prodest, locupletibus aeque, aeque neglectum pueris senibusque nocebit* [it advances among poor people just as it does among rich, the thing neglected will bring about injury in like manner among young boys and old men].

The comparison with *tamquam* [just as] is one of those means of comparison discussed in the text with supplementary correction *tam* [to such a degree], *quam* [in what way]; *quasi* [just as, or as if] has come from the question *qua?* (or *quam*) meaning *what?* [wie?] and the answer *si* [thus, yes]; *Caesar aeque ac Pompeius* [both Caesar and Pompey in the same way], actually *Caesar in the same way, and (also) Pompey* [Cäsar in gleicher Weise, und (auch) Pomp.] show the same correction as *et ... et* [both ... and], and likewise the Greek καί [and] after expressions of equality. The mutual analogic influence of the comparison with *atque* [and also] and *quam* [as, than] is transparent; and only one reference to *non aliter quam* [in no other way than], along with *melius atque* [and even better], is needed. Likewise Greek was analogically influenced: ὅμοιος [like, common] with the dative and ὁ αὐτὸς καί [together], French *plusieurs* [several], Latin *complures* [several] and *plures* [several], and German *mehrere* [several] are all without expositions, and yet with time they acquire the standard *eins* [one] from consciousness so that they are *mehr als einer* [more than one].

MHG *beide* [both], meaning *so wohl—als auch* [not only—but also] is without an exposition, for example *beide* [both] with the supplementary correction *des vater und des suns* [not only of the father but also of the son]. Likewise *er ist uns alsô leit sô dir* [not only we are sorry, but also you (are)] and NHG *als* [as], meaning *ebenso* [in the same way].

Page 158. In order not to use grossly strong language I will avoid examples which are obvious. I would simply like to refer to certain differences in the speech consciousness of generations and peoples concerning the common and vulgar elements in speech. For example, it is understandable that one would no more speak about certain parts of the body than one would expose them. The reason for this seems to be quite simply that they are connected with certain functions which arouse our disgust or which we call obscene. Ebers tells us in his travelogue, *From Goshen to Sinai*, of considerable deviation in the exposure of certain parts of a woman's body among various peoples. Are there also deviations concerning the shyness of naming these various parts of the body?

In the comparison of elevated poetic language of various peoples, deviations are also shown with regard to naming parts of the body. Thus Horace, in the most elevated style of his odes, doesn't hesitate to name the *poplites* [thighs]; for example *nec parcit inventae poplitibus* [nor does he spare the thighs of youth]. Similar examples in Virgil have been cited also. No German author would dare to speak of *Kniekehlen* [hams of the knees] in elevated style. Also to speak of the *Schienbein* [shinbone] would hardly be possible in elevated German poetry; but in elevated Roman poetry *crura* [shin] is used without hesitation. Does this deviation come from an ethical or even religious aversion, or is the reason the poetical distaste for being pedantically exact? Other parts of the body such as *heel, knee, eye, chin, mouth, tongue, fist* [die Ferse, das Knie, das Auge, Kinn, Mund, Zunge, Faust] are used a great deal and often even with the pleasant impression of the individual designation; thus with these words there must have been related thoughts which were ethically and aesthetically more elevated. And what is the relationship of the enjoyment given by the individual designation to the displeasure of the pedantically exact, if, however, the statement itself does not have the character of pedantry?

Page 161. A profitable task would be to investigate to what extent the establishment of rules has influenced the usage of language. For the Roman poets the assumption is inevitable that they learned definite rhetorical and stylistic regulations in school and applied them in their poetic creations. For example, one such rule was certainly the instruction to use the *pars pro toto* [a part for the whole] with elegant poetry. Evidently this form is well-founded in natural consciousness of speech; I do not now want to investigate how, but in the manner of its application used by the Roman authors of the Augustan period, that form became unnatural. One striking example is provided by Virgil's wooden horse in the second book of the Aeneid:

Hic trabibus contextus acernis staret equus . . . , hanc tamen immensam Calchas attollere molem roboribus textis caeloque educere iussit. . . . inclusos utero Danaos et pinea furtim laxat claustra Sinon: illos patefactus ad auras reddit equus, laetiqua caro se robore promunt. [Here might have stood a horse built of maple wood twined together . . . nevertheless Calchas ordered this immense construction to be erected of weaved oak wood and to be raised up to the sky . . . at one side, Sinon stealthily releases the Danaans enclosed in the pine den: thrown open, the horse returns them to the air, and gladly they come forth from the beloved oak.]

And in a similar manner the winds and Muses are named. Such a means of expression, which is mainly based upon conscious reflection, can, however, be mechanized like those other forms of expression and can also leave broad, deep tracks in the history of the language. This is especially true if one considers that the young generation learns its feeling for style and speech in school, especially from Virgil.

Page 182. In exactly the same way, sentence forms which designate a real fact are derived from sentences comprehended in a general way. Well-known is the combination of the Greek εἰ [would that, if] with the verbs θαυμάζειν [to wonder], ἄχθεσθαι [to be discontented], ἀγανακτεῖν [to be vexed], αἰσχύνεσθαι [to shame], μέμφεσθαι [to find fault with], etc., with the meaning of a sentence with ὅτι [that]; thus θαυμάζω [to be astonished], ὅτι ταῦτα γίγνεται [that he becomes this], and εἰ ταῦτα γίγνεται [if (would that) he becomes this].

The supplementation of reality must be supplied each time by the listener's consciousness of the situation. The same etymological development is true for the Latin sentences with *etsi, tametsi,* meaning *although* [obgleich] when it concerns a real fact; for example, *sed tamen etsi antea scripsi, quae existimavi scribi oportere, tamen hoc tempore putavi* [but nevertheless although I have written before what I deemed proper to be written, notwithstanding what I thought at this time]; also Latin *siquidem,* meaning *inasmuch* [da ja]; sentences of invocation *when I have brought thee a sacrifice, then help me* [wenn ich dir Opfer gebracht habe, so hilf mir]; and likewise in Latin and Greek.

The causal Latin *quom* [when], *cum quoniam* [when (whereas)] is also explained in the same manner. According to this, the sentence *since (when) it is raining, it is wet* [da (cum) es regnet, ist es nass], is chiefly a sentence of generality *when it rains it is wet* [wann es regnet, ist es nass], but the reality will be supplemented according to the consciousness of the situation. In this matter it is irrelevant whether we assume that the causal meaning of *cum* [when] was developed directly from the form of the question or from the application of the interrogative stem with a relative meaning, which gradually became established in the Latin consciousness of speech. In both cases, however, the basic meaning must be regarded as *when* [wann], interrogative or relative. The sentence *it is wet, when? it is raining* [es ist nass, wann? es regnet] is just as general as the sentence *when it rains it is wet* [wann es regnet, ist es nass]. Because of this the relative application of *cum,* meaning *when* [wann] must certainly already have been presupposed. It is the same with *quando.* Moreover, the origin of the subjunctive with the causal *cum* remains unclear. And the German *die weil, weil* [for this time, whilst] etymologically can only with difficulty be used in general sentences which designate the conditional.

Appendix to the Second Discussion Section XXI.

For the speaking human being, the world is mainly present only as the object of his sensations, strivings and perceptions. Everything viewed as existing externally by the person cognizant of himself, outside of himself, and thus an object; the only subject is therefore the person, himself. This manner of conception is actually the normal one, and in a sentence, for example, *my brother is going* [mein Bruder geht], the opinion is derived from the perception which the speaker has of his brother, thus actually (more fully expressed) *I perceive my brother, he is going* [ich nehme meinen Bruder wahr, er geht]; likewise with the opinions of memory and knowledge *my brother is large* [mein Bruder ist gross], actually *I know my brother, he is large* [ich weiss meinen Bruder, er ist gross].

It is the same with the sentences of desire and will: *Oh, if only brother would come, and brother should come* [o, wenn doch der Bruder käme] and [der Bruder soll kommen], actually: *I wish or I want brother, he should come* [ich wünsche] or [ich will den Bruder, er soll kommen]. The perceived tone is, of course, exactly the same as an expressed verb of desire or will. It is the same with astonishment, sorrow, and joy: in *my brother is coming* [mein Bruder kommt], the object of the concerned emotion is *my brother* [mein Bruder].

And naturally in speech which is not mechanized it is possible and common for the speaker to accent the mental process of his thought or his emotion by means of a special sentence in which the secondary subject is the object; for example *I wish from brother, that he; I hope from . . . , I think from . . . , I wonder about . . . , it distresses me about brother* [ich wünsche vom Bruder, dass er; ich hoffe vom . . . , ich denke vom . . . , ich wundere mich über . . . , es thut mir weh am Bruder]. And this form of expression is capable of even further fragmentation.

According to what was stated in the text, we would call such a form of expression a report which has obviously been formed from such cases as when the emotion could not be immediately deduced from the feeling-tone expressed, or as when the reporting and the speaking persons are not identical. With the direct communication of emotion or thought, the common form is the direct form and not the reporting form.

In the report it is now clear that the mental activity of the speaking subject has become such an indistinct element of consciousness that, in general, it no longer determines the construction of the statement. Visualized with a formula, the relationship would be the following, if we designate the subject as A, the subject of the action, which is the object for A, as B, and the action itself as x:

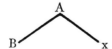

i.e., A imagines B and x or senses these objects in some way. If, on the other hand, A's mental activity recedes, then the formula would be:

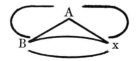

i.e., A, along with his relationships, withdraws completely into the background, and B and x are connected with one another in such a way that they appear to the listener to be completely in conformity.

It is readily apparent how this obfuscation of the consciousness took place. First, the fact of the mental activity is evident with every utterance of speech, and it is thus mechanized because of its frequency. Second, the mental process itself gives an important sign for the disclosure of the predicate only insofar as sentiment escapes; therefore, among those processes only the emotions are meaningful and valuable; objective, unemotional thought is meaningless for the inference of the predicate of value.

With this we will have to assume a gradation in the effectiveness of those mental processes on the form of the expression; the relatively strongest effectiveness will be that of the emotional processes of the speaking subject.

If we consider further, at the stage of speech in which the sentence was composed of single words only, the inclination to bring B and x together and thus to make the subject of the action and the action itself conform in words would not have been present. For this stage we would obtain this formula:

This form of expression is retained, as we have seen, in the word sentences of developed speech, for example *my boots, my coat* [meine Stiefeln, meinen Rock]; in sentences of astonishment *that man!* [der Mensch!]; in sentences of joy and sorrow such as *ah, the bird; oh, the dog* [ei, der Vogel; ach, der Hund].

Here also, with the exception of the imperative form, we constantly see the nominative; apparently, therefore, an action is thought of in connection with the object or person emotionally called or named, and this action will be sensed by the object or person as a subject.

An assimilation takes place here between the object of the emotion and the matching action, when a direct designation of the action is not present; presumably according to the pattern of the customary complete sentence.

This assimilation is neither completely necessary, nor is it actually present in all the Indo-Germanic languages. In German dialect, for example in Magdeburg, one yells: *den Minschen, sönnen Minschen* [those people, such people]. In this case, then, the *person* is obviously to be thought of as the object of the emotionally aroused subject.

The same case is very well-known in Latin—see Kuehner, *Latin Grammar*. However, in Kuehner's book the comprehension of the rule is very deficient. Wrong first of all is the assumption that special verbs like *stare, observe, look, perceive, I swear* [staunt an, betrachtet, seht, vernehmt, ich beschwöre], are thought of with *pro deum fidem* [by the faith of the gods] and the like, even if such verbs were to be completed in a fragmentary presentation. More seriously wrong, however, is the condition that Kuehner gives for the use of the accusative, that it is regularly connected with an attributive adjective or genitive. His own examples could have given him better instruction: thus without an adjective *pro fidem* [by faith], *pro deum fidem* [by the faith of the gods], *en mea malefacta* [behold my injuries], *meam en avaritiam* [behold my greed], *ecce me* [behold me], or the forms frequently used by comedians *ellum* [behold that one], *eccum* [behold him], *eccam* [behold her], *eccos* [behold them], *eccas* [behold them], *eccillum* [behold that one], *eccillam* [behold that one]. The accusative may also be used with adjectives of quality or condition *fortunatum Nicobulum* [the wealthy Nicobulus (little Nicobus)], *lepidum te* [pleasant you], *edepol mortalis malos* [indeed mortal evils], *heu me miserum* [alas unhappy me], and so on.

Although the adjectives may be thus connected as attributes, their function is nevertheless predicative; here they are exclamatory sentences with the meaning of: *miser sum* [I am unhappy]. Frequently found with this accusative are the interjections *o* [oh], *heu* [alas], *eheu* [alas], *hem* [well], *pro* [ah], *edepol* [indeed], *en* [behold], *ecce* [behold].

An expression like *me miserum* [unhappy me] shows that the predicate *miser* [unhappy] expressed by *me* [me] has conformed with the object case; the opposite was shown above when the object of the speaking subject conformed with the following predicate, as with astonishment: *the man is dying* [der Mensch stirbt].

A similar process, a similar development of the conformity of the forms, has also altered the condition of the Latin expression discussed above, except that in one example *en causam* [behold the cause] Cicero writes *en* with the nominative, and *ecce* [behold] is likewise connected with the nominative: *ecce homo* [behold the man].

This advance to conformity of the object of exclamation and the imagined action is demonstrated even more strikingly and convincingly in the German *sieh, sieh mal* [look, just look]. This imperative should always take the accusative, and this is true in the written German expression *sieh mal den Menschen* [just look at the man]; but it commonly conforms with the function of the subject thought along with it *sieh mal, der Mensch!* [just look, the man!].

The historical linguistic process is obvious: an object of the speaking subjects thought has linguistically become the subject of an activity which proceeds from the object. If we transpose this to the stage of the word sentence, then the exclamation would read first of all *den Menschen, er kommt* [the man, he is coming].

Apparently this process is identical with the so-called attraction, which appears, especially frequently in Greek, for example ἤδει γὰρ κατὰ θυμὸν ἀδελφὸν ὡς ἐπονεῖτο [For this one according to his brotherly heart toiled so]; Latin *nosti Marcellum, quam tardus sit* [Our Marcellus, how late he may be].

In this case there is also shown a competition between the activity of the main subject in reference to an object and his own activity, which proceeds from that object. In contrast to Latin, German shows an inclination similar to Greek; we happily use verbs of telling and thinking, for example, *ich stelle mir de Mittel vor, durch die* [I can imagine to myself the means by which]. In Latin it is much more customary to bring the object of the following concluding sentence in conformity, and to say: *cogito quibus rebus* [I consider the things by which].

Let us visualize that by the gradual drawing together of the sentences of cultivated speech which we are accustomed to regard as real sentences, more independent sentences have arisen. It is therefore only probable that languages themselves still offer us the remaining relationship of the object to the speaking subject, even when the conformity has long been executed. But only one more preliminary remark: in the preceding statements the expression *action* was always used intentionally, because a true subject can only be present with an action. Our Indo-Germanic languages, however, also show us subjects of condition and affliction. The grammarian rightly designates this as the logical object of an activity. True subjects of action can only be people. So much is then obvious, that with objects which cannot naturally be actual subjects, the function as a subject will also not appear, and they cannot become congruent with the function of a subject. That was only possible when the meaning of the subject was changed by certain linguistic processes in such a way that the afflicted object could also be regarded as a subject.

In the Indo-Germanic languages the fact is that whenever the groups thought of as impersonal have o- stems, they are used in the subject case with the accusative, i.e., as the object case. This is shown very clearly with the adjectives *magnum*, μακρόν [large], and with nouns like ἄντρον [man], *arvum* [meadowland], and *aratrum* [plow]. According to what has been said, it is quite obvious that objects of the speaking subject do not in general become subjects, since they could not be subjects of the action, and thus neither could they become congruent with the function of the subject as it occurs, nor congruent with the designation of the action.

These so-called neuters look like accusative masculine nouns; what is valid for their function as objects will also have to be assumed for the other neuters: *dulce*, ἡδύ [sweet], ἀληθές [true], and so on, whose function as subjects are provided in the pure stem; likewise γέρας [prize], δόρυ [wood], *munus* [duty], and γένος [race]. Characteristically enough, their function as objects is also provided by their pure stems. One says that the accusative is identical with the nominative. Obviously in this case again the designation as an object has become capable of passing as a real subject by a change in the subject's consciousness of speech.

The adjectives named clearly demonstrate how one formally differentiates the subject of the action from the object of the imagination, namely by a sentence form, i.e., by the combination with a particle, maybe *right away* [sa, sa]. Without going into this more deeply, we can nevertheless conclude that the pure stem did not originally function as a subject, but rather it designated the object of the speaking subject.

The pure stem is generally chosen as the designation of the vocative, and the vocative is an imperative which designates roughly *I want my brother* [ich will den Bruder]. But as the personal object, especially the listener addressed, the brother would supplement from this: *I should come, listen, do* [ich soll kommen, hören, thun], and thus the vocative becomes so extraordinarily similar to the nominative that the nominative itself appears as representative for the vocative, and the nominative explains the vocative in apposition.

If we were right in saying that activity or action must be supplemented and inferred in every case, then the verbal stem, which is in no way different from the nominal stem, must originally have become likewise the object of the speaking person, and λέγε [say] in the imperative must not have been any different in its function from ἄνθρωπε [man, (vocative)] but would have been used as *my cane* [meinen Stock]. This form too, however, would have been construed as a subject with *thou* [du] included.

The other forms of the verb would naturally also have been formed originally according to the pattern:

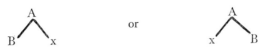

In τίθη-σι [he puts] thus the object was τίθη; σι was the object to A, and in complete agreement the stems *ma, ta* related to the first and third person, which correspondingly designate the *Casus Obliqui* and not the *Subjectcasus*.

The means of formation are thus exactly the same as with the infinitive exclamation: *eum venire* [to come to him], in which *eum* [him (acc.)] and *venire* [to come] are mainly objects of the speaking subject, exactly as they are with *dico eum venire* [I say to come to him]. However, it is in this case that conformity appears; *eum* must also be thought of as the subject of *venire* [to come], even though the infinitive retains its object case in its linguistic function. The accusative with the infinitive appears as a real object case when the passive construction demands the nominative with the infinitive, such as *dicor venisse* [I am told that I was to come]. When that is not the case, however, the accusative can then only be sensed as the subject case of the infinitive.

It is evident that we must base the relationship of the stem to the speaking subject, including all the syntactical observations, upon Indo-Germanic accidence.

Before we leave this point one more item must be cleared up. We have seen that the forms *venis, venit* [you come, he comes] were forms of reporting in which the suffix contained the exposition to the stem. The stem by itself would designate only an object of the perceptive subject, whose function would be inferred from the linguistic suggestion and the emotional tone. The form would signify approximately: *catch him, catch* [Kunft ihn, Kunft], or *get going* [Gang dich]. According to what we have stated, Latin *te venire*, *eum venire* and Greek σὲ ἐλθεῖν [to have come] would be approximately the same.

If the act of coming is not reported, but is expressed by the speaking person himself *venio* [I come[, then the expositional pronoun will be missing. If *venio* [I come] is now similar to the object *catch* [Kunft] or ἐλθεῖν [to have come] and if the speaking subject's mental process can be explained with the verbs of telling or imagining, then we would have an expression some-what like λέγω [I say], ἐλθεῖν [to have come]. However, λέγω can only be expressed at the stage of the report; thus in this case the object-subject for λέγω ἐλθεῖν is again missing, because it is the same as that of the speaking subject. If, on the other hand, this were different, then it would read λέγω ἐλθεῖν σε, αὐτόν [I say that he came]. This infinitive construction is peculiar to almost all verbs which report the mental processes of the speaking subject and his speech. The general rule was that with the same subject only the simple infinitive could be connected, but with dissimilar subjects the infinitive would be connected with the accusative. In addition to the Greek, it is also shown in the German *ich hoffe zu sehen* [I hope to see] in the isolated verbs of classic Latin such as *volo* [I want], *nolo* [I do not want], *malo* [I prefer], *cupio* [I desire], in the verbs of resolving with the simple infinitive, and in poetic usage.

We thereby see that the form of the reporting expression in the oldest periods of the Indo-Germanic languages was formed according to the same law used later in cultivated languages. The Latin constructions *polliceor me venturum esse* [I promise that I shall come] are formed according to the pattern of the reporting form and are of the same type as ἵστημι [I place] i.e., forms in which the pronoun enters according to the model of the true reporting forms ἵστης [you put], ἵστησι [he puts]. It is well-known that this analogic form also influenced the other verbs in Old Indian.

The above observation also illuminates some other cases of the old syntax, such as the Greek accusative, for example, in impressive speech: σὲ δη, σὲ τὴν νεύσουσαν εἰς πέδον κάρα [Now, stooping on the crest of a hill], in requesting: μή, πρός σε θεῶν τλῆς με προδοῦναι [By the Gods, do not abandon the suffering one (me)]; or in the lively question: τί δὲ τοὺς κινδυνεύειν μέλλοντας [But who to run the risk in the future]. In the last examples, however, it can no longer be determined to what extent the function, which was sensed in the accusative of the action, has contributed.

Certainly along with this the Greek swearing or invocation charm νὴ μὰ Δία [by Jupiter] should be included, and in connection with this probably the construction with ὀμνύναι [to swear] and ἐπιορκεῖν [to settle in a place] with the accusative, for example θεούς [Gods].

The relaxation to the speaking provides the simplest and most natural explanation for the absolute usage of the accusative, to which I add the adverbial: for example τέλος ἦκε meaning *in the end, he came* [das Ende, er kam], and τοῦτον τὸν τρόπον, *in this way, he came* [diese Weise, er kam]. And in this way the accusative of consideration also originated, for example, τὸ σῶμα ὑγιαίνει [the healthy body]. The accusative forms the object of the speaker's thought *I look at the body, it is healthy* [ich sehe den Leib an, er ist gesund]. Corresponding to these relationships the German expression *in Anbetracht, in Anseheung* [in view of, in consideration of] is formed, or verbally *sehe ich an* [I look at].

We would add to these such Latin expressions as *partim* [partly], *maximam partem* [to the greatest part], *tertium* [for the third time], *iterum* [a second time], the adverbs of the comparative such as *melius* [better], and the adverbial formations such as *singulatim* [one by one], which are the accusative of verbal nouns of the type of the Greek πρᾶξις [the doing].

Also with this usage a gradual process of conformity takes place. These accusatives become related to the action and determine it in some manner, both qualitatively and quantitatively.

I will also include here the Greek absolute participle in the accusative such as ἐξόν, and with this also, the corresponding German and Romance expressions such as *dies gesagt, dies gethan* [this said, this done]. But the principle is always abided by, that in the end all manners of construction are sensed as congruent with the function which they have for the predicate.

The especially frequent German mode of expression in common speech: *Themistokles, der siegte* [Themistocles, he conquered], reminds one clearly of one interpretation according to which *Themistokles* [Themistocles] would have a function as a sentence; compare to this the pleonastic personal pronoun of the Romance, for example *la fille donc du plus grand roy du monde elle est à toy* [indeed the daughter of the greatest king in the world (she) is yours], or the German *das Mädchen es ist dein* [the girl she is yours]. The interrogative form *ton père est-il?* [your father is he?] also belongs in this category.

Halle, Germany: Printed by Ehrhardt Karras

Bibliography

Abse, D. W. 1955. Psychodynamic aspects of the problem of definition of obscenity. *Law and Contemporary Problems* 20:572–86.

———. 1966. *Hysteria and related disorders*. Bristol: John Wright and Sons, Ltd. (Baltimore: Williams and Wilkins)

Akelaitis, A. J. 1944. A study of gnosis, praxis, and language following section of the corpus callosum and anterior commisure. *Journal of Neurosurgery* 1:94–102.

Allport, G. W. 1924. Eidetic imagery. *British Journal of Psychology* 15: 99–120.

Altshuler, K. Z. In press. Studies of the deaf: relevance to psychiatric theory. *American Journal of Psychiatry*.

Arieti, S., ed. 1959. Schizophrenia: the manifest symptomatology, the psychodynamic and formal mechanisms. *American Handbook of Psychiatry*, vol. I. New York: Basic Books, Inc.

Aristotle. On poetics. *The works of Aristotle*. The Great Books of the Western World, part 2, vol. 9. Chicago: University of Chicago Press (1952).

Balint, M. 1959. *Thrills and regressions*. New York: International Universities Press.

Balkányi, C. 1968. Language, verbalisation and superego: some thoughts on the development of the sense of rules. *International Journal of Psycho-Analysis* 49: 712–18.

Barfield, O. 1952. *Poetic diction: a study in meaning*. London: Faber and Faber.

Bartlett, F. C. 1932. *Remembering*. New York: Cambridge University Press.

Basser, L. S. 1962. Hemiplegia of early onset and the faculty of speech with special reference to the effects of hemispherectomy. *Brain* 85:427–60.

Bateson, G., et al. 1956. Towards a theory of schizophrenia. *Behavioral Science* 1: 25–26.

Bernfeld, S. 1929. *The psychology of the infant*. London: Kegan Paul.

Bernstein, B. 1964. Speech systems and psycho-therapy. In *Mental health of the poor*, ed. F. Reissman, J. Cohen, and A. Pearl. New York: The Free Press of Glencoe.

Bibring, E. 1929. Klinische Beitrage Zur Paranoiafrage, II. Ein Fall von Organprojektion. *Internationale Zeitschrift für Psychoanalyse* 15.

Birdwhistell, R. L. 1952. *Introduction to kinesics: an annotation system for analysis of body motion and gesture.* Washington, D.C.: Department of State, Foreign Service Institute.

Black, M. 1968. *The labyrinth of language.* New York: Frederick A. Praeger.

Bleuler, E. 1919. *Dementia praecox or the group of schizophrenias.* Monograph Series on Schizophrenia, no. 1. New York: International Universities Press.

——. 1918. *Textbook of psychiatry.* New York: Macmillan and Company.

Bloch, O. 1921. Notes sur le langage d'un enfant. *Journal de Psychologie* XVIII.

Bonnard, A. 1960. The primal significance of the tongue. *International Journal of Psycho-Analysis* 41:301–7.

Bram, F. M. 1965. The gift of Anna O. *British Journal of Medical Psychology* 38:part I:53–58.

Bréal, M. 1897. *Essai de semantique, science des significations.* Paris: Hachette.

Breuer, J., and Freud, S. 1895. *Studies of hysteria. See* Freud, S. *The Complete psychological works of Sigmund Freud,* vol. II.

Brown, R. 1958. *Words and things.* New York: The Free Press of Glencoe.

Bruner, J. S., et al. 1966. *Studies in cognitive growth.* New York: John Wiley and Sons, Inc.

Bühler, K. 1934. *Sprachtheorie.* Jena: Gustav Fischer.

Carnap, R. 1937. *Logical syntax of language.* New York: Harcourt, Brace, and World.

Carroll, L. *See* Gardner, M. *The annotated Alice.*

Cassirer, E. 1944. *An essay on man.* New Haven: Yale University Press.

——. 1953. *The philosophy of symbolic forms.* Vol. I, Language. New Haven: Yale University Press.

Cesbron, H. 1909. *Histoire critique de l'hysteria.* Paris: Asselin et Houzean.

Cherry, C. 1966. *On human communication.* 2nd ed. Cambridge, Mass.: M.I.T. Press.

Chomsky, N. 1967. The formal nature of language. In *Biological foundations of language. See* Lenneberg, E. H.

Church, G. 1961. *Language and discovery of reality.* New York: Random House.

Coleridge, S. T. 1812. *Lectures on Shakespeare and Milton.* London.

Critchley, M. 1939. *The language of gesture.* London: Edward Arnold.

Delicato, C. H. 1963. *The diagnosis and treatment of speech and reading problems.* Springfield, Ill.: Charles C. Thomas.

De Saussure, F. 1916. *Course in general linguistics*. New York: Philosophical Library (1959).

Deutsch, F. 1954. Analytic synaesthesiology. *International Journal of Psycho-Analysis* 35:293–301.

Dix, K. W. 1923. *Koeperliche und giestage. Entwicklung eines Kindes*. Leipzig: Barth.

Dunsdon, M. I. 1952. *The educability of cerebral palsied children*. National Foundation for Educational Research in England and Wales, publication no. 4. London: Newnes.

Edelheit, H. 1968. Language and the development of the ago. *Journal of the American Psychoanalytic Association* 16:1:113–22.

——. 1969. Speech and psychic structure: the vocal-auditory organization of the ego. *Journal of the American Psychoanalytic Association* 17:381–412.

Eissler, K. R. 1953. Notes upon the emotionality of a schizophrenic patient and its relation to problems of technique. *The Psychoanalytic Study of the Child* 8:199–251.

——. 1954. Notes upon defects of ego structure in schizophrenia. *International Journal of Psycho-Analysis* 35:141–46.

Ekman, P.; Sorenson, E. R.; and Friesen, W. V. 1969. Pan-cultural elements in facial displays of emotion. *Science* 164:3875:86–88.

Ellul, J. 1965. *Propaganda*. Tr. K. Kellen and J. Lerner. New York: Alfred A. Knopf.

Ewing, G. R., and Ewing, A. W. G. 1954. *Speech and the Deaf Child*. Manchester: Manchester University Press.

Federn, P. 1952. *Ego psychology and the psychoses*. New York: Basic Books, Inc.

Ferenczi, S. 1913. *Sex in psychoanalysis*. Tr. E. Jones. New York: Dover Publications (1956).

Flavell, J. H. 1963. *The developmental psychology of Jean Piaget*. Princeton: D. Van Nostrand Company.

Fliess, R. 1953. *The revival of interest in the dream*. New York: International Universities Press.

Flugel, J. C. 1933. *A hundred years of psychology, 1833–1933*. London: Duckworth.

Fowler, H. W., and Fowler, F. G. 1931. *The King's English*. 3d ed. Oxford: Clarendon Press.

Freeman, T. 1969. *Psychopathology of the psychoses*. New York: International Universities Press.

Freeman, T.; Cameron, J. L.; and McGhie, A. 1958. *Chronic schizophrenia*. London: Tavistock Publications, Ltd.

Freud, S. 1891–1938. *The complete psychological works of Sigmund Freud*.

Ed. J. Strachey, in collaboration with A. Freud. 24 vols. London: Hogarth Press and the Institute of Psychoanalysis, 1953-.

Project for a scientific psychology. I:295–397 (1895).

Studies on hysteria (with J. Breuer). II (1895).

The interpretation of dreams. IV and V:1–626 (1900).

Three essays on the theory of sexuality. VII:135–230 (1905).

Some general remarks on hysterical attacks. IX:227–34. (1909).

The antithetical meaning of primal words. XI:155–61 (1910).

The disposition to obsessional neurosis. XII:311–26 (1913).

The claims of psychoanalysis to scientific interest. XIII:165–90 (1913).

A metapsychological supplement to the theory of dreams. XIV:222–35 (1917).

The unconscious. XIV:159–209 (1915).

Words and things. XIV:209–15 (1891).

Introductory lectures on psychoanalysis. XV (1915–1916).

Beyond the pleasure principle. XVIII:17–64 (1920).

The ego and the id. XIX:13–66 (1923).

A note upon the "mystic writing pad." XIX:227–32 (1925).

An autobiographical study. XX:7–71 (1925).

New introductory lectures on psychoanalysis. XXII:7–182 (1938).

——. 1891. *On aphasia*. New York: International Universities Press.

Furth, H. G. 1966. *Thinking without language: psychological implications of deafness*. New York: Free Press.

Galen. *De locis affectis*, Lib. VI. Venice: Junta (1541). Quoted in Cesbron, H. 1909. *Histoire critique de l'hysteria*. Paris: Asselin et Houzean.

Galton, F. 1883. *Inquiries into human faculty and its development*. London: Everyman Edition (1907).

Gardner, M. 1960. *The annotated Alice*. (Carroll, L. 1872. *Alice's adventures in wonderland*, and *Through the looking-glass*.) New York: Clarkson N. Porter, Inc.

Gazzaniga, M. S. 1967. The split brain in man. *Scientific American* 217: 24–29.

Gazzaniga, M. S., and Sperry, R. W. 1967. Language after section of the cerebral commisure. *Brain* 90:131–48.

Gerson, W. 1928. Schizophrene Sprachnenbildung und Schizophrenes Denken. *Zeitschrift für die gesamte Neurologie und Psychiatrie* 113 (Berlin).

Gesell, A. L., and Amatruda, C. S. 1947. *Developmental diagnosis, normal and abnormal child development*. New York: Paul B. Hoeber, Inc.

Goldstein, K. 1934. *The organism*. New York: American Book Company.

Goldstein, M. N., and Joyet, R. J. 1969. Longterm followup of a callosal sectioned patient. *Archives of Neurology* 20:96–102.

Greenson, R. R. 1954. About the sound 'mm . . . '. *Psychoanalytical Quarterly* 23:234–39.

———. 1950. The mother tongue and the mother. *International Journal of Psycho-Analysis* 31:18–23.

Gregoire, A. 1933. L'apprentissage de la parole pendant les deux premières années de l'enfance. *Journal de Psychologie* 30.

Guttmann, E. 1942. Aphasia in children. *Brain* 65:205–19.

Haeckel, E. 1879. *The evolution of man*. London.

Hanfmann, E., and Kasanin, J. S. 1942. *Conceptual thinking in schizophrenia*. New York and Washington: Nervous and Mental Disease Publishing Co.

Hawkins, D. R. 1966. A review of psychoanalytic dream theory in the light of recent psycho-physiological studies of sleep and dreaming. *British Journal of Medical Psychology* 39:85–104.

Hayes, C. 1951. *The ape in our house*. New York: Harper.

Henderson, D. K., and Gillespie, R. D. 1944. *A text-book of psychiatry for students and practitioners*. 6th ed. London: Oxford University Press.

Hine, W. D. 1970. *Teacher of the deaf*. 68:129.

Hoffer, W. 1950. Development of the body ego. *The Psychoanalytic Study of the Child*. 5:18–24.

Hogarth, W. 1833. *An anecdote of William Hogarth, written by himself, with essays on his life and genius, etc.* London.

Hooker, D. 1952. *The prenatal origin of behavior*. Lawrence, Kansas: University of Kansas Press.

Humphrey, G. 1951. *Thinking*. London: Methuen.

Isokower, O. 1939. On the exceptional position of the auditory sphere. *International Journal of Psycho-Analysis* 20:340–48.

Jaensch, E. R. 1930. *Eidetic imagery and typological methods of investigation*. London.

Jakobson, R. 1942. *Child language, aphasia, and phonological universals*. The Hague, Paris: Mouton (1968).

———. 1964. Toward a linguistic typology of aphasic impairments. In *Ciba Foundation Symposium on Disorders of Language*, ed. de Renck and O'Connor, pp. 21–42. London: Churchill.

James, W. 1890. *Principles of Psychology*. New York: Dover Publications (1950).

Jesperson, O. 1925. *Die Sprache*. Heidelberg.

Jessner, L. 1931. Eine in der Psychose entstandene Kunstprache. *Archive fur Psychiatrie* 94:382–98.

Johnson, R. L., and Gross, H. S. 1966. Models of meaning and the analysis of delusional language. Paper presented at a symposium on Symbolism and Systems at the 133rd Annual Meeting of the American Association for the Advancement of Science. (The Symposium was jointly sponsored by the Society for General Systems Research, The Academy of Psychoanalysis, and the American Political Science Organization.)

Jones, E. 1953. *Sigmund Freud: life and work,* vol. I. London: Hogarth Press.

———. 1938. The theory of symbolism. *Papers on psychoanalysis.* London: Balliere, Tindall, and Cox.

Jung, C. G. 1906. *The psychology of dementia praecox.* Nervous and Mental Disease Monograph Series no. 3: New York and Washington (1936).

Katan, A. 1961. Some thoughts about the role of verbalisation in early childhood. *The Psychoanalytic Study of the Child* 16:184–88.

Kellogg, W. N. 1968. Communication and language in the home-raised chimpanzee. *Science* 162:3852:423–26.

Kellogg, W. N., and Kellogg, C. A. 1967. *The ape and the child: a study of environmental influence on early behavior.* New York: Harper.

Kleinpaul, R. 1893. *Das Leben der Sprache.* Quoted in Jones, E. 1938. The theory of symbolism. In *Papers on psychoanalysis.* London: Baliere, Tindall, and Cox.

Kraepelin, E. 1905. Uber Sprachstorungen in Traume. *Psychologische Arbeiten* 5:1.

Kris, E. 1952. *Psychoanalytic explorations in art.* New York: International Universities Press.

Kubie, L. S. 1934. Body symbolization and the development of language. *Psychoanalytical Quarterly* 3:430–44.

———. 1953. The distortion of the symbolic process in neurosis and psychosis. *Journal of the American Psychoanalytic Association* 1:59–86.

La Barre, W. 1964. Paralinguistics, kinesics, and cultural anthropology. In *Approaches to Semiotics,* ed. Sebeok, Hayes, and Bateson. Transactions of the Indiana University Conference. The Hague: Mouton.

Laffal, J. 1965. *Pathological and normal language.* New York: Atherton Press.

Langer, S. K. 1942. *Philosophy in a new key.* Cambridge: Harvard University Press (1957).

Lavater, G. C. 1789. *Essays on physiognomy for the promotion of the knowledge and the love of mankind.* Tr. T. Holcroft. London: Robinson.

Lenneberg, E. H. 1967. *Biological foundations of language.* New York: John Wiley and Sons.

Lewis, M. M. 1963. *Language, thought, and personality in infancy and childhood.* New York: Basic Books, Inc.

Lewis Committee 1968. *The education of deaf children: the possible place of finger-spelling and signing.* London: Her Majesty's Stationery Office.

Lidz, T. 1968. The family, language, and the transmission of schizophrenia. *Journal of Psychiatric Research Supplement November* 1986. 175–84.

Lidz, T., and Fleck, S. 1960. Schizophrenia, human integration, and the role of the family. In *The Etiology of the Family, ed.* D. D. Jackson. Basic Books, Inc.

Lidz, T.; Fleck, S.; and Cornelison, A. R. 1965. *Schizophrenia and the family.* New York: International Universities Press.

McCarthy, J. J.. and Kirk, S. A. 1963. *The construction, standardization, and statistical characteristics of the Illinois test of psycholinguistic abilities.* University of Illinois Institute for Research on Exceptional Children.

McNutt, S. J. 1885. Seven cases of infantile spastic hemiplegia. *Archives of Pediatrics* 2:20.

Milner, M. 1955. The role of illusion in symbol formation. In *New directions in psycho-analysis,* ed. M. Klein, P. Heimann, and R. E. Money-Kyrle. New York: Basic Books, Inc.

Minski, L., and Sheppard, M. J. 1970. *Non-communicating children.* United Kingdom: Butterworth.

Moore, J. 1962. *Your English words.* Philadelphia: J. B. Lippincott Company.

———. Talk of the Town. 1970. *The New Yorker.* 46:39:43–44 (Nov. 14, 1970).

Noble, D. 1951. Hysterical manifestations in schizophrenic illness. *Psychiatry* 14:153–60.

Osgood, C. E.; Luci, J. G.; and Tannenbaum, P. H. 1957. *The measurement of meaning.* Urbana: University of Illinois Press.

Paget, R. 1955. *This English.* London. Routledge.

Paget, R., Gorman, P.; and Paget, G. 1969. *A systematic life language.* 4th ed. London.

Parker, B. 1962. *My language is me.* New York: Basic Books, Inc.

Peller, L. E. 1964. Language and its prestages. *Bulletin of the Philadelphia Association for Psychoanalysis* 14:2.

Penfield, W. 1966. In *Brain and conscious experience,* ed. J. C. Eccles. Berlin: Springer.

Piaget, J. 1952. *The origins of intelligence in children.* New York. International Universities Press.

Piaget, J. and Inhelder, B. 1969. *The psychology of the child.* New York: Basic Books, Inc.

Preyer, T. W. 1882. *Die Seele des Kindes.* Leipzig: T. Grieben (1895).

Rainer, J. D., and Altshuler, K. Z. 1967. *Psychiatry and the deaf.* Washington: U.S. Department of Health, Education, and Welfare.

———. In press. A psychiatric program for the deaf: experiences and implications. *American Journal of Psychiatry.*

Rapaport, D., ed. 1951. *Organization and pathology of thought.* New York: Columbia University Press.

Read, H. 1943. *Education through art.* London: Faber and Faber.

Rees, J. R. 1947. *The case of Rudolf Hess.* London: William Heinemann Ltd.

Rosen, V. 1967. Disorders of communication in psychoanalysis. *Journal of the American Psychoanalytic Association* 15:3:457–90.

———. 1969. Sign phenomena and their relationship to unconscious meaning. *International Journal of Psycho-Analysis* 50:197–207.

Ruesch, J., and Bateson, G. 1951. *Communication: the social matrix of psychiatry.* New York: W. W. Norton and Company, Inc.

Ruesch, J., and Kees, W. 1956. *Non-verbal communication: notes on visual perception of human relations.* Berkeley: University of California Press.

Sapir, E. 1921. *Language: an introduction to the study of speech.* New York: Harcourt Brace and Company.

Scherner, K. A. 1861. *Das Leben des Traumes.* Berlin.

Schilder, P. 1935. In *Contributions to developmental neuropsychiatry,* ed. L. Bender. New York: International Universities Press (1964).

———. 1935. *The image and appearance of the human body: Studies in the constructive energies of the psyche.* New York: International Universities Press (1950).

Schlessinger, N., et al. 1967. The scientific style of Breuer and Freud in the origins of psychoanalysis. *Journal of the American Psychoanalytic Association* 15:2:404–22.

Scott, W., and Clifford, M. 1955. A note on blathering. *International Journal of Psycho-Analysis* 36:348–49.

Searles, H. F. 1969. A case of borderline thought disorder. *International Journal of Psycho-Analysis* 50:655–64.

———. 1965. *Collected papers on schizophrenia and related subjects.* New York: International Universities Press.

Segal, H. 1957. Notes on symbol information. *International Journal of Psycho-Analysis* 38:391–97.

Shands, H. C. 1970. Momentary deity and personal myth: a semiotic inquiry using recorded psychotherapeutic material. *Semiotica,* vol. 2, part 1:1–34.

Sherrington, C. S. 1941. *Man on his nature: the Gifford lectures 1937–1938.* New York: Cambridge University Press.

Skottowe, J. 1939. Shock therapy: a plea for proportion in psychiatry. *Proceedings of the Royal Society of Medicine* 32:843–52.

Soranus. *Gynaecology.* Tr. O. Temkin. Baltimore: Johns Hopkins Press (1956).

Sperber, H. 1912. Uber den Einfluss sexueller Momente auf Enstehung und Entwicklung der Sprache. *Imago* 1:504.

Sperry, R. W. 1966. Brain bisection and mechanics of consciousness. In *Brain and conscious experience,* ed. J. S. Eccles. New York: Springer Verlag.

———. 1968. Hemisphere disconnection and unity in conscious awareness, *American Psychology* 23:10:723–33.

Sperry, R. W., and Gazzaniga, M.S. 1967. Language following surgical disconnection of the hemispheres. In *Brain mechanisms underlying speech and language*, ed. C. H. Millican. New York: Grune and Stratton.

Spitz, R. A. 1965. *The first year of life*. New York: International Universities Press.

———. 1955. The primal cavity: a contribution to the genesis of perception and its role for psychoanalytic theory. *The Psychoanalytic Study of the Child* 10:215–40.

———. 1946. *The smiling response*. Genetic Psychology Monographs 34.

Steiner, George. 1967. *Language and silence*. New York: Atheneum.

Stekel, W. 1911. *Die Sprache des Traumes*. Wiesbaden.

Stengel, E. 1939. On learning a new language. *International Journal of Psycho-Analysis* 20:471–79.

Stern, C.; and Stern, W. 1907. *Die Kindesprache*. Leipzig.

Stone, L. 1954. On the principal obscene word of the English language. *International Journal of Psycho-Analysis* 35:1:30–56.

Strachey, J. 1957. Editor's note to Freud's Essay on the unconscious. See Freud, S., *The Complete Psychological Works of Sigmund Freud*, vol. xiv.

Stransky, E. 1929. Nature of schizophrenia. *Jahrbücher für Psychiatrie und Neurologie* 46 (Vienna).

Tausk, V. 1919. On the origin of the "influencing machine" in schizophrenia. In *The Psycho-analytic reader*, ed. R. Fliess. New York: International Universities Press (1948).

Tax, S., ed. 1960. Issues in evolution. In *Evolution after Darwin*, vol. 3. Chicago: University of Chicago Press.

Taylor, J. 1905. *Paralysis and other diseases of the nervous system in childhood and early life*. London. Churchill.

Thass-Thienemann, T. 1968. *Symbolic behavior*. New York: Washington Square Press, Inc.

Thomas, S. J. 1940. Some clinical examples of "dys-symbole": its relations to shock therapy. *Journal of Mental Science* 86:100.

Trager, G. L. 1965. Paralanguage: a first approximation. In *Language in culture and society: a reader in linguistics and anthropology*, ed. D. Hymes. New York: Harper and Row.

Tuczek, K. 1921. Analyze einer Katatonikensprache. *Zeitschrift für die gesamte Neurologie und Psychiatrie* 113 (Berlin).

Tyler, E. B. 1873. *Primitive culture*. London.

Varendonck, J. 1921. The psychology of daydreams. In *Organization and pathology of thought*. See Rapaport, D.

Veith, I. 1965. *Hysteria: the history of a disease*. Chicago: University of Chicago Press.

Vernon, M. and Rothstein, D. A. 1968. Prelingual deafness: an experiment of nature. *Archives of General Psychiatry* 19:361–69.

Vygotsky, L. S. 1962. *Thought and language.* Ed. and tr. E. Hanfmann, and G. Vakar. Cambridge, Mass.: M:I.T. Press.

Wallin, J. E. W. 1949. *Children with mental and physical handicaps.* New York: Prentice Hall, Inc.

Wegener, P. 1885. *Untersuchungen ueber die Grundfragen des Sprachlebens.* Halle: Max Niemeyer.

Werner, H. 1948. *Comparative psychology of mental development.* New York: International Universities Press.

Werner, H., and Kaplan, B. 1963. *Symbol formation.* New York: John Wiley and Sons, Inc.

Wernicke, C. 1906. *Grundriss der Psychiatrie.* Leipzig: Barth.

Wheelright, P. 1962. *Metaphor and reality.* Bloomington, Indiana: Indiana University Press.

Whorf, B. L. 1956. Language, thought, and reality. In *Selected writings of Benjamin Lee Whorf,* ed. J. Carroll. New York: John Wiley and Sons, Inc.

Wittgenstein, L., and Blackwell, B. 1953. *Philosophical investigations.* New York: Oxford Press.

Wynne, L. C., et al. 1958. Pseudo-mutuality and the family relations of schizophrenics. *Psychiatry* 21:205–20.

Young, J. Z. 1970. What can we know about memory? *British Medical Journal* 1:5697:647–52.

Subject Index

Abstraction, in the formation of models, 255

Affect: distorted expression of, 17; disclosed in figures of speech, 18

Age: effect on visual imagery, 32; effect on language, 158. See also Obscenity

Anachronisms, 199

Anna O., the "talking cure," 12, 13

Aphasia: in brain injury, 98; Freud's study of, 103; recovery from, 105

Artificial language systems: in twins, 64; in schizophrenia, 67, 71, 72, 73

Association, by similarity, contiguity, 33n

Audience, size of, affecting communication, 141

Babbling, lalling, blathering, 93–95, 99

Body awareness, 34, 128; an ingredient in speech formation, 24, 92; limitations in adult life, 35; influence on dream imagery, 36; architectural symbolism of, 36. See also Body image

Blindness, 100

Body image, 75, 83; children's, 35; continued development of, 40; interrelationship with emotions, etc., 41; in imagery and phantasy, 43. See also Body awareness

Children: language development in, 3, 6, 86, 93, 94; perceptual patterns in metaphor, 21; rejection of linguistic inheritance, 91; libidinal shifts, 92; age at acquisition of language, 107; importance in conceptualization of early input, 255

Chronological order, 205, 212; subordinate clause and tense, 211; in forming a model, 255

Coercion, an object of speech, 6, 54, 81, 174. See also Propaganda

Comparatives, 155

Condensation, 61, 63; in dreams, 48

Conversion (metaphoric aspect), 66, 68; Cäcilie M., 13; a pain in the neck, 14; revelatory nature of, 16; motor and sensory phenomenon in, 18; in schizophrenia, 65; foreshadowed in normal reference, 257

Cultural determinants in understanding, 10, 80, 108, 138, 139, 253, 254

Demonstratives, derived from imperatives, 191, 240

Derepression, 26, 46

Derision by skewed imitation, 198

Direct discourse, 149, 150

Dissociation, 17

Displacement, 42, 61; in dreams, 48

Disposition (of speaker), a clue to meaning, 137

Dominance (of cerebral hemisphere): visual, excessive, 99; in speech, 102, 104

Drama, speech in, 140, 172, 173

Dreams, 45, 61, 85; source of materials for, 30; effect of body organs upon, 35; symbol language in, 37, 38, 39, 42; sexual material in, 38; in animals, 47; dream-work, 48

Dys-symbole, 60, 70

Egoistic interests a determinant in understanding, 265

Ellipsis, 217

Empractic speech, 18, 19, 22, 54, 59

Ethical impulses: to help suffering, 53; advancement of, 101, 131; implications of courtesy in utterance, 133; purposes in speech, 175, 179

Expectation: an aid to understanding, 6, 215, 223, 225; factor in establishment of causal relationships, 226, 259;

Index of Proper Names